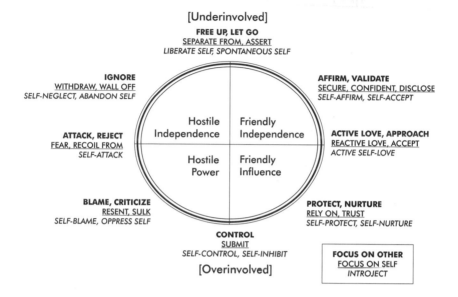

[Underinvolved]

FREE UP, LET GO
SEPARATE FROM, ASSERT
LIBERATE SELF, SPONTANEOUS SELF

IGNORE
WITHDRAW, WALL OFF
SELF-NEGLECT, ABANDON SELF

AFFIRM, VALIDATE
SECURE, CONFIDENT, DISCLOSE
SELF-AFFIRM, SELF-ACCEPT

ATTACK, REJECT
FEAR, RECOIL FROM
SELF-ATTACK

Hostile
Independence

Friendly
Independence

Hostile
Power

Friendly
Influence

ACTIVE LOVE, APPROACH
REACTIVE LOVE, ACCEPT
ACTIVE SELF-LOVE

BLAME, CRITICIZE
RESENT, SULK
SELF-BLAME, OPPRESS SELF

PROTECT, NURTURE
RELY ON, TRUST
SELF-PROTECT, SELF-NURTURE

CONTROL
SUBMIT
SELF-CONTROL, SELF-INHIBIT

[Overinvolved]

FOCUS ON OTHER
FOCUS ON SELF
INTROJECT

The Structural Analysis of Social Behavior (SASB) composite cluster model. All three circles are superimposed on the circumplex space. Labels in **boldface** type describe actions directed at another person (Focus on Other). Underlined labels describe reactions to another person (Focus on Self). *Italicized* labels describe how a person treats self and may reflect how important others have treated the person (Introject).
Source. Adapted from Benjamin LS: *Interpersonal Diagnosis and Treatment of Personality Disorders.* New York, Guilford, 1993. Copyright 1993. Used with permission.

Time-Managed Group Psychotherapy: Effective Clinical Applications

Time-Managed Group Psychotherapy: Effective Clinical Applications

K. Roy MacKenzie, M.D.
Clinical Professor of Psychiatry
University of British Columbia
Vancouver, British Columbia, Canada

Paul
Good luck in your group
work. *Roy MacKenzie*

American Psychiatric Press, Inc.

Washington, DC
London, England

Copyright © 1997 American Psychiatric Press, Inc.
ALL RIGHTS RESERVED
Manufactured in the United States of America on acid-free paper
00 99 98 97   4 3 2 1

American Psychiatric Press, Inc.
1400 K Street, N.W., Washington, DC   20005

Library of Congress Cataloging-in-Publication Data
MacKenzie, K. Roy, 1937–
    Time-managed group psychotherapy : effective clinical
applications / by K. Roy MacKenzie.
        p.   cm.
    Includes bibliographical references and index.
    ISBN 0-88048-863-8 (cloth : alk. paper)
    1. Group psychotherapy. 2. Brief psychotherapy. I. Title.
    [DNLM: 1. Psychotherapy, Group—methods. 2. Psychotherapy,
Brief—methods. WM 430 M156t 1997]
RC488.M236 1997
616.89′152—dc20
DNLM/DLC
for Library of Congress   96-21267
                                                                        CIP

British Library Cataloguing in Publication Data
A CIP record is available from the British Library.

Contents

Section III: Implementing the Generic Group

Section IV: Group Models for Clinical Service Systems

Preface

*T*his book is a successor to, not a second edition of, a previous book, *Introduction to Time-Limited Group Psychotherapy,* published in 1990 by American Psychiatric Press. The first draft of that book was written in 1988. During the 8 years since the writing of that first draft there has been a revolution in the way health care is being practiced throughout the United States. This book comes to grips with those aspects of these changes related to group psychotherapy. Over the same time period, the number of available clinical research studies concerning psychotherapy has more than doubled. There is now a firm base on which to build new approaches.

Psychotherapy developed originally around a number of schools of thought with strongly held theories. It is now clear that the subtle distinctions of technique that resulted had little impact on differential outcome. A competent clinician from any of these schools would achieve about the same results, and these results would be clearly effective compared with "no treatment" controls. These findings have been brought together in what has been called a "generic model of psychotherapy." This model identifies basic features of effective psychotherapy that cut across all theoretical approaches. These features are the known facts about what makes psychotherapy useful. Most clinicians will find that the components of the generic model sound familiar—"That sounds like what I do all the time; it's good to hear it spelled out so clearly." The generic model of psychotherapy is explained in some detail in Chapter 2 and augmented with material from the group psychotherapy literature that reinforces the idea of common mechanisms that induce change. In presenting this material, I have focused on the proper management of group dynamics as separate and distinct from psychodynamics.

This book is organized around the idea that the small interactive group is an ideal format in which the common therapeutic mechanisms of the generic model can be realized. The small group can be used as a vehicle to deliver many different theoretically based treatments. An interactive group environment automatically provides many properties of supportive psychotherapy. Specialized techniques can be built upon this base. This approach forms the structure of this book and provides a framework for implementing the use of groups in healthcare delivery systems.

Section I addresses the healthcare delivery scene from the standpoint of the group psychotherapist. Chapter 1 makes it abundantly clear that an increasing portion of psychotherapy is now being delivered in a group format and that this percentage is rapidly growing. The outcome evidence that is reviewed suggests that this is not a bad thing. The results with group formats are about the same as those with individual therapy. Groups are being used to treat a wide variety of syndromes, with a major emphasis on preventive or early-intervention treatment. This requires a flexibility in adapting the group format to a wide range of theoretical models. Historically, the group psychotherapy community has been concerned with the provision of longer-term psychodynamic psychotherapy. This perspective must be widened to meet the legitimate expectations of service systems that serve a broad range of patients. The use of time-limited techniques will be adequate for the majority of these patients. But the entire service system needs to be considered in order to achieve the optimum management of time as implied in the title of this book. Chapters 2 and 3 lay the theoretical foundation for effective use of groups by presenting clinically important basic principles that guide many aspects of therapeutic technique.

Section II is devoted to an extended discussion of assessment, group composition, and preparation of patients. The discussion begins, in Chapter 4, with a review of the DSM-IV categories and the implications for specialized psychotherapy approaches. Axis II is critically reviewed, and a dimensional model is introduced for understanding personality disorders. Assessment is expanded even further in Chapter 5, in which interpersonal diagnosis is discussed in depth. Special attention is paid to a relatively new model called the Structural Analysis of Social Behavior (SASB). The SASB system provides a map of the interpersonal terrain on which many diverse findings can be located. It also indicates what therapeutic maneuvers are likely to be most successful. All this attention to Axis II and personality is directly and specifically related to group psychotherapy, in which interpersonal behavior is the principal focus. Some of the material in Chapters 4 and 5 will be relatively new to many clinicians. An attempt has been made to explain these ideas in simple, direct terms with what I hope is an absence of jargon. The section is completed, in Chapter 6, with a consideration of how to apply the assessment material to the tasks of pretherapy preparation and group composition.

Section III is organized around the structure of group development and represents a meta-theory for tracking group events. The material in these chapters continues to be true to the principles of the generic model and can be applied to all types of groups, from behavioral to psychodynamic. Several protocols are outlined for ensuring that the basic tasks of each stage are addressed. There is an extended discussion of managing termination that emphasizes the therapeutic power of addressing the purposeful setting of a time limit. Because a majority of groups in service systems will be time limited and probably of closed membership, conceptualizing group development as occurring in stages, including termination, has broad application. The material in this section offers a new perspective for clinicians who have primarily run longer-term "slow open" groups and who, consequently, may have had few opportunities to begin and end a whole group. In these time-limited techniques, the therapeutic focus is compressed in an effort to elicit the maximum effect from a briefer course of treatment.

Most practitioners now find themselves interacting with a larger service organization in some manner. The larger flow of patients coming through these systems provides an ideal context for the use of groups, but the organizational structure for these groups must be developed and maintained. Section IV addresses an approach to the development of group programs in service systems. A series of group models provides examples that cover most common approaches. Many of the models can be adapted to other special populations without too much difficulty by incorporating different content into the structure. These models range from very brief crisis intervention groups to ongoing community maintenance groups and involve a wide range of goals, from the psychoeducational to the intensive interpersonal/psychodynamic. Throughout all of the examples, I have attempted to illustrate how to manage the available clinical time most effectively and efficiently. These models put into concrete terms the basic approach of the book. First, one must learn how to manage the small interactive group using the principles of group dynamics and the generic model. Then, this small-group format can be adapted to fit the needs of special populations.

The major issue I have faced in writing this book is how to effectively integrate the interpersonal/psychodynamic concepts of my training into other formats and blend other more structured techniques into an interpersonal framework. Two perspectives have been of great help in this process. First, I have relied on the use of the generic model as representing an atheoretical way of understanding the therapeutic process. All types of therapy can be included under its basic concepts of what is most helpful. It was not difficult to adapt this model to the group context because of the long history of group therapeutic factors. Second, I have placed greater emphasis on the concepts of supportive psychotherapy. Supportive techniques have been broadly misunderstood as simplistic encouragement. In fact, they provide a somewhat structured way to get at psychological phenomena central to both cognitive-behavioral and interpersonal/psychodynamic treatments in a manner that is less likely to get out of control and less likely to produce negative effects. Comparative outcome studies suggest that these techniques are as effective as, if not more effective than, more exploratory techniques for most patients. It became clear to me in reviewing this material just how central the supportive mechanisms are to the small-group format. These perspectives underlie the major move toward an integration of psychotherapy traditions, something most experienced therapists do much of the time.

Therapists learn most from their patients. I have used numerous clinical examples throughout the book. All names are fictitious, and the events are analogous, drawn from similar group incidents. I have used the term "patient" throughout the book because most of my experience has been in medically oriented settings. Please translate this into "client" or whatever term you commonly use in your work. Group psychotherapy comes from a multidisciplinary tradition.

This book has been a delight to write. The effort to understand how to integrate various theoretical viewpoints has been challenging. I have had the opportunity to put most of the models described here into clinical practice over a period of several years. The result, I believe, provides some indications about where group psychotherapy is headed. My overall sense is one of broadening perspectives and more opportunities to treat diverse patient populations. I hope other group therapists will share my enthusiasm at facing the challenges that lie ahead of us in these endeavors.

During the preparation of the book I have had the opportunity to try out ideas and solicit feedback from a number of valued colleagues. A short list includes Lorna Benjamin, Greg Crosby, John Livesley, David Orlinsky, Denise Wilfley, and of course all the residents, trainees, and workshop participants who were the unknowing participants in the testing of ideas. I would also like to thank the three anonymous reviewers who provided many helpful comments.

My considerable involvement in the activities of the American Group Psychotherapy Association, including a recent term as president, has provided a unique opportunity for professional validation and for appreciating the great diversity in the use of groups across the land. In particular, as initial Chair for the development of the National Registry of Certified

Group Psychotherapists, I had a thorough introduction to both federal healthcare politics and the managed care industry. The structure of this book reflects the influence of those experiences on my practice as a group clinician.

K. Roy MacKenzie, M.D.
Vancouver, September 1996

SECTION I
Understanding Small Groups

CHAPTER 1

The Psychotherapy Landscape

*C*linicians know the importance of maintaining a focus on the "here and now" of the present session and have experienced the constant struggle to stay with "the moment" and not slip too far into the past or reach too far forward into the future. In this introductory chapter I focus on the present, here-and-now state of group psychotherapy, considering it from a number of perspectives. First, I discuss the changes in the health-care service delivery system that have taken place and how these have affected or will affect the psychotherapy service delivery system, particularly in relation to group treatments. Then, I address the effectiveness of group treatments. Finally, I discuss how clinicians adapt to these changes. Opening this book with a discussion of the demands made by the evolving healthcare service delivery system, although it may seem like a somber way to begin, is testimony to the scope of changes occurring in professional practice and their impact on delivery of treatments. Within this new world of health care, group psychotherapy has an increasingly central role.

The Healthcare Service Delivery System

Healthcare costs in different countries are frequently compared. In the United States at present, nearly 15% of the gross domestic product is devoted to health care. In Canada, by contrast, less than 10% of the gross domestic product is devoted to health care, and in other comparably developed Western countries the proportion is considerably lower. There is little evidence to suggest that, overall, Americans are getting better coverage for this expenditure. Rather, the distribution figures suggest a dichotomized system, with services of high excellence being delivered in parallel with services of questionable quality. The latter services generally are the only ones provided to the 40 million people in the United States with no healthcare insurance coverage, primarily on the basis of social class. The hidden costs of advertising, management, and utilization of specialists and increasingly specialized technology are all considerably higher in the United States than elsewhere. These financial issues are driving fundamental healthcare reform. Although the long-term outcome is still to be determined, the process of change is likely to be irreversible.

The principal change in orientation of American health care may be understood as the response to providing care for a defined population base. The questions typically asked are, for example, What are the health services required by a given number of people, and what will the total cost of these services be? How will expenditures be apportioned within this cost limit? The population to be covered may be a corporation, an industry, or a geographic area. Insurers have become increasingly selective about whom they will register. As a result, more people find themselves without effective coverage. This situation has eroded the original insurance principle that risk should be spread evenly across a large population. The political response to this situation has been to develop a defined basket of basic benefits that must be made available to all.

This change in orientation stands conventional practice on its head. The problem facing healthcare delivery, once defined as how to attract enough patients to fill the available service capacity, is redefined as how to reasonably meet the needs of a given population with the available financial resources. This redefinition forces a painful review of what constitutes necessary medical treatment and how such care can be provided most effectively for the general betterment of the population as a whole. This reorientation of healthcare delivery might be described as a broadening of the healthcare practitioner's duties from private responsibility to public accountability, a major paradigm shift.

Although reliable figures are difficult to obtain, it has been estimated that as of early 1996, approximately one-half of medical care is now being provided through some form of managed care system. In fact, the major conceptual shifts have already occurred and are currently being enacted in clinical practice, long before any federal, or even much state, legislation is passed. As the "Jackson Hole" group has pointed out, "The medical cottage industry of individualists is giving way to organized structures demanding uniformity at the expense of autonomy, but promising to deliver quality more equitably and more efficiently" (1).

The most ominous feature of this new healthcare paradigm is that there will be limited dollars available to fund the programs. Cost-containment pressures are not likely to go away. Inevitably, restrictions will be placed on the extent of coverage provided. This is the here-and-now context in which mental health care, psychotherapy, and group psychotherapy must exist. It is not immediately clear just what type of service delivery system will emerge from the present rapidly changing models.

The Psychotherapy Service Delivery System

What are the implications of these changes in health care for the practice of psychotherapy? Psychotherapy services will be in direct competition with other medical care for finite funding resources. The idea of considering psychotherapy as a treatment within a medical service delivery system goes against the grain of many psychotherapists. Because psychotherapy involves a close and personalized relationship with the patient, the thought of regarding it as a service with possible limitations is difficult to accept.

Perhaps a perspective one step removed would be helpful. Think of a satellite view of North America, with the Mississippi coursing down the middle, the Great Lakes penetrating deep inland, and the white-capped mountains to the west. Clearly, a satellite map does not tell us much about specific cities, and it tells us even less about districts within cities and nothing at all about individuals. However, it does provide an important orienting overview of what to expect. A "satellite" view of the psychotherapy landscape is represented by the dose-response relationship in Figure 1–1, which portrays how psychotherapy was actually practiced before the managed care revolution. You might compare the dose-response relationship for your own practice setting with the one depicted in Figure 1–1. Be sure, however, to include everyone who is assessed, not just those you remember well because you saw them over a longer period of time.

The term *dose-response relationship* is adopted from the language of pharmacological studies. The best measure of dosage in psychotherapy is the number of contact hours. The composite graph in Figure 1–1 summarizes an extensive database of nonpsychotic patients attending mental

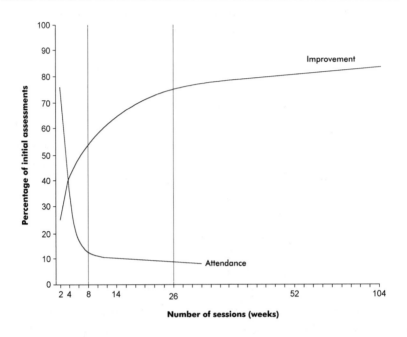

Figure 1–1.   Psychotherapy dose-response relationship.
Source.   Reprinted from MacKenzie KR: "Rationale for Group Psychother-apy in Managed Care," in *Effective Use of Group Therapy in Managed Care.* Edited by MacKenzie KR. Washington, DC, American Psychiatric Press, 1995, p. 9. Copyright 1995, American Psychiatric Press. Used with permission.

health centers or general hospital outpatient departments. It is a snapshot view of what happens to unscreened patients coming in the "front door" of the mental health system. The patterns represented in the graph may be used as a general map of the psychotherapy utilization terrain, as the results of virtually all formal psychotherapy outcome studies, individual and group, fall into these patterns.

The upper curve in Figure 1–1 is based on a database put together by Howard and his colleagues (2) and represents a measure of improvement as determined by objective assessment by an independent rater. This mea-sure is conservative because patient or therapist ratings are usually more positive than those made by an uninvolved clinician. The curve shows a rapid improvement in 50% of patients over the first 2 months, followed by con-tinuing strong improvement in another 25% of these patients over the next 4 months. The curve then rises much more slowly for the remaining time (i.e., up to 2 years). The final response rate is approximately 85%, a figure quite in keeping with several meta-analytic studies of the psychotherapy literature. It might be noted that even patients who are still in treatment 1 or 2 years later, in keeping with this curve, will have reported an early symptomatic response. This outcome curve reflects significantly greater improvement compared with that of untreated control patients.

In drug studies, the concept of a 50% response rate is used as a criterion of effective exposure to the therapeutic agent. If this criterion were adopted for psychotherapy, these curves suggest that six to eight sessions could be considered as a measure of the patient's being effectively exposed to a minimum dose of treatment.

Just as a satellite picture does not deal with the differences between, say, San Francisco and New York, so these dose-response curves do not deal with specific patient populations. For example, depressed patients appear to respond at an earlier point than patients with anxiety disorders, whereas patients with major personality disorders have a slower response pattern. The curves certainly cannot be used to predict the course of any single patient. However, they are sufficiently stable that they do form a basis for designing service programs (3). Given a particular population to be served, these curves allow one to predict with reasonable accuracy the service load that will be encountered. Therapists tend to remember those patients they have seen for a substantial period of time. Those patients who pass through quickly are just as quickly forgotten. From the patient's standpoint, however, even a brief encounter over a handful of sessions is sometimes described as a point of significant change in how the patient approaches life's challenges.

The lower curve in Figure 1–1 is based on an equally large database of actual number of sessions attended. The great majority of patients, over 80%, are seen for fewer than eight sessions. Fewer than 15% are still in treatment by 6 months. After that, there is an increased likelihood that attendance will continue for many months more. This curve appears to be quite constant across many different service systems. The exact point of the sharp bend followed by a flattening depicted in the figure as occurring at eight sessions may vary a little, but the rapid initial falloff is universal. This curve holds even for programs that are designed to provide long-term intensive psychotherapy (4).

This view of the healthcare delivery system has some direct parallels to our familiar conceptualization of the *group-as-a-whole*. We know logically that there are really only a number of individuals in the group room.

Yet, the concept of the total group is a powerful technique that seems to be particularly useful during the early stages of a group when one is trying to promote cohesion and universality. The effectiveness of the conceptualization of the total group is one of the stronger arguments for homogeneous groups. This perspective is commonly used in the advanced group to underscore common group themes (e.g., "The group has begun to act as if it believed it will continue forever, perhaps because it is uncomfortable to address the fact that we have only four more sessions left"). If we can think of the group as an entity, perhaps we can find some value in thinking of the healthcare system as an entity. Consider a "nation-as-a-whole" interpretation—for example, "The system is behaving as if everyone needs long-term treatment, perhaps because of a belief that change cannot occur outside of therapy."

Three distinct time segments are represented in Figure 1–1, as demarcated by the vertical lines at session 8 and session 26. These phases—crisis intervention, time-limited therapy, and longer-term therapy—correspond quite closely to the major outlines of clinical practice.

1. **Crisis intervention (1–8 sessions).** During this period, the task is to help the patient achieve immediate mastery by focusing on specific, but limited, goals related to promoting a return to usual functioning. Supportive techniques are used almost exclusively. Interpersonal or psychodynamic goals may be addressed but in a focused and perhaps more directive manner. It can be predicted that about one-half of the unscreened population presenting to psychiatric outpatient settings will derive benefit from this brief therapy and that an even larger percentage will terminate by the eighth session. A demoralized state of mind can be rapidly reversed for many people with a small number of psychotherapy sessions. Because a sizable percentage of patients can be expected to respond quickly and because the falloff in attendance is so steep, it has been the custom to use individual therapy in this segment. Some innovative programs have been applying group techniques during this period as well, either alone or in conjunction with individual sessions. An example of a Crisis Intervention Group is presented in the last section of this book. Early intervention might also be seen as a preventive measure to detect and address difficulties before they become entrenched.

2. **Time-limited therapy (8–26 sessions, up to 6 months).** During this period, one covered within the usual theoretical framework of time-

limited therapy, there is continuing major improvement. A broader range of goals can be addressed, and a more complex and intensive combination of supportive and exploratory strategies is more likely to be used. The increased time allows the accommodation of higher levels of distress and an opportunity to address problems related to more severe trauma or stress. This approach can also be used to treat patients whose presentation involves a greater component of longer-standing issues of a psychological nature. In short, more ambitious goals can be entertained. The majority of current psychotherapy falls into this time range, which is likely to become the "default mode" for delivering intensive psychotherapy in both individual and group formats.

3. **Longer-term therapy (more than 26 sessions, or longer than 6 months).** Beyond 6 months we move into what can be statistically defined as longer-term treatment. Patients who are still in therapy at this point tend to continue for many more months or years. Improvement continues, but the pace of change slows. The balance between active change and maintenance functions begins to shift toward the latter. During this period, a greater amount of time is spent per patient, so that the use of a group format has major economic advantage. For example, some groups are designed for long-term maintenance functions where major change is not likely but where support and containment are quite helpful. The goal for patients in these groups is to prevent decompensation and to obviate hospitalization. Groups are an ideal format for attempting to achieve this goal, providing a support system that goes far beyond that available through individual sessions. An example of such a longer-term group would be a community program for patients with schizophrenia. Other longer-term programs are designed for ongoing active treatment of patients with relatively severe problems, such as major personality disorders, who will, it is anticipated, eventually be discharged. Even in this category, the containing effects of ongoing treatment may result in a considerable cost-benefit effect because of a reduction in the use of emergency room and inpatient bed resources.

This time-segmented model is a sound starting point for planning time-managed psychotherapy. There are three critical decision points: 1) at the time of initial assessment, when a preliminary decision must be made as to the likely nature of the time contact that will be required so that the patient can be promptly directed to the most appropriate resource; 2) after a handful of sessions (e.g., six or eight), when the patient is moving beyond a crisis intervention mode; and 3) after 4 to 6 months of treatment, when the likelihood of therapy lasting longer is higher. The last decision point has more serious resource utilization implications. It is helpful when looking at a service delivery system to incorporate these sequential decisions into standard operating procedures. Even for the solo practitioner, it may be helpful to be thinking of treatment expectations in terms of these phases. Most clinicians are surprised to find that the actual distribution of their initial assessments corresponds to this breakdown into time categories.

It is important to bear in mind that the utilization curves in Figure 1–1 are based on a large number of clinical encounters and thus are useful in thinking at the programmatic level. However, they must be applied with clinical judgment in the care of an individual patient. It is clear that a sizable percentage of patients do well with only a few sessions and that a substantial minority need long-term approaches. The challenge for the clinician is in determining what patients fall into the middle zone of more intensive but time-limited therapy. This segment is not well represented in many managed care settings, in part because of fear that such treatment will evolve into longer-term treatment. Patients who would benefit from more intensive approaches are in danger of being undertreated. As treatment moves beyond the crisis intervention phase, it is predictable that more resistance will be mobilized in patients as they address maladaptive patterns. This process requires more clinical skill, and it often appears initially that continued progress will be slow. An important shift for clinicians is to understand that significant change can occur within this time frame and that, therefore, fewer patients will require longer-term treatment. The research literature summarized graphically in Figure 1–1 clearly establishes the efficacy of psychotherapy in which quite carefully monitored treatment techniques are used. Less is known about the effectiveness of psychotherapy as it is practiced in a clinical setting. The use of protocols in this book is designed to encourage the clinician to use those techniques that have been demonstrated to be effective.

The Effectiveness of Group Psychotherapy

Of special relevance, given the changes in the psychotherapy delivery system necessitated by the evolving healthcare delivery system, is whether there are advantages to using a particular modality. Is group therapy any better or worse than individual therapy? When does family therapy offer special advantages? Group techniques have historically been seen as a secondary treatment modality, certainly not on the same level as the "gold standard" of individual therapy. This opinion tends to be shared by patients. Fortunately, there is a substantial literature comparing the two approaches. In the first major meta-analytic study of psychotherapy effectiveness, approximately half of the 475 studies were taken from the group literature (5). The outcomes for patients treated in groups were the same as those for patients receiving individual treatment, and the pattern of outcomes for both groups corresponded in large part to the upper improvement curve in Figure 1–1. Recent review articles have looked at studies in which patients were randomized into group or individual treatment with the same theoretical approach. Few differences in outcome were found between these two groups, with no major trend one way or the other (6). Similarly, no statistical difference in outcome was found between group and individual therapy in several contemporary studies that were designed to meet rigorous criteria for research design (7). If anything, the results of group treatment appeared a bit more satisfactory than those of individual approaches, in part because once patients became engaged in a group they tended to drop out at a lower frequency than in individual treatment. These studies do not take into account individuals who refused to participate because of the possibility of receiving group treatment. This attitudinal issue is addressed in Chapter 6.

The research results suggest at the very least that group therapy is clearly not a second-rate treatment. The efficacy indicated by the data above, combined with the relative efficiency of the group modality, makes a powerful argument for more extensive use of groups in service delivery settings. Justification for the use of psychotherapy must, in the current clinical atmosphere, be based on empirical findings, not just personal statements of belief. The data quoted above indicate that it is reasonable to suggest that group treatment be the preferred default modality, with special justification for the use of extended individual formats. At first glance, this might seem to be an extreme statement that flies in the face of most current clinical practice. However, an extensive base of clinical research suggests that the more important decision is whether or not an individual is suitable for psychotherapy. After that decision has been made, the results with the use of individual or group modalities appear to be largely indistinguishable.

Adaptation to Change in the Healthcare Delivery System

The ultimate challenge to the practicing clinician is how to find professional satisfaction in a healthcare system that seems to be in continuous change (8). This section might be entitled "Heraclitus Won." Aristotle, you will remember, held that form and structure were eternal and that change was passing. Heraclitus of Ephesus (d. 480 B.C.) developed a theory of the soul and described its creative resources, emphasizing the importance of self-exploration—clearly born to be a group therapist. He believed, in contrast to Aristotle, that change was constant and that form and structure were ephemeral: "An individual cannot step into the same river twice." We are currently knee-deep in a swiftly flowing river of healthcare change.

The first principle of managing change is that what is being lost must be faced and mourned. This process entails an acceptance that change is occurring or has occurred. Indeed, a number of valuable and important aspects of the traditional delivery system have been or are going to be lost. Practicing in an independent manner without considering the larger healthcare system is likely to become impracticable for all but a handful of clinicians.

Current changes in the healthcare system may not bring about the end of private practice, but they will effect a major change in how private practice operates. Caps on fee schedules and on the total amount of money available for health care will likely be instituted. The setting of such caps will exert painful pressures on professionals, who will find themselves in more stringent, competitive positions than now exist. Practice guidelines will become standard for all larger healthcare systems, and the practice profile of the individual clinician will be reviewed. Individual variation will not end, but there will be less leeway for unorthodox practices. Clinicians will be expected to add time limits and targeted groups to their clinical armamentarium. Participation in some manner in larger organizational structures, at the very least through membership in provider panels, will likely be necessary. A trend toward practicing under the aegis of some type of larger healthcare consortium seems likely. These changes are becoming the current reality and are not dependent on future legislative decisions. All of these developments will initially be felt as undue intrusions on the individual clinician and will elicit escalating reactions of resentment and bitterness. Such reactions are understandable, but adaptation to these developments, however difficult, is necessary. Discussion of the future cannot be effectively conducted without gaining closure on the past.

Adapting to change inevitably entails a time of confusion and uncertainty. Nothing seems resolved or predictable. This period can be seen as a negative and destructive experience, or it can be visualized as an opportunity for creative solutions. At present, the healthcare system is clearly in turmoil, with multiple and varied solutions being recommended or being tried. It might be helpful to consider that an enormous healthcare industry, accounting for 15% of the gross domestic product in the United States at the time of this writing, has been fundamentally altered in little more than a decade. This transition has been marked by some very questionable clinical practices as well as by some innovative and successful programs. As the new models settle into place, concern about practice standards becomes more evident. As professionals, we need to be active in promoting ethical, effective, and efficient solutions.

A Historical Perspective

Historically, the use of group methods has waxed and waned. Before World War II, the systematic use of groups in psychotherapy was rare. The need to treat large numbers of service personnel experiencing stress reactions led to the widespread development of group methods. Not coincidentally, the American Group Psychotherapy Association (AGPA) was formed in 1942. W. C. Menninger, as chief of military psychiatry in the United States, felt that the development of group psychotherapy was one of the major contributions of military psychiatry to civilian practice (9).

The 1960s and 1970s saw another surge of interest in the use of groups, in part related to the passage of the Community Mental Health Center Act in 1963, with its promise of a "Third Mental Health Revolution." Parallel with these developments was the unprecedented explosion of group-based modalities in the community referred to as "encounter groups" or "T-groups." This blurring of approaches between the reasonably well functioning population and the population of individuals with identified dysfunctional illness resulted in a general discrediting of group psychotherapy. Groups came to be seen as having little specific value in terms of formal treatment expectations. Indeed, the use of therapy groups in clinical settings began to decline. This process was accentuated by the major swing of organized psychiatry into biological models of etiology and treatment.

The role of groups in mental treatment is again increasing in prominence. We are entering the third age of group psychotherapy. The first was driven by wartime necessity, and the second, by a general social swing toward experiential events. The current age is the result of more sober considerations of a scientific and economic nature. A window of opportunity exists here to influence how treatment systems develop. Groups are seen as an important resource by the managed care industry. Our job as clinicians is to work toward rational and effective implementation of group programs. We must recognize that a spectrum of services is required: some quite brief, some time-limited, and some longer term. We as clinicians should be the ones making those decisions. Providing such care will mean augmenting our present skills and adapting our present practices but will not entail a wholesale abandonment of our past. It will also mean we must be on our guard to ensure that group methods not be trivialized by setting of inadequate time limits or the use of poorly trained clinicians. We must be designers, not simply defenders. The models provided in this book may offer some ideas and guidelines.

Group psychotherapy may be coming full circle. The two founding fathers, Samuel Slavson and Jacob Moreno, began their careers on the streets of New York and Vienna, respectively. They saw groups as a way to bring therapeutic services to the common people. The current movement toward universal healthcare coverage presents an opportunity to broaden the impact of group methods. The task for us as clinicians is to prepare ourselves for this challenge and let healthcare administrators know that proper practice patterns are necessary to achieve effective treatment for our patients.

Enough of politics! This book is designed to provide the clinician with a comprehensive look at the potential of group psychotherapy and an appreciation of time management in its utilization.

CHAPTER 2

A Generic Model of Psychotherapy

*I*t has been estimated that there are more than 200 varieties of psychotherapy. Many claim unique and powerful clinical techniques related to their theoretical position. Yet virtually all comparative studies of psychotherapy find that there is a large common effect mediated through active ingredients that are found in all reasonable and planned therapeutic endeavors. These findings have been pulled together in what is known as a *generic model*. This model should not be mistakenly construed as a "lowest common denominator." The generic model identifies powerful mechanisms that underlie all types of psychotherapy.

Clinicians are increasingly using the results of clinical research to guide their practice. At one time, such mention of clinical application of research findings was greeted with either dismissal or irritation in many psychotherapy circles. This attitude stemmed from the earlier days of the development of psychotherapy in the United States. As the field grew rapidly in the years after World War II, many "turf wars" occurred, with superior efficacy being asserted by each of the various theoretical orientations. Such assertions were accompanied by testimonials but scant documentation of effectiveness, and certainly no comparative studies were available. That situation has now changed radically. The fourth edition of the *Handbook of Psychotherapy and Behavior Change,* published in 1994, summarizes controlled studies of outcome, the results of which, when taken as a whole, establish beyond reasonable doubt that psychotherapy is effective (10). The overall effect size, a statistical measure of change, is in the range of 0.85, meaning that the average treated person is better off than 80% of the untreated sample. This response rate is in the same range as that reported for most psychopharmacological treatments. The psychotherapy dose-response relationship represented by the graph in Chapter 1 (see Figure 1–1) reflects these findings. The positive results obtained with psychotherapy have led to a surge of interest in understanding how this modality works.

The *Handbook of Psychotherapy and Behavior Change* reports on no fewer than 2,354 findings dealing with the connections between process events and outcome change. This number of studies represents a doubling of the available studies in the 7 years since the previous edition. The psychotherapy research field can now be said to be entering a mature phase, and clinicians are increasingly expected to follow generally accepted criteria for the provision of clinical services. The development of practice guidelines by professional organizations is one manifestation of this process.

The present book is structured around the idea of a set of powerful common factors in psychotherapy that can be used to enhance the delivery of a variety of theoretically different treatments. A generic model for group psychotherapy is based on universal features found in all psychotherapy regardless of theoretical orientation. The general features of the model are found to be correlated with outcome for behavioral, cognitive, interpersonal, psychodynamic, and psychoanalytic therapies. The model applies equally to primarily supportive therapy or primarily interpretive therapy, a subject discussed at more length in Chapter 11.

The concept of a generic model has been comprehensively developed for individual psychotherapy (11). Because individual and group psychotherapy overlap in many ways, the dyadic treatment model will be discussed in detail first, and then the necessary adaptations for the group format will be addressed. Because most group psychotherapists also do individual treatment, this material should be doubly applicable. The model identifies common therapeutic ingredients that account for a large part of the effectiveness of diverse psychotherapies.

A Generic Model of
Individual Psychotherapy

The generic model of psychotherapy fits the cumulative results of empirical research into a coherent framework that provides guidelines for the clinician on treatment practices that are particularly helpful or harmful. In the discussion that follows, I stress only those therapeutic findings that have been found in numerous well-conducted investigations. These findings can now be considered as established facts regarding the ways to make psychotherapy most effective. Although other clinical techniques are reported in the literature as having positive evidence, there are not enough replication data to justify firm inclusion of these techniques in the generic model. In many cases, these additional techniques may be helpful for some patient populations, but may not be helpful, or may even be harmful, for other patients. Some of these techniques have simply not been adequately studied. A schematic outline of the generic model for individual psychotherapy is shown in Figure 2–1 and on the inside cover.

Input Conditions

Several ingredients are brought into the psychotherapy situation (top portion of Figure 2–1). The patient and the therapist each enters with issues related to sociodemographic status such as age, sex, family status, and social class. Each has a relationship history and interpersonal style as well as a self-definition. The patient also brings a personal treatment history that may have a major impact on attitudes about the current clinical experience. The clinician has a role definition related to professional status, theoretical orientation, and level of expertise. All of the tensions associated with differences in these attributes or beliefs will be activated within the first interview and must be effectively mediated. As we shall see later in this section, the nature of the early interpersonal relationship between patient and clinician is one of the more important predictors of outcome.

The general sociocultural context and the treatment systems in which both patient and clinician are operating directly or indirectly influence the course of psychotherapy. This overall context includes attitudes about mental illness and the range of acceptability or skepticism regarding a "talking" approach to treatment. Attitudes about mental illness in general and psychotherapy in specific vary greatly among geographic regions and social classes. Ethnic influences may preclude the expression of anger or proscribe the patient's talking personally to those outside the culture. Legal or work constraints will greatly influence the nature of therapy. Family beliefs may reinforce the importance of family secrets, or, based on these beliefs, there may be strong pressure to maintain family role expectations. Some clinicians espouse a single frame of reference for understanding pathology and consider clinicians with differing viewpoints to be "in the enemy camp." What are patients to make of diametrically opposed viewpoints about their condition? Is depression caused by a chemical imbalance or by a problem in adapting to specific sorts of stressors?

More overt pressures may be connected with the healthcare system within which the patient and therapist function and may affect their entry attitudes. Are fees required before treatment can take place? Are there restrictions on what type of service can be offered? Is the clinic setting welcoming or hostile? What are the therapist's orientation and experience, and are these appropriate to the nature of the patient population? Is the clinician being forced to offer very brief group psychotherapy by administrative fiat, and, if so, is she personally angry at these constraints?

Another input variable is the patient's previous experience with mental health resources. Does the patient, based on that experience, bring a high degree of skepticism, if not outright hostility?

All of these input conditions are in operation even before the first clinical contact and will greatly influence the shape of the therapeutic process.

Process Conditions

The most complex element of the generic model is the *process* of psychotherapy (middle portion of Figure 2–1), the various components of which are in constant interaction with one another. A formal initial focus on the *therapeutic contract* creates the frame within which therapy occurs. *Therapeutic operations,* comprising the technical aspects of psychotherapy, form an interactional loop between patient and therapist. The *therapeutic bond* describes the nature of the actual interpersonal relationship established within the context of therapy. *Self-relatedness* refers to the degree to which the patient, as well as the therapist, is open and accessible. Finally, *in-session impact* denotes the immediate experiencing of interpersonal critical incidents within the therapy session.

Each of the principal areas in the process portion of the model has been identified based on well-substantiated findings in the clinical investigational literature. These are the features common to all the psychotherapies that make psychotherapy effective. Note that the terminology is of a general nature and does not refer to specific theoretical perspectives. Also, as shown in Figure 2–1, there are numerous feedback loops between the different categories of events. Psychotherapy process is now understood as a set of complicated interactions among these variables. Because of these interactive patterns, the study of single variables in isolation is unrealistic.

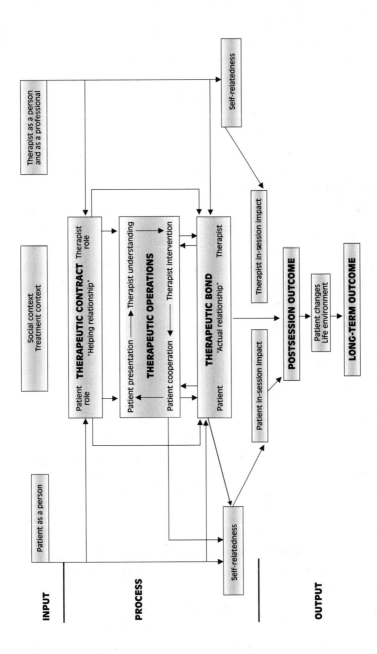

Figure 2–1. The generic model of individual psychotherapy.

Source. Adapted from Orlinsky DE, Grawe K, Parks BK: "Process and Outcome in Psychotherapy—Noch einmal," in *Handbook of Psychotherapy and Behavior Change*, 4th Edition. Edited by Bergin AE, Garfield SL. New York, Wiley, 1994, p. 362. Copyright 1994, John Wiley & Sons, Inc. Reprinted by permission of John Wiley & Sons, Inc.

Therapeutic Contract

The development of the basic therapeutic contract centers on how the "helping relationship" will be constructed and on what the roles of patient and therapist will be and how they will carry out their roles. First, formal contractual provisions such as setting, format, frequency of sessions, fees, and duration of therapy are addressed. Few significant findings have emerged regarding which formal aspects are optimum, and this suggests that various formats and schedules can be effective. However, stability of treatment arrangements and therapist adherence to a treatment model are important. That is, the presence of a consistent overall frame for the therapeutic experience is supported in the process literature, but the frame may contain different kinds of process material.

A broader view of the therapeutic contract includes several general aspects of the structure of therapy that are powerful predictors of outcome.

The therapeutic frame.   A clear knowledge of what one can expect to happen in therapy is important. This is best achieved as a consensus decision between patient and therapist, often obtained through discussion of goals for treatment and strategies for how these goals might be met. It is important that there be some collaborative agreement about such matters early in treatment. The proposed procedures need to be acceptable to the patient as well as professionally and ethically appropriate for the therapist.

Role induction.   Preparing patients for the therapeutic experience has a consistently positive effect. Such preparation is sometimes referred to as "role induction" about how to get the most from therapy. It has long been a standard practice in group psychotherapy but is uncommon as a formal procedure in individual treatment. The data suggest that this approach would be very useful in all formats of psychotherapy.

Appropriate selection of treatment.   A patient who is selected as being suitable for the specific treatment to be provided has a strong chance of being helped by that treatment. The criteria for suitability will of course vary considerably among different theoretical approaches. The important factor is to screen patients according to established criteria, which often involve cognitive and behavioral dimensions. The identification of a differential effect of some treatments for some patients has become an important focus in current psychotherapy studies.

Therapist skill.   Therapists who are able to provide their chosen form of treatment in a skillful and competent manner, not surprisingly, have good results. Both a general quality of professional competence and effective implementation of specific techniques are necessary. Increasingly, these skills are being fostered in practical clinical terms through treatment manuals.

All of these general structural dimensions of therapy are helpful across different theoretical orientations. That is, no matter what kind of therapy one does, these general procedural tasks will predictably enhance the outcome. Psychotherapy that has been well selected for the patient and is conducted in a planned manner with an openness to discussion of the plan between the patient and a skilled therapist is more effective.

Therapeutic Operations

Therapeutic operations comprise the technical procedures involved in the patient-therapist dialogue and are conceptualized in terms of an interactional loop: 1) how the patient presents a clinical problem, 2) what the therapist makes of this problem, 3) what the therapist then does about it, and 4) how the patient reacts to the therapist's intervention. Because these components interact with one another in a loop, each component is essential if satisfactory results are to be obtained. The therapist will, of course, be influenced by theoretical orientation to focus on selected aspects of the patient presentation. These aspects may or may not be those of relevance to the patient. Any significant differences in how this process is understood will need to eventually be reconciled if therapy is to proceed satisfactorily.

Patient presentation.   Two aspects of how patients present their problems consistently correlate with more positive outcome.

1. *A focus on important life circumstances and core personal relationships.* The act of specifying particular issues helps to concentrate the action so that the focus is on actual problems, not just vague generalities.
2. *An ability to express oneself in an organized and clear manner.* The correlation of this factor with better outcome may be a reflection of the general finding that patients who are higher functioning are able to gain more from their therapeutic experience. This does not mean that lower-functioning patients do not improve; however, it is harder work for both patient and therapist.

Therapist understanding.   Therapists are likely to understand the problems presented by the patient in accordance with the training and experience they have had. However, it is important that the therapist focus on the problems presented by the patient, including the affective component occurring within the session. Note that this entails following the patient's lead, though perhaps with subtle guiding of the issues. During this process, the viewpoints of the patient and the therapist may need to be reconciled. Failure to do so predicts a less satisfactory outcome.

Therapist intervention.   It is in the area of intervention strategies and techniques that there is the greatest difference among schools of psychotherapy. The empirical literature suggests that three types of interventions have a particularly powerful effect.

1.   *Cognitive understanding.* Strong empirical support is provided for the use of interventions that promote greater understanding. Providing the patient with this type of cognitive feedback appears to be very important. The exact framework used to generate this understanding is less important than that a systematic rationale be used. Some negative effects are reported with this process, especially when the patient is not open to such input.
2.   *Experiential confrontation.* Identifying, addressing, and promoting the experience within the treatment setting is strongly supported in the literature. Therapy is conducted through an actual relationship from which to learn. Some negative effects are reported with the more active involvement implicit in this intervention.
3.   *Support.* The provision of general emotional support by the therapist has a positive effect, though not as much as do the two more active techniques described above. It should be noted that, unlike the two more active techniques, a supportive intervention has virtually no negative effects.

Patient cooperation.   The nature of the patient's response to therapist interventions is a highly critical component in effective psychotherapy.

1.   *Cooperation.* A response of cooperation and alignment, as opposed to a response of resistance and defensiveness, is strongly predictive of positive outcome.
2.   *Affective response.* Strong affective quality in the response of the patient is also predictive of better results, especially when the affective quality is positive.

3. *Negative affect.* The measurement of negative affect in patient responses in a large number of studies reveals quite mixed results. In one-third of these studies, negative affective responses correlated with less satisfactory outcome. However, one-quarter of the studies found that such responses correlated positively with outcome, and the remainder found no significant association. The relationship between negative affective responses and outcome clearly stands out as an area for further study. It may be that issues of personality style and therapist timing and the nature of the therapeutic bond are implicated in the lack of consistency of these findings.

Overall, these technical procedures show some consistent patterns. Focusing on life problems and core personal relationships and experiencing the affective quality of these appear to be central to effective psychotherapy. Interestingly, a focus on here-and-now process events does not stand out as a strong predictor of outcome. An exception to this is in group psychotherapy, where a here-and-now focus appears more effective. In general, active therapist interventions appear important and support is benignly helpful. A key component is an affectively charged and cooperative response from the patient. A somewhat provocative finding is that patient measures of self-understanding and self-exploration have a relatively low correlation with outcome. In determining outcome, the evidence would suggest that the experience of being actively involved in psychotherapy carries more weight than does the specific content that is discussed.

Therapeutic Bond

The quality of the therapeutic bond has been one of the most intensively studied areas of the therapeutic process. The therapeutic bond reflects the personal qualities of the real emerging relationship between the patient and the therapist. It is independent of transference or countertransference qualities. Indeed, the implication is that a strong therapeutic relationship will prevent such transference distortions from sabotaging the treatment effort when they inevitably occur.

Several overlapping terms have been used in the literature to describe the therapeutic bond. A common designation is that of the *therapeutic alliance.* The more recent literature describes three separate, though related, qualities that together constitute the therapeutic bond: the personal bond between the participants, a joint agreement concerning the goals of therapy, and a positive collaboration in regard to how the task of addressing problems might best be approached. Of these three dimensions, the last-mentioned, also referred to as the *working alliance,* tends to be the best predictor of outcome.

Although the therapeutic bond is conceptualized as a separate feature of the psychotherapy process in the generic model (and thus accorded a separate box in Figure 2–1), certain features of the actual relationship may overlap with those of the other two main areas of the psychotherapy process discussed previously. For example, agreement regarding goals may be part of the therapeutic contract or may be an early focus during therapeutic operations. Collaboration regarding the tasks of therapy occurs during therapeutic operations.

The nature of the therapeutic bond may be examined from several perspectives: the patient's, the therapist's, an independent observer's, or one based on technical analysis of the transcription of the sessions. The patient's perspective is consistently the best predictor of outcome. Indeed, for some dimensions, the therapist's perspective is a relatively weak predictor.

The overall strength of the therapeutic bond is the best single predictor of therapy outcome. Early positive measures of the therapeutic bond, at the third or fourth session, are particularly strong predictors of a positive outcome. Presumably, this is because a constructive and collaborative process is in place early in therapy. Both the patient's and the therapist's contributions to the therapeutic bond are important, with the patient's being the more significant. Experiencing a positive, constructive therapeutic bond appears to be a rather specific antidote to the demoralized state in which patients entering psychotherapy frequently present.

The measurement of the therapeutic bond has involved a number of different dimensions across more than 100 studies. Both the patient's and the therapist's roles in establishing a strong therapeutic bond have been examined. Each of the therapeutic bond qualities listed in Table 2–1 has been found independently to predict outcome. Although clearly overlapping to some extent, these dimensions alert the clinician to the complex nature of the relationship that is evolving within the therapy setting (12).

Self-Relatedness

Self-relatedness refers to an intrapersonal trait: the way the individual manages thoughts and feelings and defines self. It might also be described as

Table 2–1. Dimensions of the therapeutic bond that have been found independently to predict outcome

Patient dimensions
  Motivation to enter into and to continue in treatment
  Engagement in the role of patient
  Collaboration in the treatment process vs. exhibiting either excessive
    dependence or excessive control
  High degree of expressiveness, as measured by participation rates
  Attitude of positive affirmation of the therapist

Therapist dimensions
  Attitude of engagement vs. detachment
  Collaborative approach vs. either a directive or a permissive stance
  Firm and credible presentation vs. unsureness and uncertainty
  Empathic understanding of the patient's experience (i.e., being "on the same
    wavelength")
  Attitude of positive affirmation of the patient by the therapist

Dimensions involving both the patient and the therapist
  An overall quality of communicative attunement ("We understand each other")
  Presence of reciprocal affirmation, with respect and autonomy

"relationship with self" or "how one behaves toward self." Self-relatedness commonly is conceived of in terms of a continuum ranging from psychological openness/exploration/flexibility to defensiveness/externalization/constraint. On the positive end, self-relatedness has been referred to as a sense of centeredness regarding self, a sense of self-responsiveness, an attuned and articulated self-awareness. A modulated sense of self-esteem and flexible self-regulation would be elements of this positive self-relatedness. On the negative end, self-relatedness is characterized by inhibiting self-control or, conversely, excessive loss of control, as well as self-punitive attitudes, self-alienation, excessive and inhibiting shame, and a closed attitude toward self.

The degree of self-relatedness is correlated with psychotherapy outcome. High self-relatedness in the patient is highly correlated with positive outcome. Low self-relatedness makes it difficult for the patient to absorb what might be offered in the therapy context, and the therapeutic experience may only confirm the patient's original negative perceptions of himself or herself or of the world. Patients with a higher initial level of self-relatedness stand to gain more from the psychotherapeutic process.

Often, self-relatedness is correlated with patient cooperation in therapeutic operations and with patient contribution to the therapeutic bond. Therapist self-relatedness is also correlated with outcome, although not as strongly as patient self-relatedness.

In-Session Impact

The processes described above have a cumulative negative, neutral, or positive impact on the patient within a single session. Elements of this impact are sometimes thought of as occurring in specific segments of a session, referred to as *critical incidents*. Positive micro-outcomes include a sense of relief derived from emotional catharsis, a sense of self-efficacy arising from confrontation of irrational attitudes, a feeling of empowerment through effective problem solving, an experience of success through learning a new skill, and a sense of mastery following psychological insight. These kinds of reactions are likely to induce a sense of hope that change is possible. The impact within a session may also be in a negative direction, such as confusion from overwhelming affect, embarrassment at self-disclosure, a sense of failure to resolve issues, or an experience of rejection or criticism. It is useful to resolve in-session experiences during the session to the extent possible so that the in-session impact is constructively understood and contained. A positive therapeutic bond also contributes directly to in-session impact, presumably by improving morale and increasing motivation.

Output Conditions

In the generic model, the outcome of therapy is conceptualized as an ongoing process. The effects of therapy are experienced following each session and have an impact on internal thoughts, attitudes, and emotional states. Behavioral changes in how one interacts with others in the outside world may also result. However, these developments exist in the context of the individual's current life. If the patient's environment outside therapy is not supportive or is actively destructive, then the impact of a session may be quickly dampened or completely overturned. On the other hand, in a facilitating environment, the impact may be augmented. The accumulation of postsession outcomes creates more enduring states of change. In this way, over time, individuals become better equipped to manage themselves and to determine the shape and direction of their life. This process has been described by Orlinsky and colleagues as "the activation through the process of interpersonal communication of a powerful endogenous therapeutic system" (13). Such an internal transformation can be expected to continue long after treatment has ended.

Important Interactions Within the Generic Model

Several feedback loops occur within the generic model of individual psychotherapy (Figure 2–1). Therapeutic operations are continuously influenced by the nature of the therapeutic bond. Conversely, the quality of the therapeutic bond is affected by the success or failure of the technical interventions. Similarly, the sense of self-relatedness interacts continuously with the therapeutic bond. Patient cooperation with therapist interventions also has an impact on self-relatedness. That there are multiple interactions among components of the psychotherapy process will come as no surprise to the experienced clinician. Indeed, the empirical literature is, in general, very supportive of usual clinical practice. However, conceptualizing the various components as discrete qualities of the treatment process can be helpful in addressing problematic situations. The generic model contains three critical screening processes that act as filters for the effectiveness of therapy:

1. *Patient cooperation with therapist interventions.* Frequently, patient cooperation models the interpersonal response style that has caused difficulties in relationships and thus lies behind the patient's seeking treatment in the first place. Skillful technique may be required to manage difficulties at this level.
2. *Self-relatedness.* Openness allows the assimilation of information, the acceptance of the developing therapeutic bond, and the capacity to absorb new perspectives. Thus, self-relatedness provides the patient access to the potential benefits of the therapeutic experience.
3. *The therapeutic bond.* The therapeutic bond is a central feature in the therapeutic process, being part of numerous feedback loops. The extent to which the therapeutic bond is positively developed is the single most powerful predictor of effective therapy. The state of the bond will determine whether the therapeutic context can function as a holding environment that will accommodate opportunities for incremental change. The therapist's role in the development of the therapeutic bond is directly in the Rogerian tradition, characterized by qualities of nonpossessive warmth, accurate empathy, genuineness, and unconditional positive regard.

The generic model suggests that the impact of the technical aspects of therapy is strongly influenced by the nature of the therapeutic bond. It is clear, based on the overwhelming evidence of process-outcome studies, that a strongly developed positive therapeutic bond is necessary for effective therapeutic work. In the absence of a positive and constructive therapeutic bond, successful results are unlikely. As can be seen in Figure 2–1, the therapist is in a position, through skillful interventions, to effect patient cooperation and, through expression of certain personal relationship qualities, to influence the therapeutic bond. Both of these strategies will also contribute to increased patient self-relatedness, which in turn will augment the therapeutic bond and will contribute directly to in-session impact. Technical, theory-based interventions are seen as important, but only if they succeed in altering the relationship existing between the patient and the therapist.

The foregoing discussion is based on investigations that have included many different types of therapy, spanning the range from relatively non-directive psychoanalytic techniques to very directive behavioral techniques; from vigorously interpretive techniques to primarily supportive techniques. These principles appear to be the basic ingredients that contribute to successful outcome in all theoretical orientations. They form the foundation on which specific theory-based strategies are superimposed. Consequently, constant attunement to the process of therapy is an important clinical guideline.

Specifically, the therapist is well advised to attend constantly to the patient's state of receptivity to interventions (i.e., patient cooperation), to monitor the quality of the personal relationship that is evolving between patient and therapist (i.e., therapeutic bond), and to assess the patient's personal state of openness (i.e., self-relatedness). Failure to see positive developments in these three spheres means that the therapist needs to take corrective action to focus on them. At the same time, the therapist would do well to regularly reflect on his or her own role in the process in regard to maintaining the therapeutic bond and his or her own state of self-relatedness during the sessions. This emphasis on the nature of the relationship between therapist and patient puts into interpersonal language many of the ideas found in the transference-countertransference literature. Bordin (14) suggests that the major goal of therapy is to constantly repair threatened ruptures of the therapeutic alliance.

Generic Principles of Group Psychotherapy

You have probably already been thinking about how the generic model for individual psychotherapy applies to groups. The input and output conditions apply to group psychotherapy in the same general manner. However, considerable modification in the psychotherapy process section is required to adapt the generic model of individual psychotherapy to a group context. The following discussion may be seen as an "addendum for group" to the preceding material from the individual literature.

In individual treatment, the therapeutic ingredients arise from the interventions of the therapist and the nature of the relationship between therapist and patient. In group psychotherapy, the situation is radically different. The individual patient is interactionally engaged with each member of the group. The individual also experiences the atmosphere of the whole group that results from the mix of all contributions. An understanding of this more complex field of action must take into account the principles of small-group psychology that are listed in Table 2–2 and that are discussed at length elsewhere in this book.

The qualities specific to group processes create an interactional field that is considerably more complex than that in the individual therapy setting (15). Technically, these features apply mainly to the nature of the interventions and of the therapeutic bond, which now involves the entire group membership and not just the therapist. This multidirectional interaction significantly alters the entire model. The main effects of a group setting on each segment of the psychotherapy process in the generic model of individual psychotherapy are briefly addressed below. To provide you with a fuller appreciation of these effects is the task of this book.

Therapeutic Contract

The basic components of the therapeutic contract of group psychotherapy and individual psychotherapy are similar. However, some of the components are significantly modified for the group setting.

The group therapist is in a position to significantly affect the nature of the group through composition decisions. In particular, a high degree of homogeneity will determine, to a major extent, the focus for group work and also is likely to promote and more rapidly effect group cohesion.

Table 2–2.   Generic principles of group psychotherapy

1. Therapeutic contract

   Group composition
   Closed groups
   Interpersonal goals
   Pregroup preparation

2. Therapeutic operations

   Presentation of personal problems
   Process of understanding the nature of problems
   Consideration of the whole group when determining intervention strategies
   Multidimensional feedback

3. Therapeutic bond

   Group cohesion
   Multiple relationships

4. Self-relatedness

   Modeling
   Social pressure

5. In-session impact

   Critical incidents involving several members

Homogeneity may, however, interfere with more confrontational patterns as patients reinforce their mutual blind spots. Conversely, it may enhance group members' ability to see the defenses of others. When group members have widely discrepant levels of coping, the group may be doomed to continual renegotiation of what is to be addressed in the sessions. In brief, the therapist's decisions have a great impact on the nature of the operating contract that will emerge during the early stages of the group.

Time-limited group psychotherapy is commonly conducted in groups that have a closed membership and a predetermined ending point. Such an approach entails more complex organizational arrangements and certainly affects the nature of the termination process, which becomes a major issue as the entire group together deals with the impending termination. Clinical experience suggests that the setting of a definite time limit encourages patients to finish the "course" of treatment. Closed groups provide this format automatically.

Many patients are less than enthusiastic about the idea of group therapy. Consequently, a careful exploration of attitudes and expectations is required. Therapy groups are particularly well suited for addressing the interpersonal manifestations of psychological difficulty. Therefore, goals established prior to therapy are usually couched in interpersonal language, such as dealing with the loss of a developing relationship, or learning to be more assertive. Greater emphasis is placed on the importance of using the group environment as a focus for experiencing typical reactions involving one's relationships with others. To facilitate this process, the therapist must lay the groundwork for an understanding of constructive group norms. The basic nature of the roles of patient and therapist in the dyadic thera-peutic relationship is well understood. For groups, however, it is useful to fully explore the role of the leader and how member input forms an im-portant therapeutic component. Because of these additional requirements, the preparation for group psychotherapy must be carefully organized and applied and is usually more extensive than for individual psychotherapy.

Therapeutic Operations

Therapeutic operations in group psychotherapy are substantially different from those in individual psychotherapy. It was noted earlier in this chapter that in dyadic psychotherapy a here-and-now focus has not been found to be a major predictor of outcome. In group therapy, however, such a focus is essential. Groups provide a distinctly more "real" relationship environ-ment in which the complex reactions of the individual may emerge through interaction with a host of protagonists, not just the authority figure of the therapist. The group context affects all components of therapeutic opera-tions and their interactions, as follows:

1. The presentation of personal problems generally results in greater in-itial anxiety in a group than in individual therapy because of concerns about the response of other members. This anxiety will be greatly in-fluenced by the overall group climate. A positive and receptive atmo-sphere often results in active self-disclosure early in a group as members model on the behavior of more open members. In addition, each member must to some extent vie for group time. Consequently, the role that the individual occupies in the group—a role that may change over time—will influence the ease or difficulty of self-disclosure. Similarly, the evolving level of group cohesion and the impact of group norms will influence the nature of members' presentation of their problems to the group.

2. To understand the nature of personal problems, the patient must consider the responses of other group members in addition to those of the leader. This process of mutual recognition of issues tends to be accelerated in groups because of the presence of therapeutic factors such as universalization and altruism. Indeed, some therapeutic factors are found only in the group situation, and others, although part of dyadic treatments, are quite different when experienced in a group context. Once started, therefore, the process of self-disclosure and feedback often moves quickly in early group sessions. An opinion or reaction of one member stimulates a variety of responses within the group, promoting the need to integrate diverse opinions. This situation creates a more flexible learning environment than in individual therapy. Despite the therapist's attempts to appear nondogmatic, the opinion of the therapist represents that of the dominant member in dyadic therapy. The working atmosphere of the group will also change perceptibly as the group develops, with each stage offering a different interactional climate within which to address issues.

3. Intervention strategies must be considered on two levels in group therapy. By far, the greater number of interventions are made by other group members, not the therapist. Group members express numerous interpretations, ideas, suggestions, and common experiences. This provides each member with a wealth of feedback for consideration. Often the spontaneous human responses of a peer are a more acceptable source of feedback than the more technically filtered views of the clinician. In addition, interpersonal confrontation happens automatically and early, so the individual is immediately forced to challenge accepted rationales or logic. Groups are able to mobilize powerful support through mechanisms of identification and understanding. Such support is of quite a different quality than that experienced in individual psychotherapy. The role a member plays in the group will be a major determinant of the type of interventions that are directed his or her way. For example, someone in the scapegoat role will receive more negatively tinged comments than will the sociable role members.

   The overall nature of the interactional climate will be affected by the developmental stage in which the group is functioning and the kind of interactional norms that have become established. During the engagement stage, supportive factors are heavily mobilized. Later, in the working stage, a more challenging process is anticipated. The interventions of the group leader often are directed at group-level issues and are intended to affect the group climate rather than individual members. Thus, the role of leader tends to be less direct in group therapy than in individual therapy. Therapy is conducted at one step removed, through the group itself.

4. The individual's receptivity to feedback is generally actively addressed at an early point in a group. Often, patients who have been unresponsive to individual treatment approaches find themselves melting before the supportive but persistent pressures from the group members for participation. The patient may be able to give up a skeptical and resistant attitude if there is active modeling of openness by other group members. The polarization of power that is inherent in dyadic therapy is greatly diluted in a group. This may allow patients to soften their defensiveness because they feel less need to justify their positions against authority figures.

Therapeutic Bond

The nature of the therapeutic bond, as noted earlier in this chapter, is the strongest single predictor of outcome in individual psychotherapy. A similar trend is also found in the group literature. However, the concept of therapeutic bond is more complicated. The closest analogy to the therapeutic bond in dyadic therapy is that of *group cohesion,* a property of the entire group. The group literature suggests that this group quality is indeed related to better overall group outcome. However, group members may not all share the same view of the group. Some evidence suggests that the opinion of the individual member is a better predictor of outcome. A sense of belonging or of being accepted is an individual reaction that may be independent of the overall level of group cohesion. Obviously, highly cohesive groups are likely to have more members who feel positive about their involvement.

It was noted that the therapeutic bond refers to the real relationship between the patient and the therapist. In therapy groups, there exist numerous relationships that have a very strong sense of reality. Thus, the individual patient has available a broad array of opportunities for positive affirmation and support as well as for challenge and confrontation. In many situations, the group therapist will purposefully refrain from such involvement and, rather, will respond at a group level, with the objective of building a sense of group cohesion. Thus, the nature of the therapeutic bond affects the choice of technical strategies, which may vary considerably.

Self-Relatedness

One would anticipate that the findings on self-relatedness in group therapy would be similar to those in individual psychotherapy. The main difference is the opportunity in groups for members to respond to modeling by other members. A cohesive group is able to exert considerable social pressure on individual members to join the group. In short, the task of addressing defensiveness is spread far beyond the therapist.

In-Session Impact

The principal difference between individual psychotherapy and group therapy is that in the latter, critical incidents usually involve several members. Thus, the interactional working climate of the group has a major effect. Here again, the therapeutic factors may contribute actively to a change-inducing experience. At the same time, a member who is the butt of criticism from or rejection by other members or by the group as a whole is subject to a potentially damaging experience. As in the literature on individual psychotherapy, a negative interactional tone needs to be directly addressed.

CHAPTER 3

The Nature of the Small Group

*T*he first challenge for the group psychotherapist is to make the transition from the individual to the group environment. Rather than experiencing the familiar context of two people interacting, the therapist must now consider what is going on in a room with a number of interacting patients. In this chapter, I discuss a number of perspectives that can be applied to understand the group system (16). These ideas form the basis for understanding group dynamics (Table 3–1). The phenomena described will occur in all groups that are allowed to proceed through the development of the interactional process. These include cognitive therapy groups and longer-term support groups, as well as groups in which the intention is to focus specifically on the group process. Group dynamics are not the same as psychodynamics. Clearly, the nature of group participation will be shaped by the internal issues of each member. However, group dynamics need to be attended to in all groups, and they also need to be considered in tandem with psychodynamics in process-oriented groups.

Structure of the Small-Group System

The basic structural elements of a therapy group form a number of important boundaries (Figure 3–1). A boundary can be thought of as a physical structure. For example, closing the door of the therapy room is a statement about the external boundary of the group. The number of members selected to join the group also establishes the number of individual member boundaries that will be present. However, in group therapy, a more important way

Table 3–1.   Theoretical concepts of group dynamics

Group structure

Group norms

Group size

Group development

Group social roles

Group cohesion

Group therapeutic factors

of thinking about boundaries is to regard them as psychological dimensions within the group space. From this perspective, a boundary is present when there is a clear sense of differences across the boundary. For example, during the early sessions in a new therapy group, the members begin to share their experiences and to appreciate that the process of self-disclosure within the group contrasts with many of their attempts to speak of their distress outside of the group. This recognition of a different interpersonal climate within and outside the group helps to consolidate the idea of an external group boundary.

The identification of specific boundaries within the group constitutes the first step in an important therapeutic strategy. The therapist is in a position to identify what boundary is in focus at a given point in time. By focusing on that boundary, the therapist can in many cases promote useful dialogue around the issues that are represented across the boundary. The therapist primarily has to be persistently interested in what differences appear to be present, thus activating the thematic material. For example, it might be observed that two members are exchanging frequent glances across the room. In a session early in the course of the group, this might represent a process of mutual identification that could be usefully reinforced to promote group cohesion. By innocently inquiring about the glances, the therapist may promote an open discussion of the sense of common issues between the two members. This approach would technically represent construction of a small subgroup that could then be used as a base for extending the inquiry to other members in the group. At this stage in the group, the intent is to reinforce a process of universalization that would strengthen the external group boundary. In later sessions, the same observation may lead to the exploration of a subgroup process that is working against group openness.

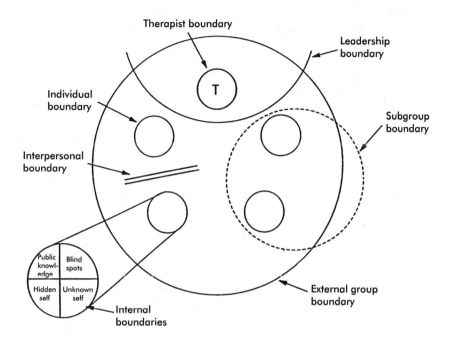

Figure 3–1. Structure of the group system.
Source. Reprinted from MacKenzie KR: "The Group System," in *Introduction to Time-Limited Group Psychotherapy.* Washington, DC, American Psychiatric Press, 1990, p. 37. Copyright 1990, American Psychiatric Press. Used with permission.

This theoretically simple technique of identifying boundary issues and promoting a discussion about them constitutes a group systems approach to managing the group interaction. The idea of "massaging" a boundary captures the idea of working that particular territory to understand the tensions and, by expressing them, to promote resolution and tension relief. This approach is atheoretical in the sense of its not being tied to an established theoretical orientation, such as cognitive-behavior or psychodynamic therapy, and thus is applicable to the group process in many different types of groups. Of course, this technique is not really atheoretical; it enacts an understanding of the group based on systems theory (17).

It is useful to practice superimposing the schematized group system in Figure 3–1 onto the group under consideration. This exercise will alert one to seven important boundary structures:

1. *External group boundary.* The external group boundary is the frame of the group that encompasses all participating members and the leader(s). An aggregate of individuals is not really a group until there is a clear recognition that it has become a unique social system with its own boundary. The first overriding task of the group therapist is to create this sense of groupness. It may sound trite, but group therapy cannot be conducted without a group. This sense of uniqueness within the group room creates a feeling of groupness. In Chapters 9 and 11, I discuss ways to conceptualize the group-as-a-whole. That discussion will revisit the importance of the external group boundary. The external boundary is closely connected with the initial development of the therapeutic contract in the generic model.

2. *Leadership boundary.* The leadership boundary is a specific interpersonal boundary that has particular importance in therapy groups. There may be one or two, or occasionally more, leaders within the leadership boundary. The leadership boundary extends beyond the external boundary of the group, because the leader(s) may also represent a larger organizational or administrative structure. For example, in a mental health clinic, decisions about the type of treatment offered may be influenced by administrative policies. The therapist will be seen as representing those policies, particularly if those policies have evoked negative feelings within the group. The leadership boundary often is the focus of important work for the group members. Groups offer the potential advantage of having many more interpersonal boundaries for interpersonal learning. Therefore, the leadership boundary, although important, is not as central to the group process as it is to the less complex system of dyadic therapy. Issues involving the leadership boundary pertain to the therapist's experiences and interactions in the generic model presented in Chapter 2 (see Figure 2–1, right side of diagram).

3. *Therapist boundary.* Therapists will be revealing to the group, both through words and through behaviors, many things about themselves, including their own state of self-relatedness. The group will respond to the leader as a real person, as a professional, and as a representative of the class of authority or parental figures.

4. *Personal boundary of the individual member.* Members in a new group are particularly aware of their personal boundary. They are likely to have a strong sense of the possible difference between how they are feeling inside and how other group members may see them. Self-disclosing statements move across this personal boundary, and nonverbal messages

also speak with greater or lesser clarity about the internal state of the member. The therapist often will encourage early self-disclosure in the group to make the individual feel more included. Feedback to the member must also cross this boundary. Awareness of the importance of the personal boundary and of its state of permeability is a useful guideline for the therapist, closely connected with the category of self-relatedness in the generic model.

5. *Interpersonal boundary.* An interpersonal boundary occurs between two group members. The number of interpersonal boundaries within a group is determined by the size of the group. Much of the work of therapy will occur across these boundaries. When the group has cotherapists, an interpersonal boundary exists between them. The importance of the relationship between cotherapists will be discussed in Chapter 11.

6. *Internal boundaries.* Internal boundaries refer to hypothetical boundaries within the individual. Clinicians trained in different theoretical traditions will use different concepts, involving different terminology, to understand internal states (i.e., therapist understanding, a component of therapeutic operations in the generic model, as depicted in Figure 2–1). In Figure 3–2, the internal divisions are conceptualized by use of the *Johari Window,* which has some value in terms of promoting useful, insightful work. The Johari Window is based on a two-dimensional model of things known and unknown to self and others. It is included in the pretherapy preparation material as one way of conceptualizing interpersonal issues and is discussed in more detail in Chapter 9.

7. *Subgroup boundary.* It is not uncommon for some group members to form a particularly close sense of identification with each other. Such a development may be a positive supportive event, or it may interfere with effective group work. In either case, it is useful to note such developments. The boundary for the subgroup extends beyond the external boundary of the group because subgrouping phenomena often occur outside of the group session.

Implicit within these boundary definitions is the idea of organizational levels. Four such levels are particularly useful for the group clinician: 1) the whole group, 2) subgroups involving two or more members, 3) interpersonal events between individual members in the group, and 4) internal processing within each group member. Of course, activity takes place at all of these levels simultaneously. The therapist has the option of deciding which level would be most appropriate for intervention. Early in the group in particular, interventions at the whole-group level might be advantageous so as to consolidate the sense of group identity. Later, if there is discord between members, the interpersonal boundary, or perhaps the subgroup boundary that involves several members, would be a more effective level for intervention. As the group moves into deeper work, more interventions might be made at the internal level. Because all levels are in process simultaneously, it is to be expected that an intervention at any level will have reverberations at the other levels. Thus, if the therapist is in doubt as to which level is most appropriate for intervention, there would be some justification for intervention at the highest level (i.e., the whole group) in the expectation that such an intervention might be most effective for the most members.

Group Norms

Group norms, another important quality of the small group, refer to the implicit or explicit rules or expectations that the members have regarding how things should be done in the group (18). Norms can be conceptualized in two ways. One way is to conceptualize group norms as what actually happens in a group. From this perspective, norms reflect to some extent the expectations that the group members have about how one should behave. A second, and perhaps more useful, way of conceptualizing group norms is to consider them to represent what the members think the others in the group believe should happen. Viewed in this way, norms reflect a process of conformity to group expectations.

A useful way to think about group norms is presented in Figure 3–2 (19). This matrix is based on what behaviors members feel would be acceptable and what behaviors they think will actually take place. *Positive norm regulation* involves high-frequency behaviors related to positive expectations, such as self-disclosure, provision of support, and efforts toward solving problems. *Risky behaviors* are actions that most people would consider suitable for the group but that do not occur because they entail risk. Identifying such behaviors and promoting a discussion about them may shift them into the positive norm regulation category. A common example of a risky behavior would be a member's being emotionally open in the group; that is, is crying (or showing anger, shame, or joy) acceptable? *Deviant behaviors* are those actions that occur in the group that are not welcome (e.g., con-

		EVALUATION	
		Consensus considers acceptable	Consensus considers NOT acceptable
EXPECTATIONS	Consensus expects to occur	POSITIVE NORM REGULATION (permissive)	DEVIANT BEHAVIORS (conflict)
	Consensus expects NOT to occur	RISKY BEHAVIORS	NEGATIVE NORM REGULATION (conformity)

Figure 3–2. Model of norm regulation in small groups.
Source. Adapted from MacKenzie KR: "The Group System," in *Introduction to Time-Limited Group Psychotherapy.* Washington, DC, American Psychiatric Press, 1990, p. 23. Copyright 1990, American Psychiatric Press. Used with permission.

sistently arriving late, monopolizing the group by engaging in monologue). Through group discussion, these behaviors would be clearly labeled as undesirable. *Negative norm regulation* involves lower-frequency behaviors that disrupt the integrity of the group, such as physical violence or breaches of confidentiality. Often, an open discussion about what members agree should not occur may be helpful in regulating adherence to these group rules, which are few in number.

Generally, there is consensus about the acceptability or unacceptability of any particular behavior. The importance of considering group norms specifically is to identify and label those behaviors that can be encouraged and those that are problematic and should be addressed. Failure to address unacceptable behavior will result in diminished group cohesion and lower morale. Failure to address behavior that is inhibited because it seems too risky will result in less effective treatment.

Group Size

Changing the number of participants in a small group affects the group interactional process in predictable ways (20). The number of possible interactions is a function of group size (Figure 3–3). As a group becomes larger, the potential complexity increases. The formula provided in Figure 3–3 allows you to calculate how many directions of interaction are possible in a group you are currently conducting.

Increasing group size will predictably result in the following:

1. An increased search for leadership to combat the sense of being swallowed in the mass
2. A greater likelihood of subgrouping as a way to find a sense of personal connection
3. Skewed participation rates, as some members come to dominate and others participate less
4. Less emphasis on personal matters and personal responsibility
5. Paradoxically, a greater likelihood of less inhibited behavior, because members can hide within the larger collective, often in subgroups

This information is helpful in deciding how many members to include in a group. If the goal is to use the interactions between members as a major therapeutic focus, then a group size of from 5 to 10 members is ideal. As

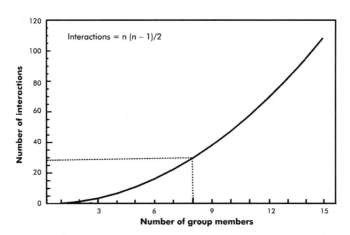

Figure 3–3. Potential number of interactions between members of a group as a function of group size.
Source. Reprinted from MacKenzie KR: "The Group System," in *Introduction to Time-Limited Group Psychotherapy*. Washington, DC, American Psychiatric Press, 1990, p. 24. Copyright 1990, American Psychiatric Press. Used with permission.

groups drop in size to fewer than 5 members, more specific control issues often emerge and are resolved by a pattern of focusing on one person at a time rather than using the whole group. As groups grow in size to more than 10 members, the increasing complexity of interactions makes it more difficult to focus on the individual and on the interactions between individuals. The use of more group-level interventions is one way of dealing with this situation. Once a group moves beyond 15 members, the ability to respond to individual needs drops sharply and the atmosphere becomes more like a classroom. This context might be appropriate for more structured activities such as psychoeducational programs but makes interpersonal work difficult.

Stages of Group Development

Stages of group development have been demonstrated in many different kinds of groups. An appreciation of the phenomena of group development provides the clinician with a powerful perspective in making sense of group events (21). Conceptualizing group development as occurring in stages is one way of describing the group-as-a-whole. Each group stage can be characterized as centering around an interactional task with associated typical behaviors. The notion of group development is particularly appropriate for time-limited groups, because these groups are usually closed groups with constant membership and, therefore, the developmental stages are more readily identifiable.

As noted earlier when the group as a system was discussed, events at one level in the group will be reflected at other levels. Thus, the developmental processes within each member will parallel those of the group-as-a-whole as it proceeds through its developmental stages. It is therefore important that each member of the group participate in the activities of each stage. Attention may need to be given to members who are either too far behind or too far ahead of the group so that the entire membership can move more or less together through the developmental process.

The model of group development presented here is limited to four stages (Table 3–2). This is the most abbreviated format for understanding group development. Other authors have described up to nine stages. However, for use in closed time-limited groups, the context in which developmental ideas are most relevant, the four-stage model is adequate.

Table 3–2. Group developmental stages

Stage	Boundary focus	Group task	Threat to individual	Resolution to threat	Individual task vs. attendant danger	Resolution of group task
Engagement	External group	Group identity; cohesion	Unacceptability	Universality; self-revelation	"We're all the same" vs. isolation	Acceptance of membership; commitment to participate
Differentiation	Individual member interpersonal	Conflict resolution	Conflict exploration	Assertion; cooperative unrealistic	"I'm somewhat different" vs. collaboration in polarizations	Tolerance of difference; resolution
Interpersonal work	Intrapsychic; interpersonal	Understanding the individual; relationship patterns	Self-esteem; rejection; inequality	Introspection; acceptance of relationship implications	"My uncertainties can be understood by others" vs. danger of openness to self or others	Toleration of self and others; openness and equality
Termination	External group	Close in the presence of separation/autonomy	Aloneness	Internalization of group; acknowledgment of loss/aloneness	"I can exist even though I'm alone" vs. nihilism	Acceptance of self-responsibility; acknowledgment of group's importance

Source. Adapted from MacKenzie KR, Livesley WJ: "A Developmental Model for Brief Group Therapy," in *Advances in Group Psychotherapy: Integrating Research and Practice.* New York, International Universities Press, 1983, p. 113. Copyright 1983. Used with permission.

Engagement

The foremost task of the beginning group is for members to become engaged in the group process. Until the members appreciate that they are actively part of the group, group therapy is difficult. Two basic mechanisms underlie this process of engagement.

The first is a search for common issues and interests. This process of universality makes the group safer because the members have some means of relating comfortably to one another. The process is driven primarily by a desire to find similarities.

A second mechanism is a recognition that the group is a special place with unique features that make it different from outside situations. In a technical sense, this process is a firming of the group external boundary. This boundary can be reinforced by comparisons between events within group and those without. For example, it is not unusual for members in a newly formed group to experience a sense of uniqueness at being able to share information about personal worries. This ability to share with group members may be contrasted with the difficulty in doing so with family or friends. The use of limited self-disclosure is essential for this process. Generally, in this first stage, the leader takes a more active role to orient the group, as the members seek guidance and support in how they should participate in the group.

The tasks of engagement can be considered to have been met when all members have a firm sense of commitment to participate and when each member has, at least to a limited extent, participated in the discussion with some degree of important self-disclosure. This process is generally accompanied by a rapidly rising sense of group cohesion and individual self-esteem.

Differentiation

The positive and collaborative atmosphere of the first stage is followed by a shift to a more negative and confrontational tone. Evidence of disagreements and potential conflict emerges. The essential task during this stage is for the group to develop patterns for resolving tension and conflicts that arise. Development of such patterns is a cooperative process in which problematic matters are openly addressed. The underlying pressure driving this stage is the need for members to assert themselves as unique individuals. During this stage, the emphasis shifts from common issues, the characteristic focus of the first stage ("We are all the same"), to differences between members.

At the same time, each member is also beginning to address aspects of self that may be problematic and associated with negative, angry, or shameful feelings. The intensity of the more challenging atmosphere eventually results in an increase in self-definition as members begin to sense themselves as more complex beings in the group.

The differentiation stage is often, perhaps always, accompanied by a challenge to the group leader. Such a challenge may be understood as the need for the collective membership to differentiate itself from the control of the leader. In this process, the group has an opportunity to forge a renewed definition of group norms. This process often has an adolescent quality to it; challenge is more for challenge's sake than for real change. Frequently, in groups that are having difficulty resolving tension between the members, the members need to turn their attention to what their thoughts are about the leader.

The group acquires important operational features during these two early stages of development. During the engagement stage, the group develops a sense of itself and each member attains a sense of belonging. During the differentiation stage, the group assists in putting into place a mechanism by which to address issues in a *positively* confrontational manner. Thus, the group is ready to move into more vigorous interpersonal work. These two stages, although occurring early in terms of group development, provide opportunities for important therapeutic experiences. The development of trust in the group and of the capacity to speak up in disagreement addresses core features of difficulty for many people seeking therapy. For the average weekly outpatient psychotherapy group, these first two stages are usually traversed in about 4 to 8 weeks. If the tension of the differentiation process has not emerged by the sixth week, there is need for concern that the group is, for whatever reason, stuck.

Interactional Work

The group is now equipped to begin addressing problematic issues for each member in a more vigorous manner. The onus for initiation of group work shifts increasingly toward the members. During the first two stages, the members have, of course, actively engaged in dialogue. Now it is expected that the group, through this interactional process, will address more specifically the issues that each member has brought into the group. The capacity to be both supportive and confronting fosters an environment in which interpersonal patterns can be identified and challenged. For the individual member, a parallel process of challenging self and being open to a more introspective examination is triggered. Initially, this process generally assumes a person-centered focus as members begin to explore with the group issues that are of deeper personal concern to them. The emergence of the individual, a process that began in the differentiation stage, is thus consolidated.

The personal nature of this work increases the level of closeness among the members. This increased closeness provides members with further opportunity to look at the nature of relationships. A growing sense of intimacy, sometimes of a romantic nature, brings the threat of possible rejection by members who have become quite close. Issues of self-esteem and trust are central to this process of risking rejection. By examining relationships, members become increasingly aware of issues of independence versus overinvolvement. Features related to dependency and control are central to this interactional work.

This progression from introspection to intimacy to equality, although commonly encountered, really only describes the evolution of increasingly important relationships. Often, themes fluctuate during the course of a given session. The therapist is perhaps better guided by attending to the issue of the moment rather than trying to superimpose too rigid an expectation of sequential development of the themes.

Termination

The final task for the group involves the termination process. Although listed as the fourth stage, in fact, termination may occur at an earlier point in the group's development. Later in this book, I discuss groups that are intentionally kept in the engagement stage until termination (e.g., a crisis intervention group).

Addressing termination issues is an important task and is particularly central to closed time-limited psychotherapy groups when the entire group ends together. Several important issues are brought into sharp focus in the process of dealing with ending the group. Members may feel that they have not gotten enough out of the group, perhaps just as they feel they have not received enough out of life. They must address the ending of relationships that may have become quite important to them. This triggers a sense of loss that frequently contains echoes of previous losses. In addition, members must now face the necessity of managing for themselves. Thus, termination raises many existential themes of responsibility for self and dealing with loss. These powerful psychological issues are all central to the maturational task. Paradoxically, the intentional imposition of a time limit provides an opportunity to address such matters directly. This work is difficult for both the group members and the therapist but must not be avoided. The intensity of the termination process will be directly related to the amount of time the members have spent together and the degree of interpersonal exchange.

This discussion of group developmental stages is intended as an overview. The developmental perspective informs many of the clinical applications discussed throughout this book in terms of helping the therapist make sense of group process and determine therapeutic strategies.

The Designated Leader

The social psychology literature places great emphasis on the role implications of official leadership. For the clinician, this designation brings with it a host of expectations that both provide opportunities and create problems for effective therapeutic work.

Designation as therapist of a psychotherapy group automatically places one in the sociocultural role of the "healer." This position carries with it expectations that the therapist has appropriate knowledge and skills and will uphold ethical standards. It is anticipated that the individual who takes on the role of leader will be helpful and positively motivated toward the members and will assume responsibility for preventing damaging experiences.

In the model of the group system discussed earlier in this chapter, the *leadership boundary* separates the therapist(s) from the other group members (see Figure 3–1). The "differences across the boundary" that form this boundary are heavily influenced by the expectations members hold concerning the designated leader role. These expectations may have little to do with the actual person or behavior of the leader. Every group leader (or committee chair) has been amazed at the powerful reactions elicited simply by sitting in the leader's chair. The image of the "throne" produces strong reactions, both positive and negative. Many group psychotherapists are quite egalitarian in their worldview and feel uncomfortable at the expectations projected onto them by group members and the members' subsequent reactions. Group therapists also are often concerned about the question of responsibility for initiating group activity. Both of these themes will be taken up in Chapter 11.

As was suggested in the foregoing review of group development, a certain amount of therapist initiation is appropriate in the early stages of the group. During the engagement stage, the therapist has a responsibility to promote the development of an effective and cohesive system. This responsibility can then be gradually shifted from the therapist to the group members so that they may feel confident of initiating leadership challenge during the differentiation stage. The process may be assisted through systematic pretherapy preparation, as discussed in Chapter 6, and by continual reinforcement of patient initiative during the early sessions. One therapist goal is the development of a working group that will assume much of the leadership function for promoting therapeutic change. This theme—that of the therapist's using the group as the agent of change—runs through much of this book.

At the same time, the role of designated leader carries with it distinct powers that should not be neglected. By virtue of the role, the leader is in a position to influence group events. Usually this can be done with subtle reinforcement, but, if necessary, a firm management stance can be taken. The leader is in a position both to view group events from the perspective of stage-appropriate challenges and anxieties and to conceptualize longer-term change effects. An understanding and accepting therapist who can tolerate group events without exhibiting overt anxiety exerts an enormously stabilizing effect on the group and allows the group to proceed with its work.

The role of designated leader will stimulate responses from members that are characteristic of their relationship with parental and authority figures. Material directed specifically to the leader needs to be considered as comprising a special and powerful class of interactional events within the group that may offer unique opportunities for therapeutic insight. It is a technical challenge for the therapist to encourage the use of this material without at the same time downplaying the importance of or detracting from the learning that can occur through interactions between members.

Some diversity of opinion exists regarding how best to respond to reactions to the leader that are above and beyond the real relationship, that is, reactions influenced by the role of designated leader. Some therapists view the group as a setting in which most, if not all, member behavior should be understood in terms of its relationship to the leader. Such therapists spend much time interpreting parental/authority themes. Other therapists view the group in a more egalitarian light and downplay the prominence of the therapist while promoting the importance of member interactions. Some of the implications of these positions are addressed in Chapters 9 and 11. In all cases, the role of designated leader must be treated with care, and thoughtful attention must be paid to its implications.

Social Roles

Another way of thinking about the group system is in terms of social roles. The concept of *social role* forms a bridge between the personality of the individual member and the function of the member within the group and is central to understanding social functioning. By definition, people with significant personality difficulties tend to adopt rather polarized role positions. For example, they may be excessively dependent on others or excessively suspicious of others. By understanding the function of social roles in the group, the therapist can attempt to differentiate between what is being driven by the personality of the member and what is needed by the group. The clinical literature contains numerous and sometimes colorful descriptions of group roles. In the social psychology literature, four basic social roles have received the most extensive discussion, resulting in a more succinct and operational set of definitions (22) (Table 3–3). Each role has both positive and negative features.

Sociable Role

Someone who assumes the sociable role has long been referred to in the literature as the "socioemotional leader." People who tend to assume this

Table 3–3.   Group social roles

Sociable role

Structural role

Divergent role

Cautionary role

role are friendly and supportive. They seek to maintain their relationships in a positive tone. They enjoy relationships and rapidly develop a sense of trust in others. They are eager to help others, often to their own disadvantage. These features make it easy for them to become group members. They play an important function for the group in promoting cohesion and engagement. At the same time, their naive quality may lead to their being taken advantage of by other group members. In addition, they may actively resist any tendency in the group to deal with negative or angry material. Members assuming this role generally have an important constructive function in the group and often appear aligned with the therapist. Their supportive functions are particularly useful during the engagement stage.

Structural Role

The structural role is closely connected to the classical definition of the "task leader." Members who assume this role are active in organizing the group. They tend to emphasize cognitive understanding and are concerned that the group stick with its task. They thus will appear to have a leadership style that may at times appear to be in competition with that of the designated leader. Members assuming this role are continuously concerned with having a sense of control or mastery of the group process. This concern for control may at times show itself through rigid intellectualizations and excessive attention to factual details. These members may provide advice to others but often have difficulty in receiving advice themselves. Their focus on cognitive mastery prevents them from feeling comfortable with spontaneity and emotional disclosure. They are able to provide the group with a focusing activity that assists the therapeutic task and are generally positive participants. A group therapy situation is frequently more effective than individual therapy in helping these people address the emotional side of their lives.

Divergent Role

The role of the "scapegoat" has been well recognized, particularly in the family literature. The term *divergent* has been chosen to highlight the function of members occupying this role in the group. Such members tend to be challenging and questioning; they often take a position contrary to the majority opinion or to the group norms. These members tend to be quite active in the group, perhaps impulsive, and to have considerable influence on the group process. This activity often forces the group to come to grips with important issues. Members who assume the divergent role have an intuitive ability to appreciate emotional issues and are not reluctant to bring them to the fore. Thus, they are helpful in promoting group interaction. At the same time, they run a danger of becoming isolated in the group and attacked by other members; they often become the repository of negative tensions existing in the group.

A group member who assumes the divergent role plays a crucial part during the differentiation stage of the group. If a group is having difficulty addressing the issues faced during this stage, there will be strong pressure for someone to take on the divergent role. Such members have an important function in the group, even though the therapist may at times have difficulty appreciating this. If a scapegoat is lost, you can be sure the group will find someone else to appoint to that function.

Cautionary Role

The cautionary role has not been discussed as extensively in the literature as the other social roles. Members occupying this role tend to be reluctant group members; they participate minimally and are not eager to reveal much about themselves. Sometimes this distancing is accompanied by an angry or dissatisfied tone. These members may appear to be defying the power of the group to get them involved. Because of their low activity level, they are in danger of being ignored in the group or of being criticized as not trying hard enough. At the same time, they may model for the group the importance of autonomy and the need to address the dangers of over-involvement. They may be helpful in promoting a realistic discussion of how to apply learning outside the group and how to deal with termination.

These four social roles provide a succinct vocabulary for characterizing the functions that group members may play in the group. These role descriptions also capture important characterological features. The therapist will often find that a review of group roles promotes a helpful discussion of individual problematic patterns. One might conceptualize one of the purposes of therapy as the modification of excessively rigid role dimensions. At the same time, recognition of who is providing the most influence in the group at a particular point in time may reveal important group dynamics at work. (See discussion of the Structural Analysis of Social Behavior in Chapter 5.)

Group Cohesion

The term *group cohesion* is used to describe the general emotional tone of a group (23). It is, unfortunately, a rather global term that is subject to many interpretations. At the same time, we can all recognize when there is a sense of "groupness," "togetherness," or "esprit de corps." Such terms can be applied to all small groups, whether a sports team, an administrative committee, or a therapy group. The important point is that the term *cohesion* applies to the functioning of the group-as-a-whole and not specifically to interactions between individual members.

Cohesion suggests that the members are committed to the goals and work of the group. They can identify with one another in their common task and have a sense of compatibility with the group activities. Generally, such identification with a common task also includes positive identification with the group leader, although this is not, perhaps, a necessary component. (A group can be quite cohesive around an internal leader and polarized against the designated leader.) Cohesion is generally considered to be an important condition for change, a group analogue to the therapeutic bond (see Chapter 2). It is most reliably assessed by monitoring actual group behavior. Members in a cohesive group attend regularly and are punctual. Few members drop out of the group. Cohesive groups are characterized by high levels of participation, and there is a sense of involvement and arousal in the sessions. Members tend to be open in their participation and to have a low level of defensiveness.

Cohesive groups are also characterized by a high level of acceptance of the members. It is possible, of course, for groups to be cohesive around a particularly pressing task or around a strong charismatic leader. In such situations, the actual relationships among the members may be of less importance in terms of determining the degree of group cohesion. Generally, cohesive groups are seen as supportive and as having high levels of compatibility among the members. This support is reflected in strong evidence of trust, spontaneity, and an eagerness to learn. At the same time, cohesive groups also show higher levels of challenging, confronting, and risk-taking behaviors. The overall result, therefore, is that the members of a cohesive group have access to a broad range of group experiences that are likely to be therapeutic. Indeed, the empirical literature indicates that there is a strong correlation between cohesion and outcome. A systematic way of measuring group cohesion has been developed by Budman and colleagues (24) (Table 3–4).

Table 3–4.   Group Cohesiveness Scale

Low cohesion	High cohesion
−5 −4 −3 −2 −1	+1 +2 +3 +4 +5
Global evidence of fragmentation	Global evidence of cohesion
Evidence of withdrawal and self-absorption	Evidence of interest and involvement
Evidence of mistrust	Evidence of trust
Evidence of disruption of therapeutic work	Evidence of cooperation toward therapeutic goal
Evidence of being unfocused	Evidence of being focused
Evidence of being abusive	Evidence of expressed caring

Note. Each of the six dimensions is given a score in a 10-point range from −5 to +5.
Source. Adapted from Budman SH, Demby A, Feldstein M, et al.: "Preliminary Findings on a New Instrument to Measure Cohesion in Group Psychotherapy." *International Journal of Group Psychotherapy* 37:75–94, 1987. Copyright 1987, American Group Psychotherapy Association, Inc. Used with permission.

Cohesion is particularly important in the early phases of a group, where it indicates that the group has established a constructive working atmosphere. This parallels the individual psychotherapy literature, in which early measures of the therapeutic alliance are a good predictor of final outcome. The salient message to the group therapist is that group cohesion is an important group property and should be constantly monitored. Group cohesion will vary over time as the group develops, responding to important group events such as a change in membership. Cohesion should be considered a necessary precondition for the enactment of many of the therapeutic factors that are discussed next.

Therapeutic Factors

Small groups provide a number of process events—referred to as "therapeutic factors"—that promote group cohesion and are specifically helpful to the members (25). Therapeutic factors are mechanisms available within the group that are independent of the theoretical orientation of the leader. These factors are mutually reinforcing, with the enactment of one promoting the emergence of others. A reciprocal relationship exists between group cohesion and the presence of therapeutic factors. Group cohesion significantly enhances the therapeutic factors, and promotion of the therapeutic factors increases group cohesion. It is useful to describe the various therapeutic factors separately to make them more recognizable. These factors, derived from a long group psychotherapy tradition, have been grouped into four clusters—supportive factors, self-revelation factors, learning factors, and psychological work factors—for easier recall (Table 3–5).

Supportive Factors

Supportive factors—universality, acceptance, altruism, and hope—promote a sense of involvement and membership in the group and help the member to regain a sense of mastery. They are specifically effective in addressing the demoralization and low self-esteem that are commonly found in patients presenting for psychotherapy.

Universality.   Members quickly find that others in the group have had similar experiences. The resulting sense of commonality is a powerful reinforcer for group membership and is particularly relevant in early sessions, because the individual may have begun the group with strongly negative self-attitudes. The process of universalization is a specific antidote to a sense of isolation from others. The sense of commonality and shared experience gained early in therapy frequently reappears at times of group tension to reinforce a sense of group membership.

Acceptance.   It is a powerful experience for a patient who is experiencing distress and a sense of alienation to be accepted into a group. This experience is quite different from the nature of acceptance in individual therapy,

Table 3–5.   Therapeutic factors in small groups

Supportive factors	Learning factors
Universality	Modeling
Acceptance	Vicarious learning
Altruism	Guidance
Hope	Education
Self-revelation factors	**Psychological work factors**
Self-disclosure	Interpersonal learning
Catharsis	Insight

in which the patient expects the therapist to have an attitude of basic concern. In a therapy group, acceptance must be earned. Therefore, the experience of acceptance by the group provides a strong boost to self-esteem. It is rare for a patient not to be accepted, especially in early sessions. The therapist can promote and reinforce the experience by ensuring that all patients participate in early sessions so that each member has specific opportunities for a response from other members.

Altruism.   Many patients report that it was helpful for them to experience an opportunity to be of help to another member. They may have offered support, made a helpful suggestion, or shared their experience with a similar problem. This process of altruism, which is unique to the group setting, reinforces self-esteem and helps to create a sense of self-worth.

Hope.   Most patients decide to come for therapy not specifically because of symptoms but because they have reached a point of futility and hopelessness. An important early effect of group therapy is the restoration of self-worth that comes from a sense of acceptance and support in the group. This restoration of self-worth rekindles a sense of hope that improvement is possible. Seeing improvement in other members or speaking constructively about their situation also promotes hope for one's own improvement. With hope that improvement is possible, the patient typically is strongly motivated to continue in the difficult work of treatment. Thus, it is important for the clinician to reinforce the instillation of hope, particularly in early sessions.

Supportive factors emerge spontaneously early in group interaction. Universality promotes a sense of linkage and acceptance. The patient's helping others encourages others to help the patient. These factors promote a sense of hope that change might be possible. Through these mechanisms early in therapy, the group develops a sense of cohesion. Interactions of this nature will occur automatically if not impeded. The therapist can encourage them by subtle reinforcement and by staying out of the way so that they can emerge.

Although particularly crucial early in a group's life, supportive factors continue to be important throughout the course of the group. Whenever the sense of group cohesion is decreasing, these factors can be promoted to help sustain the group through the difficult period. As noted above, these factors also increase the patient's motivation to continue in therapy.

Supportive factors are found in all types of groups. Self-help groups, for example, often provide these supportive functions very effectively.

Self-Revelation Factors

The self-revelation factors, self-disclosure and catharsis, generally occur together. The purpose of describing them separately is to encourage the recognition of those situations where only one is in evidence. For example, important personal information may be disclosed, but without the expected affect. Or, conversely, states of high affect may be present without a clear indication of the nature of the underlying issues. Self-disclosure and heightened affect, although found in all therapy settings, take on extra meaning in a group context. In the move from a private atmosphere to a group environment, self-revelation will be open to the opinions and evaluations of one's peers and thus will produce more anxiety. At the same time, it provides a realistic opportunity to understand how others see one and to experience their acceptance of material that often has carried with it reactions of shame or guilt. More important learning takes place when self-disclosure and catharsis occur together. The clinician therefore needs to monitor the process of integration between information and the associated affective tone.

Self-disclosure.   Self-disclosure of personal information is necessary for the group process to proceed. But apart from this procedural aspect, the act of putting personal information into words serves to externalize that information. Describing past critical events, presenting current problems, and revealing hidden thoughts encourage a thoughtful and more objective review. With the decision to place important information before the group, the patient is giving implicit permission for this information to be used in further exchanges. Self-disclosure is thus an acknowledgment that the disclosed information is associated with issues that need to be looked at. Self-disclosure deepens cohesion in the group.

Catharsis.   Catharsis, from the Greek *kathairein* ("to cleanse"), involves the expression of deeply felt emotion, especially feelings that are not usually revealed. Often, more negative affect states, such as anger, sorrow, or guilt, are involved, but on occasion positive feelings that are not normally shown, such as affection, play a part. This simple process of ventilation brings with it a sense of relief and promotes a feeling of greater mastery. It also generally results in stronger interactional bonds between the group members.

Learning Factors

The learning factors represent different ways by which patients learn from the group process. These factors tend to be downplayed in the group literature as being of less importance. However, they play a role during group sessions, and group members regularly report that these are quite useful. Since these types of learning are going to be present in any case, it is useful for the group therapist to consider how they might be most effectively used.

Modeling. Copying the behavior of others is a major learning strategy used both with children and with adults ("Follow me and try it out"). In therapy groups, members will be very alert to what the therapist does and will emulate those behaviors. Therapists therefore need to be aware of exactly what they are providing for modeling purposes. Patients will also use as a model actions of other group members that they feel are worthwhile. Modeling between members might be explicitly introduced as a good topic for discussion.

Example

A group for patients with severe characterological problems had several members dealing with management of extremely volatile emotional responses. One of them reported that she had tried out some relaxation techniques to keep herself under control. Indeed, she had just done the same thing in the group when challenged by another member, and it had worked. The therapist acknowledged this as a new skill she was applying and identified other group members who had mentioned similar problems. This generated a useful discussion and mutual attempts among the group members to apply such self-mastery efforts.

Vicarious learning. The process of vicarious learning is related to modeling in that members see what others are doing and use this experience to think privately about their own issues. Here again, the therapist may promote this process by being interested in what others have taken from specific group incidents. Taking such an interest promotes the idea that everything that happens in a group can be used for therapeutic purposes. Often, members will later relate the impact such experiences had on them— for example, "After I saw you two really confronting each other and actually learning something from it, I got thinking about how I never dare to do that with someone who is important to me. So last night I took a deep breath and told my husband we needed to sort some things out, and he actually listened to me." Vicarious learning may derive its effectiveness, in part, from a process of identification with another member, an aspect closely connected with universalization.

Guidance.   Advice and guidance will be offered continuously by the members during group sessions. Members often use such comments as a way to gain an alternative perspective on their own situation. This process between members can sometimes be more effective in opening up issues for exploration than direct confrontation by the therapist. Because guidance invariably will occur, it is helpful for the therapist to have some guidelines regarding the process. Of most importance is that all advice and guidance need to be seen as tentative and for consideration only—that is, as alternatives to be considered, not necessarily as imperative directives to be followed. The therapist needs to be particularly alert to suggestions that are given as commands or that seem potentially damaging. Often, such suggestions reflect important issues for the person giving the advice and may reflect that person's own difficulties. Opening up the advice-giving process for group reflection may therefore help both the giver and the intended recipient and encourage a recognition of an altruistic experience.

Groups that are designed to have primarily a supportive function, such as self-help groups, as well as groups that are based primarily on cognitive-behavioral principles, utilize advice and guidance quite liberally as part of the procedures. In these types of groups, it is important to strike a reasonable balance between the usefulness of advice from an authority source and the importance of patient self-initiation and autonomy. Generally, guidance and information have a useful function in most groups as long as they do not become the primary mode of discussion. As psychodynamic groups develop over time, the incidence of advice-giving usually decreases.

Education.   Some group formats are based specifically on educational principles. This approach may be a useful way for patients with specific illnesses to begin their group experience. For example, psychoeducational groups are often used as the first intervention for patients with bulimia nervosa. Similarly, some forms of psychotherapy for patients with major depression begin with a detailed review of the depressive syndrome. Groups designed to focus on a particular skill, such as anger management or assertiveness training, are primarily educational in nature. Many group programs have a routine pretherapy preparation program through which future members are educated about how to get the most out of their group experience. Overall, a learning paradigm is very appropriate for the practice of psychotherapy. It has a positive growth orientation that promotes mastery rather than focusing solely on negative affect or perceived deficits.

Psychological Work Factors

Interpersonal learning.   Interpersonal learning is fundamental to group psychotherapy, although, interestingly, it came rather late to the forefront of group theory. Early in the history of group psychotherapy, the focus of treatment was on the interactions between the individual member and the leader, almost to the exclusion of other processes. Now, in contrast, interpersonal learning is seen as a useful component because it dilutes the importance of the role of the leader. Interpersonal learning takes place through an interactional loop of self-to-others and others-to-self. This interactive process leads to the "corrective emotional experience" that is basic to psychological change. Attempts to isolate output learning (behavior) and input learning (feedback) have not proven realistic; the interactional loop, as an ongoing cycle, has no beginning and no end.

In the group the member has the opportunity to reveal typical interpersonal behaviors, get solicited or unsolicited feedback on them from other members, and try out new strategies. Issues can be clarified and understood, affect expression can be increased or dampened, assertiveness can be attempted, and intimacy can be experienced. The member can learn to soften defensiveness, accept criticism and learn from it, and be more sensitive to the reactions of others. The therapist is in a position to promote interpersonal learning, knowing that this "here and now" experience is a critical component of the process. The topic of interpersonal learning is discussed at length in Chapter 11.

Insight.   Insight, the internal component of the interpersonal learning process, primarily involves making connections between, on the one hand, feelings, thoughts, and behaviors and, on the other hand, recent or remote interpersonal events. The change may result from the experiencing of self in a different way, in identifying recurrent unrealistic negative thought processes, or in understanding typical interactional patterns that lead to problems. Interpersonally focused groups emphasize learning connections between earlier patterns and the present, detoxifying ancient images of parental figures. Such internal insight can have an impact on external behavior and on the internal sense of self-esteem and self-worth. These changes are harder to measure than external behavior, and one must usually rely on patient self-report to understand their nature. Genuine insight should be accompanied by evidence of more adaptive interpersonal and social functioning.

Implications of the Therapeutic Factors

It is clear that the list of therapeutic factors contains many overlapping threads. Certainly those within each cluster have a lot in common. But by teasing them apart this way, one can more easily see them in action within the group and specifically reinforce them. Many of these same processes occur in individual therapy as well. One possible way of comparing the two modalities is presented in Table 3–6. This way of comparing the therapeutic factors, although somewhat arbitrary, captures some sense of those factors that are unique to, or at least vastly different in, the group setting. For example, acceptance is found in the dyadic context but is of a very different nature than acceptance in a group setting. Interpersonal learning takes place in individual therapy, but in a much more restricted sense. Even most

Table 3–6. Therapeutic factors exclusive to, or very different in, group therapy and those common to both group and individual therapies

Exclusive to, or very different in, group therapy	Common to both group and individual therapies
Acceptance	Instillation of hope
Universality	Self-disclosure
Altruism	Catharsis
Modeling	Guidance
Vicarious learning	Education
Interpersonal learning	Insight

of the therapeutic factors common to both group and individual therapies are manifested quite differently in groups. The broadened interactional context makes most of these factors more complex and realistic.

The importance of each cluster of therapeutic factors generally shifts over time in a group. The supportive factors are clearly critical at the beginning but become less important, or perhaps just taken for granted, as the group proceeds. The self-revelation factors are important throughout the life of the group, although probably they are emphasized more frequently early on. The learning factors are operating all the time. The salience of the psychological work factors tends to increase as the group moves into more intense interpersonal work.

In this chapter, I have reviewed a number of perspectives for understanding the group system and group process. It is helpful for the group psychotherapist to become familiar with these concepts, because they are the basic building blocks of small-group function. At first, one may need to focus intentionally on these processes to develop the observational skills to identify these group qualities. One good method is to review audio- or, preferably, videotapes of group sessions. Often, such observation is enough to draw attention to features of the group that may have been missed during the action in the group room. Similarly, observation of groups run by others with a chance for a discussion following the session provides another effective way of sharpening group observational skills. The concepts presented in this chapter emerge regularly in applied situations throughout this book.

SECTION II
Assessment and Pretherapy Tasks

CHAPTER 4

Assessment of the Patient

*T*he assessment of patients for group psychotherapy is an important and complex task. The assessment process is useful not only for diagnostic purposes but also as a method for increasing awareness of issues that might be relevant to therapy. In this chapter, therefore, I discuss this pretherapy work in considerable detail. In the subsequent chapters in this section, I address how the information obtained from assessment of the patient is drawn on to establish a focus for therapy, to make group composition decisions, and to prepare patients for the group experience.

Review articles on the ability to predict how patients will behave in psychotherapy and how much they will benefit have yielded relatively few consistent findings (26). This lack of consistent evidence for the capacity to predict stands in contrast to most clinicians' belief in their ability to identify suitable and unsuitable candidates for psychotherapy. The empirical evidence suggests that an attitude of cautious skepticism is warranted. In Chapter 6, I discuss a pregroup workshop format that gives the clinician an opportunity to see how the potential group member actually participates in a semistructured group exercise. Such a format may be a more useful way to determine the patient's capacity to participate in a group setting.

The assessment process has several goals. First, and foremost, the clinician needs to identify specific contraindications for psychotherapy. Related to the first goal, it is then important for the clinician, after correctly diagnosing the condition(s), to determine whether there are specific treatment techniques available. When psychotherapy is indicated, the clinician must decide on an individual or group format for the psychotherapy. If group psychotherapy is determined to be more appropriate, the clinician must choose a particular type of group psychotherapy. Group composition decisions must be addressed. Finally, the results of the assessment process may be used as a component of the pretherapy preparation process for the patient. All of these goals are dependent on a sensitive and informed diagnostic approach.

DSM-IV

The *Diagnostic and Statistical Manual of Mental Disorders,* Fourth Edition (DSM-IV), published in 1994, is the current basis for formal diagnosis in most mental health treatment systems in the United States (27). The disorders included in DSM-IV are similar, though not identical, to those in the 10th revision of the *International Classification of Diseases* (ICD-10), published in 1992 (28). The discussion that follows concentrates on common and important diagnostic issues related to psychotherapy groups and is not intended to replace a working knowledge of DSM-IV.

The DSM-IV system contains five axes (Table 4–1), each of which refers to a different domain of information related to treatment planning and prognosis. This multiaxial approach prompts the clinician to take a broad view of the evaluation task.

The five axes of the DSM-IV multiaxial system are reasonably compatible with general clinical practice. The area of most controversy involves the relationship between Axis I and Axis II conditions. This controversy reflects, in part, a formal diagnostic problem related to overlapping descriptions. However, it also has a philosophical component, in that Axis I

Table 4–1.   DSM-IV multiaxial classification

Axis I:	Clinical Disorders
	Other Conditions That May Be a Focus of Clinical Attention
Axis II:	Personality Disorders
	Mental Retardation
Axis III:	General Medical Conditions
Axis IV:	Psychosocial and Environmental Problems
Axis V:	Global Assessment of Functioning

Source.   American Psychiatric Association 1994.

categories, unlike personality disorders on Axis II, are considered by some to be discrete diagnostic illnesses comparable to other medical diagnoses such as pneumonia. The ongoing evolution of Axis II is testimony to the difficulties surrounding the unrealistic hope of applying this degree of diagnostic precision to personality assessment. These issues will be addressed in the discussion of personality later in this chapter. Axis I and Axis II are discussed in greater detail later in this section.

Axis III prompts the clinician to consider the impact of other medical conditions, many of which have a considerable influence on cognitions, behavior, and mood.

In DSM-IV, the rating of psychosocial stressors found on Axis IV in the revised third edition of the *Diagnostic and Statistical Manual of Mental Disorders* (DSM-III-R) (29) has been dropped and replaced with a list of possible psychosocial or environmental problems. This list is a convenient way to identify problem areas and is conducive to establishment of a corresponding list of target goals or focus areas. Axis IV is best limited to current sources of stress so that psychosocial or environmental problems are not confused with the effects of earlier stress that may now have been internalized.

Axis V, the Global Assessment of Functioning (GAF) Scale, has a lengthy psychometric history as one of the more solid measures of the outcome of treatment. More recently, the GAF Scale has been modified, with the items separated into two categories—symptoms and psychological functioning, and social and occupational functioning—each of which is rated independently (30) (see Appendix 1). In DSM-IV, social and occupational functioning is assessed with the Social and Occupational Functioning Assessment Scale (SOFAS), which appears as an appendix in DSM-IV but is here integrated into the modified GAF Scale in Appendix 1. Also included in DSM-IV is a scale for rating the nature of relationships, the Global Assessment of Relational Functioning (GARF) Scale (see Appendix 2). These scales are useful additions to the DSM diagnostic system because they provide more opportunity for the clinician to register global evaluations in a semistructured manner. They make allowance for a patient who continues to function reasonably well despite significant symptoms, a patient who functions poorly but without major psychological symptoms, or a patient whose main difficulties are limited to the nature of his or her intimate relationships. It is most practical to use Axis V to rate the patient's current level of functioning. In some settings, a longer time frame might be appropriate to capture the level of decompensation the patient has undergone; when this is the case, the time frame should be clearly specified.

DSM-IV provides a simple, comprehensive report form whose use might be considered in a clinical program (see Appendix 3).

Axis I

The major DSM-IV Axis I diagnostic categories are listed in Table 4–2.

Categories 1–5. The first five categories are not discussed in depth here. This is not to say that patients with diagnoses falling within these categories might not receive group psychotherapy, but the diagnostic issues are relatively straightforward. In any diagnostic assessment, it is important to rule out problems with cognitive, behavioral, or affective states that might be related to organic features, to other medical illness, or to substance use. Similarly, the presence of psychotic symptoms plays a major role in determining the type of treatment indicated. Approaches to many of these conditions are addressed later in this book when models of group psycho-

---

Table 4–2.   DSM-IV Axis I diagnostic categories

1. Disorders usually first diagnosed in infancy, childhood, or adolescence
2. Delirium, dementia, and amnestic and other cognitive disorders
3. Mental disorders due to a general medical condition not elsewhere classified
4. Substance-related disorders
5. Schizophrenia and other psychotic disorders
6. Mood disorders
7. Anxiety disorders
8. Somatoform disorders
9. Factitious disorders
10. Dissociative disorders
11. Sexual and gender identity disorders
12. Eating disorders
13. Sleep disorders
14. Impulse-control disorders not elsewhere classified
15. Adjustment disorders
16. Other conditions that may be a focus of clinical attention

Source. American Psychiatric Association 1994.

therapy are described. The important diagnostic message is for the clinician to be alert to these possibilities.

Category 6: Mood disorders. Depressive symptoms are found in the majority of patients presenting for psychotherapy. Often, it is not easy to decide whether the symptoms meet the criteria for a formal diagnosis of depression. It is likely that clinicians favoring a biological understanding of behavior will make a diagnosis earlier than will those favoring a psychological approach. The situation may be complicated by the fact that depressive symptoms often, perhaps almost always, occur in combination with anxiety symptoms. With the advent of effective specific treatments for depression of both a pharmacological and a psychological nature, however, the importance of identifying major depression has increased. It should also be noted that there is considerable scope for clinician bias in assessing DSM-IV criteria for major depression such as "depressed mood most of the day" or "diminished ability to think or concentrate." Generalized anxiety disorder shares a number of criteria with major depression (e.g., restlessness, fatigue, poor concentration, irritability, sleep disturbance), and this feature makes diagnostic overlap inevitable.

Dysthymic disorder encompasses a category of patients who have chronic low-grade depressive symptoms associated with more general features such as low self-esteem, difficulty in making decisions, and feelings of hopelessness. There is controversy over whether this picture should be seen as a form of mood disorder or as a manifestation of personality disorder. In DSM-III-R, "depressive neurosis" was given as an alternative label for dysthymia. This label has been quietly dropped and replaced with frequent references to the common association of dysthymic disorder with other personality disorders. In truth, the issue is appropriately unclear. There is some evidence in dysthymic patients of physiological measures commonly associated with depression, often a family history of depression, and sometimes a response to antidepressant medication. These patients are certainly at risk for superimposed major depression.

Two specific categories of depression must be identified. The first category is a history of manic or hypomanic episodes. A positive history would identify patients with a bipolar disorder that might require specific pharmacological intervention either for acute treatment or for longer-term prevention. The second category is severe depression, the symptoms of which are listed in Table 4–3. Psychomotor retardation or extreme agitation detected during the assessment interview is the single most important core

Table 4–3.   Features of severe depression

Delusions or hallucinations

Catatonic features
  Motoric immobility
  Excessive motor activity
  Extreme negativism or mutism
  Peculiarities of voluntary movement
  Echolalia or echopraxia

Melancholic features
  Loss of pleasure in all, or almost all, activities
  Lack of reactivity to usually pleasurable stimuli
  Distinct quality of depressed mood
  Depression regularly worse in the morning
  Early morning awakening (at least 2 hours before usual time)
  Marked psychomotor retardation or agitation
  Significant anorexia or weight loss
  Excessive or inappropriate guilt

Source.   Adapted from American Psychiatric Association 1994.

feature. This endogenous symptom complex constitutes a strong indication for antidepressant medication.

Category 7: Anxiety disorders.   Anxiety symptoms, like depressive symptoms, pervade the entire spectrum of patients presenting for psychotherapy. However, within the general category of anxiety disorders, four conditions stand out for specific consideration. Recent empirical studies indicate that these four disorders respond more readily to cognitive-behavioral therapy (CBT) than to other forms of psychotherapy. They also respond to medications. However, there is a much higher relapse rate after discontinuing medications than after CBT. In short, patients with these conditions should receive competently delivered CBT, with or without medications. This may be delivered in an individual or group format (31).

1. *Panic disorder.* The diagnosis of panic disorder requires not only the presence of panic attacks but also concern or worry on the part of the patient to such an extent that a significant change in behavior results. Panic attacks may also occur in other anxiety disorders or as a result of a general medical condition such as hyperthyroidism or use of drugs such as amphetamines.

2. *Agoraphobia.* Panic disorder is often accompanied by agoraphobia, a fear of being in places or situations from which escape might be difficult or embarrassing or in which help may not be available. Agoraphobia reinforces the patient's concern about the possibility of panic attacks. A housebound state with major restriction in social functioning may result. Panic attacks with or without agoraphobia, in the absence of other anxiety diagnoses, respond to both psychotherapy and medication. The greater the role of specific stressors or specific relationship contexts in triggering such attacks, the more likely it is that psychotherapy will be effective. A group model for patients with panic disorder is discussed in Section IV of this book.
3. *Specific phobias.* Patients with specific phobias, such as those related to animals, heights, or flying, respond well to behavioral interventions, which may be administered either individually or in a homogeneous group format.
4. *Obsessive-compulsive disorder (OCD).* OCD of a long-standing nature does not respond well to insight-oriented psychotherapy. OCD is often found in combination with major depression. The newer class of serotonergic antidepressant drugs may be useful for both components.

Categories 8–15. The remaining Axis I categories often have associated depressive and anxiety symptoms leading to a generally upset state. In all of these categories, situational stress and interpersonal difficulties are common. Group approaches have been reported for virtually all of these categories, with the principal issue being whether there should be homogeneous groups for a particular disorder. The question of group composition is addressed later in this chapter.

Category 16: Other conditions that may be a focus of clinical attention. It is worth noting that this final category includes psychological factors affecting medical conditions, relational problems, and problems related to abuse or neglect. These conditions have now been fully incorporated into the Axis I diagnostic system. They are often found in combination with other Axis I and Axis II diagnoses.

Before finishing this discussion of Axis I, a word is in order regarding the combined use of medications and psychotherapy. In the early days of psychoanalysis, there was concern that medications would interfere with the proper development of a therapeutic working alliance and that symptomatic relief would decrease the motivation to address underlying problems. One still hears echoes of that belief. There is now abundant evidence that these fears were groundless. In fact, there is an emerging consensus that the combination might offer specific advantages. Medication often has an early effect, particularly on physiological problems such as insomnia and physical tension. Psychotherapy tends to have a longer delay before the onset of recognizable effects. These phenomena have been studied primarily in the treatment of depression and anxiety conditions.

Studies that have reported better outcome with the combination of drugs and talking may tend to be ignored in the enthusiasm for a contest about the most effective approach. No data suggest, in any systematic way, that the combination of psychotherapy and drugs interferes with effective treatment. This does not mean that in specific situations, when the two approaches are played against each other, there may not be complications. It is more likely that such complications are related to clinical management issues rather than to actual treatment effects. The great majority of Axis I categories are associated with interpersonal difficulties and negative views of the self. These aspects tend to respond less readily to pharmacotherapy. The patient can, and should, be reassured that attacking a problem with two effective treatments will enhance the results by addressing different levels of the system.

Axis II

Salient personality issues are found in most patients who seek psychotherapy. These issues may be the primary focus, or they may play an important background role in shaping how the individual adapts to particular circumstances. Because personality issues are omnipresent in psychotherapy and because they are currently the focus of much contemporary research, an extended discussion is warranted.

In DSM-IV, as in DSM-III-R, Axis II is organized into specific diagnostic categories. These categories are unchanged from DSM-III-R, except that passive-aggressive personality disorder has been designated a "category for further study" and shifted to an appendix. The current Axis II personality disorder diagnostic categories are listed in Table 4–4, with the disorders organized into the three clusters used in DSM-IV.

Table 4–4.   DSM-IV Axis II diagnostic categories: personality disorders

Cluster A: Odd or eccentric
  Paranoid personality disorder
  Schizoid personality disorder
  Schizotypal personality disorder

Cluster B: Dramatic, emotional, or erratic
  Antisocial personality disorder
  Borderline personality disorder
  Histrionic personality disorder
  Narcissistic personality disorder

Cluster C: Anxious or fearful
  Avoidant personality disorder
  Dependent personality disorder
  Obsessive-compulsive personality disorder

Personality disorder not otherwise specified

Source.   Adapted from American Psychiatric Association 1994.

   A personality disorder is diagnosed only when it is established that the patterns of functioning are of a long-standing nature. Certainly, these patterns must have been evident by early adulthood, and generally they are recognizable during adolescence, if not childhood. Personality pathology should not be diagnosed if dysfunctional symptoms first emerge at any time beyond early adulthood. In such circumstances it would be particularly useful to search for some important source of stress or adaptational change. A careful search for evidence of substance abuse also would be useful. It is possible for personality issues to be uncovered because of changing circumstances—for example, when death of a spouse reveals dependency—but an unresolved grief reaction may itself have features similar to those of some personality disorders. It is also dangerous to diagnose personality disorder in the context of acute stress. Everyone regresses to some extent at such times and may appear almost as a caricature of their normal selves. Similarly, patients who are experiencing major depression or a chronic anxiety state may appear to have a personality disorder until the condition is effectively treated.
   The problematic patterns should be evident in all aspects of a person's life and not be selective to specific situations or persons. The personality qualities must be inflexible and maladaptive and must lead to significant functional impairment. The general DSM-IV diagnostic criteria for a personality disorder are listed in Table 4–5.

Table 4–5.   DSM-IV general diagnostic criteria for a personality disorder

---

A. An enduring pattern of inner experience and behavior that deviates markedly from the expectations of the individual's culture. This pattern is manifested in two (or more) of the following areas:

 (1) cognition (i.e., ways of perceiving and interpreting self, other people, and events)

 (2) affectivity (i.e., the range, intensity, lability, and appropriateness of emotional response)

 (3) interpersonal functioning

 (4) impulse control

B. The enduring pattern is inflexible and pervasive across a broad range of personal and social situations.

C. The enduring pattern leads to clinically significant distress or impairment in social, occupational, or other important areas of functioning.

D. The pattern is stable and of long duration and its onset can be traced back at least to adolescence or early adulthood.

E. The enduring pattern is not better accounted for as a manifestation or consequence of another mental disorder.

F. The enduring pattern is not due to the direct physiological effects of a substance (e.g., a drug of abuse, a medication) or a general medical condition (e.g., head trauma).

Source. Reprinted from American Psychiatric Association: *Diagnostic and Statistical Manual of Mental Disorders,* 4th Edition. Washington, DC, American Psychiatric Association, 1994, p. 633. Copyright 1994, American Psychiatric Association. Used with permission.

The reliability of personality categories was improved (i.e., there is better agreement about identifying them) in the latest two versions of DSM (DSM-III-R and DSM-IV). However, there have been few studies of the use of Axis II under usual clinical conditions, and it is suspected that clinicians do not use the formal criteria or decision rules in a systematic manner. Clinicians have to face situations on a daily basis in which patients' presentations do not neatly fit into any specific diagnostic category even though a clinical diagnosis of personality disorder is warranted on the basis of significant dysfunction.

These practical diagnostic issues arise because the specific items within any given Axis II category do not hold together very well (i.e., there is poor internal consistency). This lack of consistency suggests that more than one concept is being measured. Of even more importance, there is major overlap between categories. If a patient's clinical presentation meets the criteria for one Axis II diagnosis, then it is highly likely that it will meet those for one or more other categories. Patients meeting the criteria for borderline personality disorder have a clinical presentation that often is found to meet the criteria for several other categories. This problem of overlap is particularly prevalent for categories within a given cluster, but cross-cluster overlap is also quite common (32).

Important connections occur between Axis I and Axis II diagnoses as well. The characterological aspects of dysthymic disorder have already been discussed. Similarly, there is major overlap between avoidant personality disorder on Axis II and social phobia on Axis I. Panic attacks with agoraphobia often are related to dependency issues. The entire range of anxiety diagnoses may be related to an underlying personality tendency to emotional overreactivity (see discussion of neuroticism later in this chapter). Many of the features of depression have much in common with Cluster C categories of personality disorder. Borderline personality disorder has been considered by some to be a variant of a mood disorder. There are some highly suggestive data that schizotypal personality disorder is on a continuum with schizophrenia. These areas of overlap bring into focus the question of state-versus-trait disorders. In general, Axis I diagnoses are thought of as illness states to be treated and made better, whereas Axis II disorders clearly derive from the domain of personality traits. Unfortunately, many of the common Axis I psychiatric disorders do not behave as if they were states, but, instead, present frequently relapsing courses that pose all of the ongoing management problems of trait disorders.

This diagnostic fragmentation often seems to the clinician to obscure rather than clarify the problems of the individual. A formal diagnostic decision may be useful in ruling out particular treatments but often is of limited use when one is attempting to determine the optimum approach. For example, most comparative treatment studies of the depressive and anxiety disorders indicate limited differential effect between psychopharmacological, psychodynamic, and cognitive approaches. It is generally believed that patients with character disorders from Cluster C, the anxious or fearful cluster, tend to respond best to psychotherapy. For many of the Cluster B disorders, patients also respond to this modality, but their treatment presents more challenges to the therapist. Patients with Cluster A patterns appear to respond least satisfactorily to psychotherapy.

A Dimensional Model of Personality

Given that the present Axis II system is less than satisfactory, is there an alternative approach to understanding characterological problems? DSM-IV makes passing reference to the *dimensional model of personality*. This approach has a lengthy history in personality research but historically has been ignored in the development of the psychiatric nomenclature. It is particularly pertinent to the interpersonal focus that lies at the heart of group psychotherapy. The present Axis II system does incorporate a basic dimensional component through its organization of the disorders into three clusters. These clusters correspond roughly to Eysenck's dimensions of psychoticism (disorders of thought), extraversion (disorders of behavior), and neuroticism (disorders of affect) (33).

The dimensional model is based on the idea that all people have discernible personality traits. Because several dimensions can be used to describe a given individual, the dimensional model allows the complexity of the personality to be more fully recognized than is possible when categories are used. The concept of personality represented by this trait model offers one hopeful alternative to obviate some of the problems mentioned in the previous subsection. To apply the dimensional model, the clinician must first come to grips with the need for a major paradigm shift. The model is based on dimensions, that is, taxonomic traits that are descriptive, not etiologic, in nature. Most clinicians have been trained to think of dysfunctional patterns as stemming from unfortunate early learning experiences. The psychodynamic clinician conceptualizes these patterns as centering around conflictual issues or a failure to master developmental tasks. The cognitive clinician thinks in terms of learned patterns of thinking about self and others. It is somewhat of a culture shock to consider personality as something that one simply has and must live with, like being excessively tall.

For a given personality trait, there is as much likelihood of dysfunction with too much of a given trait as with too little. That is, like blood pressure, personality traits tend to have a normal distribution in the population, and pathology lies at both extremes. This conceptualization contrasts with usual diagnostic methods, which are based on the assumption that if one has received a diagnosis, one is ill, and that if one has not, one is healthy. Similarly, in many of our therapeutic approaches, there is a tendency to assume that better function lies only in one direction. For example, an engaging, extraverted interpersonal style might be assumed to be "better" than a quiet and reserved pattern, which might be seen as defensive and reflective of low self-esteem. However, a patient with major extraversion characteristics tends to have difficulty with intimate relationships and may need stimulation to such an extent that self-destructive patterns emerge.

Several aspects of a dimensional model are worth considering:

1. The use of the personality trait model encourages the clinician to be a neutral observer. In the trait approach, the individual is considered to have a particular predisposition that, for most personality dimensions, has genetic origins rather than being the result of learning experiences per se. What is of greater interest is how such characteristics have interacted with both the patient's rearing environment and her current interpersonal world to produce more or less effective functional adaptation. The emphasis is on how the patient can learn to adapt more successfully. Such an emphasis can be helpful in allowing the clinician to differentiate between the long-standing style and the person underneath who must mediate between the style and a particular set of circumstances. The value of also viewing a patient in terms of personality style is to encourage therapeutic efforts to manage a style as well as to resolve a conflict (34).

2. An understanding of how the patient "is" in terms of trait terminology helps the clinician to understand the individual's inner reality, in terms of the model the patient uses when interacting with others. This approach falls under the original meaning of "phenomenological": one's psychological experience of the world. Such an understanding is likely to enhance empathy as the patient comes to feel that his own view of self is understood by the clinician. This idea of understanding the patient's perspective is closely aligned with personal construct theory (35). Constructs are conceptualized as the criteria by which individuals assess and create their interpersonal worlds. This orientation provides a bridge linking personality dimensions with the use of cognitive strategies as well as with interpersonal theory.

3. The recognition of trait qualities may contribute to the choice of therapeutic strategies. In particular, such recognition may be of considerable value in determining the mix of the less structured approaches that fall under the interpersonal/psychodynamic label, and the cognitive or behavioral self-control techniques, in which a more structured approach is used. This is not to say that various techniques cannot be combined. The trait perspective may, however, be illuminating as to how to balance the mix.

4. The trait perspective also may temper the clinician's judgment as to what is likely to change during the course of therapy and how the therapeutic alliance will evolve. Traits are not going to disappear or turn into their opposites, however much the clinician and the patient may want this to happen. In practice, patients usually find it helpful to know that they are not going to have to stop being themselves entirely. The task, rather, is for the patient to determine how to come to grips with being more adaptive given her personality traits.

Six personality dimensions have particular relevance (Table 4–6). These terms will not be unfamiliar to the reader, because they represent concepts that are thoroughly built into our language and our thinking. Three of these dimensions—emotional reactivity (neuroticism), conscientiousness (compulsivity), and openness—deal with self-management characteristics of the individual that are reflected in relationship situations. The other three—quality of relationships, extraversion, and agreeableness—are active ingredients of relationship development. Five of these six dimensions—emotional reactivity (neuroticism), conscientiousness (compulsivity), openness, extraversion, and agreeableness—are the Big Five personality dimensions that have recently been the subject of considerable research (36).

1. *Emotional reactivity (neuroticism)* refers to a tendency to react to circumstances with symptoms of psychological distress. People with high levels of neuroticism experience strong reactions to relatively minor stressors and may have excessive cravings or difficulty in tolerating the

---

Table 4–6.   Personality dimensions

1. Emotional reactivity (neuroticism)[a]
2. Conscientiousness (compulsivity)[a]
3. Openness[a]
       Psychological mindedness
4. Quality of relationships
5. Extraversion (vs. introversion)[a]
6. Agreeableness (vs. distrust)[a]
       Conduct disorder

---

[a]A Big Five personality dimension (see note 36 to this chapter).

frustration caused by not acting on one's urges. Symptoms of anxiety, depression, anger, vulnerability, and self-consciousness are common. People with low levels of neuroticism may appear phlegmatic and stoic, bland in the face of stress.

2. *Conscientiousness (compulsivity)* refers to the degree of organization, persistence, control, and motivation in goal-directed behaviors. People with high levels of conscientiousness tend to be organized, reliable, hardworking, self-directed, punctual, scrupulous, ambitious, and persevering. People with low levels of conscientiousness tend to be aimless, unreliable, lazy, careless, lax, negligent, and hedonistic.

3. *Openness to experience* refers to the individual's capacity to experience his or her own emotional and spontaneous states. Individuals with high openness are curious, imaginative, and willing to entertain creative and novel ideas and often espouse unconventional values. They seem to experience the whole gamut of emotions vividly. They are very open to self. By contrast, individuals with low levels of openness tend to be conventional in their beliefs and attitudes, conservative in their tastes, dogmatic, and rigid. They tend to be set in their ways and emotionally unresponsive. They are quite closed to self.

Psychological mindedness has long been used as a rationale for selecting patients for psychodynamic psychotherapy. It shares some of the same general domain as openness. Despite a lengthy history of interest in psychological sophistication, the actual measurement of psychological mindedness has been difficult to achieve. This difficulty is directly related to the fact that people interpret psychological mindedness in quite different ways (e.g., insightfulness; introspectiveness; capacity for self-observation or self-awareness; effortful cognitive endeavors; motivation).

A recently developed measure can be used to assess the patient's ability to identify dynamic (intrapsychic) components and to relate them to her own or another person's difficulties. When psychological mindedness is defined in this way, the result is directly related to the capacity to work within a psychodynamic model. The Psychological Mindedness Scale (see Appendix 4), developed by Piper and colleagues, reflects basic assumptions of psychodynamic theory (37). Higher levels of psychological mindedness represent a tendency to elaborate a complex understanding of the person, with more sophisticated and elaborate explanations. The scale also reflects a temporal sequence that is consistent with psychodynamic theory: that anxiety develops before defensive maneuvers are deployed.

For clinical purposes, the critical transition point appears to be at midlevel: the recognition of inner tension around conflicting issues. Patients who function at a level lower than this have an increased likelihood of dropping out of interpersonal/psychodynamic psychotherapy groups. Thus, this specific measure of psychological mindedness appears to support the clinical wisdom that psychological sophistication is an important predictor of the course of therapy. However, the situation is more complex. If patients who are rated as low in psychological mindedness manage to complete the course of therapy, they do as well as patients with higher scores. This suggests that patients rated as low in psychological mindedness simply do not speak the same language as the therapist and other group members and so, in many cases, drop out. The language is not what they expected or are accustomed to. However, they seem able to use an interpersonal group environment effectively once they get used to the language style.

4. *Quality of relationships* refers to the nature of a person's important relationships, a dimension that is clearly a marker of psychological health and maturation. Technically, we could call this "quality of object relations." It is a basic assumption of psychological development that internal structures are modified and mature through the experiences of a healthy interpersonal world in early years. During pathological development, these interpersonal expectations and anticipations become rigidified. Thus, they tend to be applied in an inflexible manner as new adult relationships are formed.

    The Quality of Relationships Scale (see Appendix 5), developed by Piper and colleagues (38), encompasses a spectrum from mature interpersonal functioning to primitive. The scale is based on the idea that self-worth is influenced by the nature of relationships and that emotional states are triggered by relationships. The scale assumes that a person strives, both unconsciously and consciously, both in fantasy and ultimately in actions, to reduce anxiety and experience gratification through satisfactory relationships. The nature of how this is done represents a measure of the quality of relationships.

    In the course of an assessment interview it is common to learn about the nature of a number of important relationships. As these interpersonal vignettes are being described, the clinician can think of where they could be located on the Quality of Relationships Scale. It is to be expected that not all relationships will be the same. And in any given relationship, there will be periods of higher functioning and lower functioning. However, by applying the five levels from the scale, the clinician can arrive at a general level of functional capacity. This assessment of relationship capacity is not directly related to symptom status or general adaptation as measured by Axis V in DSM-IV.

5. *Extraversion* refers to the quantity and intensity of preferred interpersonal experiences, activity level, and need for stimulation. People who have high levels of extraversion tend to be sociable, active, talkative, person oriented, optimistic, fun-loving, and affectionate. People with low levels of extraversion (i.e., introverted) tend to be reserved, sober, aloof, independent, and quiet, though not necessarily unfriendly.

6. *Agreeableness* refers to a continuum from compassion to antagonism in interpersonal relations. People with high agreeableness tend to be nonassertive, soft-hearted, good-natured, trusting, helpful, forgiving, and altruistic. They are eager to help others and are responsible and empathic. People with low agreeableness tend to be cynical, rude or even abrasive, suspicious, uncooperative, and irritable. They may be manipulative, vengeful, and ruthless. People with low agreeableness are good at taking advantage of people with high agreeableness.

People with low agreeableness may exhibit a pattern of behavior that fits the description of a *conduct disorder*. A person with conduct disorder violates expected behavior norms, ignoring social expectations and standards and, perhaps, engaging in negative activities, often of a destructive nature. This pattern may be accompanied by, but should be seen as independent of, substance abuse. Many patients with substance abuse appear much different after they have achieved sobriety.

At the extreme end of the conduct disorder dimension, there is a clustering of people who must be identified in an assessment interview if at all possible: persons who meet the criteria for a psychopathic personality. The diagnostic category of psychopathic personality, which has a long history, has been described as consisting of two major components: 1) selfish, callous, and remorseless use of others and 2) social deviance as manifested in a chronically unstable and antisocial lifestyle. DSM-III-R was criticized for an almost exclusive focus on social deviance characteristics. DSM-IV has addressed some of these concerns. The criteria have been simplified, taking the form of more general principles rather than descriptions of specific behaviors, and pathological lying, conning/manipulative behavior, and lack of remorse have been included.

Other personality qualities that have been historically associated with the diagnosis of psychopathic personality include those that overlap with narcissism, such as glibness, superficial charm, a grandiose sense of self-worth, shallow affect, callousness and lack of empathy, and failure to accept responsibility for actions. These qualities result in an incapacity to form deep or meaningful interpersonal relationships and a failure to learn from experience or punishment. A stimulus-seeking quality also is often present. This expanded definition goes beyond that included under antisocial personality disorder in DSM-IV (39). It is interesting to note that studies of incarcerated criminals yield a psychopathic diagnosis in only about 20% of persons when the full definition is applied. That is, the individual with psychopathic personality stands out even within a criminal population.

The detection of features of a conduct disorder is an important function of a diagnostic interview. Behavior that meets the social deviance criteria is relatively easy to detect, but the more subtle features of personality may at first not be so evident because they may be masked by social charm. These personality qualities are relatively resistant to therapeutic efforts. The most hopeful approach is with homogeneous groups, in which the members can use their well-honed skills to confront one another about their deception and dissembling. It is likely that with these patients the pressures of group norms are more effective than individual therapy. Such patients are not likely to benefit from a regular therapy group, and they may wreak havoc with other members. There is controversy regarding the capacity of persons with truly psychopathic personality disorders to respond to any kind of treatment. The clinician might be alerted to the possibility of psychopathy by a combination of low conscientiousness, low agreeableness, and high extraversion (especially a component of stimulus-seeking behavior).

These six personality dimensions will go a long way in describing personality features and have the advantages of being grounded in a substantial research tradition and of being described in readily understandable, clinically useful terms. These dimensions will be used throughout this book as a systematic way of describing and understanding relationship issues.

Example

Patients referred to an antidepression group with treatment-resistant depression and dysthymia tend to have a predictable profile. Many are high on conscientiousness, low on openness, low on extraversion (i.e., introverted), and high on agreeableness. These characteristics would predict some difficulty in using a group environment. This potential difficulty may be counterbalanced with a homogeneous group composition and with early structure around psychoeducational topics and cognitive definition of interpersonal patterns to develop engagement. As the group progresses, particular attention is given to the passive niceness of high agreeableness and the need to develop more assertive capacity.

Structuring the Assessment Process

The assessment process has two principal goals: 1) to assess the patient adequately to make a diagnostic decision and decide on a preferred treatment course, and 2) to use the diagnostic information obtained to help the patient to develop a reasonable focus for the treatment. It is strongly recommended that such an assessment procedure be allocated a minimum of two interviews. This is not an unreasonable time expectation for most service settings, especially when the outcome is a decision to enter the patient into a treatment program that entails a significant expenditure of time, energy, and expense.

The patient is assessed in a standard diagnostic interview lasting approximately 1 hour. Through this interview, a DSM-IV diagnosis is established and a general formulation is developed pulling together past development, current stress, and relevant psychological issues. The interviewer must therefore be selective in obtaining information related primarily to the diagnostic task. On the basis of this interview, a decision about the most suitable treatment program is made. The patient is given a written handout about group therapy, as discussed in a later chapter of this book (see Chapter 6), and then he or she may complete a set of questionnaires appropriate to the program to be entered. The process of answering some paper-and-pencil questions is helpful in preparing the patient for treatment. It stimulates an introspective process and helps to identify important issues that can be realistically addressed in the proposed treatment.

The second meeting, also approximately 1 hour, consists of a detailed feedback session based on the conclusions from the diagnostic interview as well as the responses on the questionnaires if these were used. In the next chapter, I describe strategies for helping to develop a focus for treatment and for reviewing this focus with the patient.

CHAPTER 5

Formulation of a Focus and Interpersonal Diagnosis

*I*nterpersonal language is particularly well suited for use in groups. It can be used to include both behavioral and cognitive aspects under the more general heading "How I get along with others." It can also be used to describe internal attitudes (i.e., "How I behave toward myself"). This general orientation allows the therapist and the group some leeway in addressing the nature of difficulties using whatever frame of reference seems most important for a given patient at a particular time. No matter what kind of group is being conducted, interactions between the members during the sessions will provide important material for diagnostic and therapeutic use. Efforts during the assessment process to identify clearly what the major characteristics are in close relationships will alert the patient to material that can be effectively addressed in the group. At the same time, of course, the process will sharpen the clinician's view of central issues so that care can be taken that these issues will continue to be addressed.

All forms of group psychotherapy should include an attempt to formulate a focus for the treatment process. In crisis groups, the leader may encourage the development of a focus primarily during the group interaction, where a constant effort is made to deal exclusively with short-term applied goals. The time-limited group psychotherapy literature has placed major importance on the task of establishing at the beginning of the group a clear focus for treatment. When writing this chapter, I have kept that purpose particularly in mind. Longer-term groups will also want to develop directions for work, but the longer format might allow the focus to emerge more gradually during the early stage of the group. For all group treatments, it is important to keep in mind that initial goals may need to be modified in the light of therapeutic developments.

A protocol for establishing a focus in time-limited group psychotherapy—one that embodies general principles that can be used with modifications in most settings—is described below. Because of the time constraints, the therapist must constantly strive to find strategies that will compress the therapeutic process. Many of these strategies are embedded in the procedures before the group begins. After a careful diagnostic assessment, such as that described in the preceding chapter, the next task is to identify specific important issues to be addressed during treatment. This process has a double advantage. It primes the patient for therapy by identifying key issues in a highly specific manner. It also orients the therapist to the same issues so that they can be kept in focus at times when resistance is evident. In addition, developing a focus represents a collaborative process between patient and therapist that establishes a good model for the emergence of a strong working alliance.

The interpersonal focus involves pattern recognition, which can be applied at various levels. Behavior, cognitions, and relationship meaning are commonly involved. Developing a focus in conjunction with the patient allows the therapist to align with the patient's frame of reference and thus is a powerful method of enhancing empathy. A clear cognitive description of a pattern also serves to externalize the issues by implying, in effect, "This is not the total you; it is something you do or experience that can be looked at." Through this process of externalizing issues, the concept of learning new patterns is reframed, becoming part of a more objective collaborative process.

This technique of clearly identifying target areas for therapeutic focus represents a break from the older psychotherapeutic tradition. Classically, it was assumed that important material would emerge over time and that hidden issues would be discovered with patience. The role of the therapist was to wait for this process of self-discovery. Above all, to provide answers would be considered a serious technical lapse, because the momentum for therapy was to come from the patient. In time-limited approaches, however, this process is altered. The therapist makes a direct effort to work with the patient in identifying the issues up front. This process utilizes the therapist's evaluation expertise as one component. At all times, however, this knowledge is shared with the patient in a tentative manner, an approach that encourages open discussion around sensitive issues. This process is an important component of the pretherapy preparation.

Structuring the
Focus-Setting Interview

The discussion of a therapeutic focus generally takes place at the second or perhaps third meeting with the patient. It is important that the therapist have on hand and have reviewed both the initial assessment and the results of any questionnaires that were administered. Any additional information from other sources, such as referring clinician or previous medical records, should also have been reviewed. The therapist needs to be prepared for this focusing session armed with as much information as possible.

The focus-setting interview is carefully constructed. The clinician adopts a stance of neutrality, cognitive clarity and directness, and tentativeness about the meaning of the results and maintains an interest in limited exploration of what the results might mean to the patient, with a particular emphasis on eliciting real-life examples. Patients are reassured that there is no magic to the evaluation of the information that they have provided. The results are described as being simply "their own words" coming back to them in a different form. All results are presented in a speculative manner, with discussion, elaboration, and examples invited. In particular, the clinician emphasizes the patient's own role in defining the issues of importance. The therapist is available for this process as a technical resource and a generator of ideas. The intent is to use the neutral structure provided by the information to move into a serious working engagement with the patient that undercuts the expectation that the therapist will provide all of the answers. This process has a certain paradoxical quality, because the therapist may be raising sensitive core issues for discussion. The secret to avoiding resistance is to present this material in a factual manner, citing its origins either in the assessment interview or in the questionnaire results (e.g., "As you mentioned when we were talking last time" or "It looks as if you are describing yourself in this questionnaire as . . ."

Patients are deeply interested in feedback concerning how they describe important relationships and personal issues. Generally, they promptly acknowledge and elaborate on the patterns revealed. The clinician must be careful not to make absolute interpretive statements. All results are described in bland and somewhat technical language that encourages a cognitive exploration of the issues raised. The onus is placed on the patient to take the self-generated information and apply it to attitudes or patterns regarding self or others. The feedback material is couched in terms of raising ideas or perspectives that should not be accepted immediately but might be pursued further within the context of therapy.

Most patients welcome this direct and candid discussion of core issues related to their dysfunctional patterns. The fact that the information is generated directly from their own responses in the assessment interview or on the questionnaires makes the process even more acceptable. Most express relief that important issues are not going to be skirted. They often acknowledge they have known for a long time that they would have to tackle the sorts of concerns that they themselves have identified. Sometimes, new, or at least unacknowledged, perspectives are opened up by this process. It seems that often patients have an awareness, perhaps only a hunch, about what needs to be changed but might not have actually put it into words before. The assessment procedures help to make these implicit understandings more explicit. Consideration might be given to providing the patient with a copy of the assessment record. This can be another way of both ensuring a collaborative effort and reinforcing important issues.

Different types of therapy will tend to focus on different types of goals. For example, behavioral treatments will identify specific targeted behaviors to be modified. Cognitive treatments specify negative thought patterns as the target. Interpersonal psychotherapy tends to focus on relationships and recurrent patterns in them. Psychodynamic treatments focus on attitudes about self and the reactions prompted internally by events and relationships. However, a word of caution is warranted about adopting too limited a focus. Most clinicians are now interested in integrating these different perspectives into a treatment approach that may emphasize different aspects at different times. For example, a patient who at one level could be described as having problems with self-esteem may have associated with that intrapsychic state many repetitive negative thought patterns about self, as well as behavioral evidence of passivity and lack of assertion. Although one may wish to focus on a particular level of difficulty, it is wise to be sure that by adopting this theoretical approach, one does not ignore the fact that the patient experiences parallel patterns at all levels simultaneously.

Some general guidelines will help the clinician to develop appropriate goals:

1. *First and foremost, the goal must be important and relevant to the patient.* To superimpose a goal that might be useful but not accepted by the patient is courting failure.

2. *The goal needs to be realistically achievable, particularly with the type of treatment being offered.* Working through major early family trauma may be needed but would not be appropriate for an eight-session assertiveness training group.
3. *To be most helpful, a goal needs to relate to changes the patient can make rather than changes that involve someone else's actions.* The intent of the changes may be to alter other situations, but only through what the patient personally can do.
4. *The time frame of the goals needs to be considered.* Long-term objectives are helpful in setting a general direction, but shorter-term initial steps are usually required. Or, in the other direction, as short-term objectives are achieved, longer-term goals can then be entertained, and in fact may be necessary to shift therapy to a more challenging level.

Behavioral Goals

The identification of specific behaviors as target goals is appropriate in the selection of patients for groups that will be more structured and more oriented toward behavioral or cognitive-behavioral strategies (40). However, it is not uncommon that fairly specific behavioral goals also find their way into more interpersonal or psychodynamic groups as well. For example, many patients in interpersonal groups are bound to face difficulties in asserting themselves.

The identification of specific problematic behaviors, although appearing at first glance to be easy, can be complicated. In particular, it is a challenge to identify the situations in which these behaviors occur, the specific antecedents to their enactment, and the nature of the consequences that might serve as reinforcers.

Behaviors can be usefully categorized according to the following schema:

■ Behavioral excesses (e.g., compulsions, aggressive outbursts, exhibitionistic behaviors)
■ Behavioral deficits (e.g., lack of assertiveness, social isolation)
■ Behaviors under inappropriate stimulus control (e.g., phobias, panic attacks, binge-purge episodes, intense help-seeking behavior)

Cognitive-Behavioral Goals

Methods to resolve distortions of thinking are common to all of the psychotherapies. For some purposes, it is useful to focus not on the issues of meaning and general relevance, but simply on the thought patterns themselves. The effectiveness of this approach, especially in the treatment of depression and anxiety states, has been well documented (41).

The first step in this process involves the identification of dysfunctional thought patterns that produce a distorted view of life events and of the self. Cognitive distortions imply significant misrepresentation of situations or people. Everyone may get some issues out of focus, but we are speaking here of serious and persistent misreading of situations or events that ends in dysfunctional adaptation. Common types of thought distortions are listed in Table 5–1. Although the categories overlap considerably, specific identification of these subpatterns enables the patient to more accurately track their presence.

The *cognitive triad* refers to the negative or distorted views that people have about themselves, the world, and the future. In an attempt to develop a therapeutic focus, it is useful to rank the three domains along with specific examples.

1. *Cognitive distortions about oneself.* A focus on attitudes and beliefs about the self (e.g., "I have never succeeded at anything").
2. *Cognitive distortions about the world.* A focus on the reactions of others to self (e.g., "No one will accept someone with my background; my personal origins mean I will never be acceptable as a lover or as an employee").

Table 5–1.   Maladaptive thought patterns

Polarized all-or-nothing thinking ("everything in extremes")
  Magnification of problems or shortcomings and of their significance
    ("catastrophizing")
  Inflexible "should" statements about self or others ("no room for variations")
  Extremes in relationship roles ("one is either the helpless victim or responsible
    for everyone else")

Overgeneralization ("untested minimal evidence")
  Mind reading ("jumping to conclusions with little or no evidence")
  Global labeling ("one or two qualities lead to a strong opinion")
  Mental filtering ("only the negative gets through")

Personalization ("Everything others do is related to me and probably my fault")
  Emotional reasoning ("I feel this way, so it must be right")

---

3. *Cognitive distortions about the future.* A focus on what is likely to happen that interferes with what is going on in the present (e.g., "What's the use of trying to get an education now; in a few years no one will hire someone with my background").

Schemas are organizing belief systems that underlie and promote the more specific cognitive distortions discussed above. Particularly powerful schemas involve attitudinal sets laid down in early childhood that involve regarding self as bad or good and others as positive or negative figures (see discussion of categories of attachment later in this chapter). Some schemas may be dormant until activated by specific types of situations. For example, a schema that carries the message "I cannot manage on my own without someone to look after me" will be particularly vulnerable to activation at the death of a dominant spouse. When used to address these schemas, cognitive focusing activities closely resemble the approaches that interpersonal therapists might use when working with patients to address issues surrounding important relationships. Indeed, this convergence has led to a growing trend to merge cognitive and interpersonal strategies (42). The artificial separation of behavior, cognitions, internal psychological meaning, and relationship patterns has truly been unfortunate. All of these components are in continuous interaction and, in the group format, are evident early in therapy. A flexible integration seems inevitable, since the interaction between members will not be conducted according to the subtleties of professional theories.

Discussion of negative thought patterns, for example, will lead to references about how such ideas were initially generated. Usually, parental references will be present and picked up by other members, and suddenly the group finds itself exploring recurrent interpersonal patterns. Often, the focus will involve mastering the reaction to a specific event, which may be of relatively recent occurrence or may go back many years—a critical event that shaped how the patient came to see himself and his interpersonal world. Sometimes, the focus will involve coming to terms with the relationship with a specific person, sometimes a person from the distant past. All of this material contains important behavioral and cognitive aspects that can be addressed.

Interpersonal Diagnosis

Many of the descriptions in Axis II of DSM-IV make reference to interpersonal behavior. Indeed, personality disorders may be thought of primarily as dysfunctional interpersonal behaviors (43). These patterns of behaviors are recognized when they persistently disturb others, not necessarily when they disturb the patient. In gross or subtle ways, persons with personality disorders break or stretch social and cultural rules and norms. They overuse a narrow range of responses, showing either a rigidity of style or, just the opposite, a great instability of style. The responses are often expressed in an intense manner. Personality pathology is eventually far more damaging to the individual in terms of social costs, which outweigh the perceived benefits.

The nature of the interactional process should be carefully studied when there is a possibility of a personality disorder. Useful questions to ask repeatedly are "What is this person trying to do, with or to me, in this situation?" and "How is she attempting to structure our relationship?" This process might be thought of as trying to understand how the patient trains others to reinforce the patterns she desires. Consider the person with a dependent personality who expects others to be in control and to take care of him. The dependent person presents with docile conformity, solicits advice, and maneuvers others into making decisions for him because of his passive stance. In this way, the dependent person elicits a sense of pity that serves to train others to help him to remain helpless and ineffectual. A thumbnail sketch of the cognitions and strategies characteristic of the interpersonal strategies associated with various personality disorder categories is provided in Table 5–2.

The Interpersonal Circumplex

Interpersonal problems are among the most common complaints that patients report during clinical interviews. Also, interpersonal behaviors are more reliably described and reported than more general internal or intrapsychic states. There is a distinct advantage to using an established framework for describing relationships. There is a long history of describing interpersonal behavior through the use of two major dimensions. The first of these, *Affiliation,* ranges from a positive, loving, enjoying quality to a negative, cold, rejecting, nonrevealing quality. The second dimension, *Control,* ranges from domineering/controlling to nonasserting/submitting.

These two dimensions, which appear to be quite independent, can be integrated into a circular model called a *circumplex.* Though conceptually simple, this model has proven quite useful in clinical assessment. Intermediate clusters can be designated to fill out the circumplex structure.

Table 5–2.   Core cognitions of personality disorders

Personality disorder	Basic beliefs/ attitudes	Overdeveloped strategies	Underdeveloped strategies
Paranoid	I must be on guard.	Vigilance, mistrust, suspiciousness	Serenity, trust, acceptance
Schizoid	Others are un-rewarding.	Autonomy, isolation	Intimacy, reciprocity
Schizotypal	I am different, and I don't care what you think.	Detachment, unemotional, isolation	Sociability, warmth, involvement
Antisocial	I am entitled to break the rules.	Combativeness, exploitativeness, predation	Empathy, reciprocity, social sensitivity
Histrionic	Others are there to serve and admire me.	Exhibitionism, expressiveness, impressionism	Reflectiveness, control, systematization
Narcissistic	I am special.	Self-aggrandizement, competitiveness	Sharing, group identification
Avoidant	People will reject me.	Social vulnerability, avoidance, inhibition	Self-assertion, gregariousness
Dependent	I need others to survive.	Help seeking, clinging	Self-sufficiency, mobility
Obsessive-compulsive	I must not err.	Control, responsibility, systematization	Spontaneity, playfulness

Source.   Adapted from Beck AT, Freeman A, and Associates: "Theory of Personality Disorders," in *Cognitive Therapy of Personality Disorders.* New York, Guilford, 1990, p. 42. Copyright 1990. Used with permission.

For example, Intrusive is a combination of Domineering and Overly Nurturing, and Exploitable is a combination of Nonasserting and Overly Nurturing. Agreeableness and Extraversion, the two dimensions that are specifically interpersonal from our list of six personality dimensions, can be superimposed on the circumplex, as shown in Figure 5–1.

The resulting eight clusters of the interpersonal circumplex are defined as follows in terms of the problems encountered:

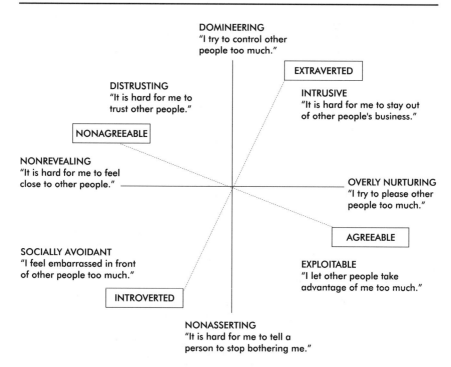

Figure 5–1. The interpersonal circumplex.
Source. Derived from Horowitz LM, Rosenberg SE, Baer BA, et al.: "Inventory of Interpersonal Problems: Psychometric Properties and Clinical Applications." *Journal of Consulting and Clinical Psychology* 56:885–892, 1988. Copyright 1988, American Psychological Association. Reprinted with permission.

1. *Domineering.* Problems related to controlling, manipulating, exhibiting aggression toward, and trying to change others.
2. *Distrusting.* Problems related to distrusting and being suspicious of others, being unable to care about others' needs and happiness, and perhaps being vindictive.
3. *Nonrevealing.* Problems related to being unable to express affection toward or to show love for another person, leading sometimes to an appearance of being cold.
4. *Socially Avoidant.* Problems related to feeling anxious or embarrassed in the presence of others and experiencing difficulty in getting into social interactions, expressing feelings, and socializing with others.
5. *Nonasserting.* Problems related to experiencing difficulty in making personal needs known to others, experiencing discomfort in authoritarian roles, and being unable to be firm with and assertive toward others.

6. *Exploitable.* Problems related to experiencing difficulty in feeling anger and expressing anger for fear of offending others and being gullible and readily taken advantage of by others.
7. *Overly Nurturing.* Problems related to trying too hard to please others and being too generous, agreeable, trusting, caring, or permissive in dealing with others and avoiding conflict.
8. *Intrusive.* Problems related to being overly self-disclosing and attention seeking and to experiencing difficulty in spending time alone.

The interpersonal circumplex can be used by the clinician as a conceptual tool to organize an understanding of a relationship. It can also be measured with the Inventory of Interpersonal Problems (IIP), a brief self-report questionnaire based on the interpersonal circumplex model (44). The accompanying items take two forms: "It is hard for me to _____" and "I _____ too much." Patients find it easy to identify with these formats. Figure 5–1 includes a representative item from the IIP for each cluster.

The results from the IIP questionnaire can be expressed in several ways. First, the overall mean item score is a reasonable summary of how persons describe themselves in terms of interpersonal problems. This score can be compared directly with the results from a symptom questionnaire such as the Brief Symptom Inventory (45) or the Outcome Questionnaire–45 (46). It has been suggested that people who see their difficulties as being associated to a greater degree with interpersonal problems than with symptoms such as anxiety or depression might be better candidates for psychotherapy. This measure, although not absolute, could be used to alert the clinician to check the patient's degree of motivation to talk about issues rather than to get symptoms medicated.

An average score of the items on each of the eight clusters can be calculated. Consideration of these eight scores gives the clinician an impression of how persons see themselves functioning in the interpersonal context. It should be noted that the questions are expressed in terms of "problems," so simply discussing the interpersonal features for which higher scores were obtained automatically leads to a preliminary idea of which interpersonal problem areas will be the focus of therapy.

An overall direction within the circle can be determined based on the elevated scale scores. For example, a person may describe himself as having problems related to Overly Nurturing, Exploitable, and Nonasserting—an indication that his interpersonal functioning is characterized by what could be called High Agreeableness, as represented in the lower-right quadrant of the circumplex model in Figure 5–1. Generally, patients find such conclusions immediately recognizable and can proceed to discuss what it is like for them to be faced with issues in that area of interpersonal functioning. Another patient may have elevated scale scores on Nonrevealing, Socially Avoidant, and Nonasserting—an indication that her interpersonal functioning is characterized by Introversion, as represented in the lower-left quadrant of the model. For most clinical purposes, identifying the most salient quadrant is adequate.

However, on occasion, the overall location vector may be misleading. It is not uncommon for patients to describe themselves as having problems drawn from opposite sides of the circle. A *Conflict Score* is introduced when scales on opposite sides of the circle are elevated. There are four possible Conflict Scores: Domineering and Nonasserting, Distrusting and Exploitable, Nonrevealing and Overly Nurturing, and Socially Avoidant and Intrusive. A Conflict Score suggests that the individual may experience some tension between the two styles. This tension may be manifested in different ways: unpredictable shifts from one style to the other, experiencing anxiety around situations involving these issues, or avoidance of such situations. Patients in general do not have difficulty recognizing competing states within themselves; they often can verbally describe these contrasting styles quite easily. One woman remarked, "I do everything for other people, but they have no idea what I'm going through" (Overly Nurturing vs. Nonrevealing). People with conflicts on the Control dimension (represented by the vertical axis in Figure 5–1) may describe sudden shifts from excessive passivity to bursts of angry, demanding confrontations. These reports may reflect clinically relevant internal states: "I always get used by people because I don't want to upset anyone. Then I get so angry at myself about the situation I decide I'll never have another relationship again."—a description indicative of a conflict along the Exploitable/Distrusting axis or between states of mind characterized by High and Low Agreeableness. Discussion of Conflict Scores also encourages psychological mindedness regarding internal tensions.

Another aspect of interpersonal behavior that may become evident when the interpersonal circumplex is being used relates to the reciprocal influence between two persons. That is, one person's actions will elicit, evoke, or invite particular types of responses from the other. The general principles of this "complementarity" process are that positive behavior tends to elicit positive behavior and negative behavior tends to elicit negative behavior, and that control behavior tends to elicit submission from the other and submissiveness elicits control behavior. This is one of the mechanisms by which persons create self-fulfilling prophecies in their relationships. A person with a helpless presentation will attract a controlling partner; indeed, the controlling person is seen as just the sort of person that the dependent person needs in order to feel comfortable.

Attachment Pathology

The circumplex model has also been used as a way of organizing problems with attachment. Group psychotherapy is concerned with the nature of relationships, and a perspective based on current ideas of attachment pathology is therefore particularly useful (47). The attachment literature suggests that children internalize basic positive/negative responses regarding whether the early attachment figures are likely to respond or to not respond to the child's needs, and whether therefore the child is the sort of person to whom anyone is likely to respond in a helpful way. First, attitudes toward others refer to the expectational set regarding how others will behave toward oneself—whether they are likely to be trustworthy and available or unreliable and rejecting. Second, attitudes toward self refer to whether or not the self is worthy of love and support—a positive/negative attitude toward self closely related to self-esteem.

The clusters of the interpersonal circumplex (Figure 5–1) can be matched with the attachment categories (Figure 5–2). The attachment schema in Figure 5–2, based on results from a study of patients with personality disorders, creates a two-dimensional space directly parallel to the interpersonal circumplex. Secure Attachment is based on basically positive views of both self and others. Ambivalent Attachment might be inferred with any of the Conflict Scores mentioned earlier.

The following are examples of assessments for group psychotherapy in which the IIP is used as a way of eliciting information from the patient.

Examples

A 36-year-old divorced woman described a series of relationships with men in which she would fall intensively in love and totally commit herself to responding to her partner's needs and requests. This pattern applied to all aspects of their relationship, including social decisions, financial contributions, and sexual compliance. As each relationship developed, her partner took increasing advantage of her complying behavior. Finally,

		Attitudes about others	
		Negative	Positive
Attitudes about self	Positive	Counterdependent Attachment: I'm all right but others are not going to be accepting, so it is best to be independent and invulnerable. Who needs others anyway?	Secure Attachment: I am lovable and others are generally accepting and responsive to my needs.
	Negative	Avoidant Attachment: I am unlovable and others are nonreceptive, so it is best to avoid everyone rather than getting hurt again.	Anxious Attachment: I am not lovable but others are positive, so I must keep trying my best to win their affection so I can feel better about myself.

Figure 5–2. Categories of attachment pathology.
Source. Adapted from Horowitz LM, Rosenberg SE, Bartholomew K: "Interpersonal Problems, Attachment Styles, and Outcome in Brief Dynamic Psychotherapy." *Journal of Consulting and Clinical Psychology* 61:549–560, 1993. Copyright 1993, American Psychological Assoc. Reprinted with permission.

she would tearfully leave the relationship, generally returning home to her parents for brief periods of time. Her referral for treatment came when she was in the throes of a major depression after the pattern intruded excessively into her first marriage. Her scores on the IIP were clustered in the lower-right quadrant: Exploitable, or High Agreeableness. She was able to respond actively to a description that she herself had provided by talking with energy and tears about her difficulty in asserting even to a limited extent her own needs or views and her realization of how totally absorbed she would become in a relationship. She also recognized these patterns in her involvement with her family. Consideration of these issues led to a general discussion of how she might therefore find herself participating in the group. She could see herself as being the sort of member who was quick to provide support for others but who would find it difficult to reveal her own distress or ask for attention to her issues. Thus, consideration of the assessment information led smoothly into a pretherapy preparation context that served to alert her to the sorts of issues she would need to attend to in the early sessions of the group. She was encouraged to tell the group at the first session about how she might reenact this pattern with them. Thus, she was able to begin to address core issues immediately by behaving in a more assertive fashion.

A 28-year-old male graduate student was referred for symptoms of depression and anxiety in the context of a pattern of energetic involvement in social activities that would regularly be interrupted by abrupt withdrawal and a period of painful isolation. In this state of isolation, the patient would meet the criteria for major depression of moderate to severe intensity with suicidal ideation, though without major melancholic features. From his descriptions of himself on the IIP, a Conflict Score emerged: elevations on both Intrusive and Socially Avoidant. He was encouraged to expand on what this conflict pattern might reflect. He described with a burst of animation his enthusiastic and positive state, in which he would find himself drawing into an intimate relationship with a woman. After a few dates, and especially if the talk turned to some mention of an ongoing relationship, he would experience rising anxiety and feel an intense pressure to stop seeing the woman. Often, he would end the relationship abruptly, without any warning or conversation with the woman involved. He would then experience severe guilt over acting in this way but could not bring himself to address the issues directly. In the course of this discussion, he became increasingly serious and acknowledged that he had not really seen the connection before between the threat of an intimate relationship with some sense of commitment and his rising anxiety. This was discussed as an area that he might explore actively in the group. It was suggested by the therapist that he might well experience a similar reaction if the group became cohesive. He was encouraged to consider bringing this issue before the group at an early point so that they would be better prepared to understand the patient's response if this were to happen.

Conducting an Interpersonal Inventory

So far, I have addressed interpersonal patterns as if the same pattern applied to all relationships. A general focus like this may serve to usefully point one in the right direction. However, it can also blur important distinctions. A person may establish quite different types of relationships with different people, in which case overgeneralization can be misleading. This overgeneralization can be addressed by eliciting specific descriptions from patients of the important intimate relationships, past and present, in their lives. This is often done implicitly in a standard interview that looks at various life stages. However, there is some value in developing an *interpersonal inventory* as a specific strategy with the apparently benign request, "Can you tell me the names of the most important people in your life, people that had an important influence on you, whether good or bad?" Sometimes patients search through their histories to identify important close relationships. One man in his late 30s said that he had gotten along with a roommate in university and they had gone to movies together, but he had not kept in touch after graduation and there had been no one any closer since then. On the other hand, a 26-year-old woman was able to quote no less than three marriages and four common-law relationships since high school. Before the list is finalized, it is useful to review specifically for marital or common-law partners and to routinely ask about any important figures from the extended family. Often, grandparents or aunts or uncles emerge who at one time provided an important counterbalance to distressing parental relationships. Sometimes other adults are found—a teacher or coach who was a source of major support during a difficult time. With such a list, the nature of specific relationships can be explored systematically. In some ways, this approach gives more relevant and useful information than reliance solely on general patterns. A simple format for conducting an interpersonal inventory is presented as the List of Important Relationships in Appendix 6.

A further advantage of this technique is that difficult relationships can be specifically identified. It is often the case that important psychological work needs to be focused on these particular "toxic" relationships. Such work sometimes deals with how these relationships have progressed and often addresses the termination of the relationships through death or separation. The area of interpersonal focus can be expanded in the interview setting by 1) establishing who the person is, 2) how the relationship ended, and 3) describing the important interpersonal themes in that relationship. Developing a therapeutic focus in this way equips the therapist with the means to look later in the group for process evidence that seems to fit the same theme. Time taken to clarify such prototypic situations is well spent. In the next section, therefore, we go a bit deeper into techniques for assessing relationship patterns. This material is particularly relevant for the assessment of patients entering an interpersonal or psychodynamic group.

Structural Analysis of Social Behavior (SASB)

The two-dimensional circumplex model of the IIP described in the previous section has been expanded in a theoretical model developed by

Benjamin (48) called the Structural Analysis of Social Behavior (SASB). SASB has been gaining recognition as a workable and reasonably comprehensive system for the clinician. This model is derived from the theoretical work of Sullivan, who emphasized human development in terms of the effects of social experiences on the developing child, as opposed to the Freudian orientation around primitive drive states. Normal development is understood as a process of increasing differentiation of the individual from parental figures. Adult behavior is seen to be a reflection of the individual's perceptions of early social learning experiences. According to this model, therapy therefore should focus on the patient's interactions with important others and the effects these have on self-concept. Relevant figures may be drawn from the past and the present and might involve anticipated relationships in the future. This theoretical orientation is particularly useful for the group therapist.

The concepts of SASB will be described in some detail because they form a coherent and practical method to locate a given set of relationship qualities within a formal structural model of interpersonal behavior. SASB provides a map on which to place the events of assessment and therapy, a way to code intuitive responses. This encourages a systematic approach to designing intervention strategies. The language of SASB will be applied to clinical situations in later chapters.

Benjamin uses a musical analogy to describe her system. The SASB "notes" form the interpersonal "scale" that is played by the patient using her own unique harmonics and rhythm, but with the recognizable melody always present. In practice, the experienced musician focuses on the creative result, almost unaware of constantly incorporating the building-block components. Similarly, the clinician automatically responds to interactional nuances without specifically identifying the component core dimensions. The ideas incorporated into the SASB system are familiar to every clinician. The structure helps the clinician organize this conventional clinical wisdom in a useful manner.

SASB is built on an interpersonal circumplex model, but with the vertical control dimension of the IIP replaced by a dimension ranging from high independence and autonomy ("So distant you are almost out of the relationship") to high involvement, interdependence, or enmeshment ("So involved that you almost lose your sense of yourself in the relationship"). Technically, this dimension represents an Independence-Interdependence dimension rather similar to the Quality of Relationships Scale discussed in Chapter 4. Note that the SASB approach suggests that too much differentiation can also lead to problems, an aspect not covered in the Quality of Relationships Scale. The two dimensions of Affiliation and Interdependence are used to form the circumplex, as shown in Figure 5–3, which also contains general labels for the four quadrants.

SASB incorporates the Domineering/Nonasserting dimension from the IIP at the lower pole of the circumplex. This placement is in keeping with the Quality of Relationships Scale, which also has relationships characterized by control issues at the lower end of the scale. I will come back to this aspect of the SASB circumplex after describing an interactional loop (Figure 5–4). The SASB model is applied to two different components of interaction: Acting-on-Other (Focus on Other) and Reacting-to-Other (Focus on Self). This idea of thinking of "actions toward" separately from "reactions within myself" takes a little getting used to. Placed in the context of the interactional loop, however, this approach starts to make sense. Consider a close relationship and work through Figure 5–4. How does that person typically relate toward you (upper part of the loop)? How do you typically experience that behavior (right side of the loop)? Then, how do you typically act toward the other (lower part of the loop)? And, finally,

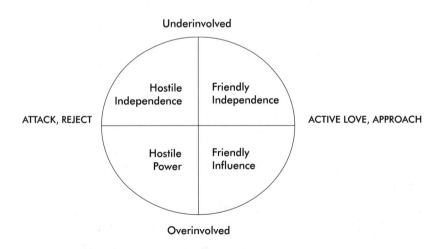

Figure 5–3. Structural Analysis of Social Behavior (SASB) system: two principal dimensions.

how do you think that person experiences your action (left side of the loop)? Your answers to these questions will succinctly describe an interactional loop. This same process can be carried out with the same relationship when the relationship is at its best and at its worst.

The SASB system uses different, and complementary, sets of descriptors for the transitive Focus on Other and the intransitive Focus on Self self-states. For example, Blame/Criticize is paired with Sulk/Resent. One can see how these would fit on the interactional loop. Control and Submit, the vertical axis on the IIP, are found at the lower pole of the circumplex as components of an interactional loop.

In addition, a different circle of eight SASB descriptors are used to describe Acting-on-Self (or the Introject concerning self), such as Self-Affirm or Self-Control.

The result is a set of three circumplex circles that can be superimposed on one another to create a composite circumplex model based on the horizontal axis of affiliation and the vertical axis of interdependence (49). These three circles will be termed *Focus on Other, Focus on Self,* and *Introject* throughout the book. This composite model has the advantage of making connections across the circles more evident and results in the basic cluster

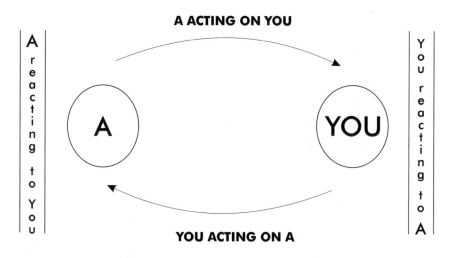

Figure 5–4. The interactional loop.

model of SASB shown in Figure 5–5. As with the IIP, each circle is completed with intermediate clusters that consist of a combination of the two main axes. Thus, a Focus-on-Other combination of Active Love and Control indicates a pattern to Protect/Nurture. A Focus-on-Self combination of Fear and Submit results in a state characterized as Sulk/Resent. The SASB composite cluster model represented in Figure 5–5 appears on the front flyleaf for convenient reference. In the following discussion, the actual labels of the SASB model will be used, even though they are at times somewhat stark. Bear in mind that each point on the circle can be expanded into a general description of the style referred to by the label.

The SASB system description of Focus on Other can also be seen as a parental orientation, and the Focus on Self, as a child dimension. Developmental theory suggests that the Introject is a reflection of the parental Focus on Other (i.e., on the child). Thus, a child subjected to a high level of Blame/Criticize from the parents is likely to internalize this as Self-Blame (see lower-left quadrant in Figure 5–5). In the interpersonal approach, current relationships are conceptualized as being driven by the power of earlier attachment patterns. These early experiences provide an organizational structure of self experience, as well as expectations of how others will behave toward self.

As a general rule, well-functioning relationships tend to be characterized by higher levels of Affirm, Approach, and Nurture, along with their complementary Focus-on-Self styles, as represented by clusters from the right side of the composite circle in Figure 5–5. On the other hand, problematic relationships are characterized by higher levels of Ignore, Attack, and Blame and their complementary styles, as reflected in clusters on the left side of the circle, or by a high degree of Underinvolved or Overinvolved, as represented by clusters at the very top or bottom of the circle.

Mature adult positive relationships marked by equality are characterized much of the time by features from the upper-right quadrant of the circle. Of course, this does not mean that other clusters might not appear given a specific context. When assessing level of dysfunction, one can consider both the style (location on the circle) and the intensity with which a given style is maintained. Intensity can be thought of as radiating out from the hub of the circle in all directions. We all utilize components from the entire circle regularly. Problems in relationships emerge when interactional patterns are particularly strong , inappropriate to the circumstances, or inflexible. For example, a passing irritable remark is quite different from loud and sustained angry critical outbursts that occur on a daily basis.

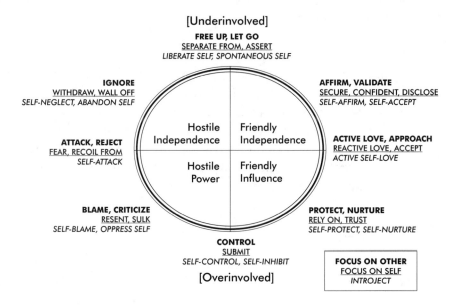

Figure 5–5. The Structural Analysis of Social Behavior (SASB) composite cluster model. All three circles are superimposed on the circumplex space. Labels in **boldface** type describe actions directed at another person (Focus on Other). Underlined labels describe reactions to another person (Focus on Self). *Italicized* labels describe how a person treats self and may reflect how important others have treated the person (Introject). *Source.* Adapted from Benjamin LS: *Interpersonal Diagnosis and Treatment of Personality Disorders.* New York, Guilford, 1993. Copyright 1993. Used with permission.

Once familiar with the SASB rating system, you can use it during a clinical interview or group session in an informal manner by following a consistent three step sequence.

1. Determine which circle from the composite SASB model is being utilized (see Figure 5–5). Is this statement designed to influence the other (Focus on Other), or does it describe what one is currently experiencing in regard to self in reaction to the other (Focus on Self), or is it a commentary or attitude toward oneself (Introject)?

2. Determine if the statement is in a positive or negative direction.
3. Assess whether the statement is toward autonomy or toward enmeshment.

This decision sequence should allow you to place the behavior, at least, within a SASB quadrant. In the process you may derive some additional ideas about the meaning of the transaction or how best to respond.

The six personality dimensions from Chapter 4 may be superimposed on the SASB model. This reveals some interesting associations and illustrates how the SASB model can be used as a framework for mapping relationship phenomena. In particular, it shows how any given personality dimension may have rather complex interactional applications. (Refer to the SASB composite model in Figure 5–5 as you work through the following descriptions.)

1. *Emotional reactivity (neuroticism),* as a largely negative state, corresponds to Withdraw, Fear, and Resent, as represented by the left side of the Focus-on-Self circle, and may also appear in the same location on both the Focus-on-Other and Introject circles.
2. *Conscientiousness (compulsivity),* primarily characterized by high levels of Self-Control in the Introject circle, can also be reflected in Control located at the bottom of the Focus-on-Other circle. There is often an associated Self-Blame and Blame component that corresponds to much of the lower-left quadrant.
3. *Openness* represents a self-state on the Introject circle that includes qualities of Spontaneity, Self-Affirm, and Active Self-Love, all of which are found in the upper-right quadrant.
4. *Quality of relationships* is concerned with the vertical dimension of the interpersonal circles. A low rating on this scale, which corresponds to the bottom of both the Focus-on-Other and the Focus-on-Self circles, reflects an enmeshed relationship in which dominance issues are prominent. A high rating of quality of relationships corresponds to Affirm/Validate and Secure/Confident in the upper-right quadrant according to the Piper scale (see Appendix 5). The SASB model suggests that extreme autonomy, as represented by Let Go and Separate From, would define an overly distant state of underinvolvement. The lowest level on the Quality of Relationships Scale (i.e., primitive) describes a state of fluctuating behaviors that might involve almost all portions of all three circles at various times.

5. *Extraversion/introversion* requires a more complex application to the SASB model. Extraversion includes Approach, Protect, and Control features that are located in the lower-right quadrant of the Focus-on-Other circle. Introversion consists of Separate From, Withdraw, and Recoil From features that are found in the upper-left quadrant of the Focus-on-Self circle. This dimension is primarily of an interactional nature and involves both of the interactional circles.

6. *Agreeableness,* which also involves both interactional circles, extends at one end from Accept, Trust, and Submit on the Focus-on-Self circle to Attack, Blame, and Control on the Focus-on-Other circle at the other end of the dimension. In both of these applications it involves a significant degree of overinvolvement with the Other.

The Axis II personality disorder categories are, not surprisingly, primarily associated with clusters from the left side of the SASB circles in various combinations. Benjamin has developed a detailed analysis of each category in accordance with DSM criteria. This analysis indicates that virtually every Axis II category has features from many different parts of the SASB space. (Borderline personality disorder, for example, involves 11 out of the possible 16 interpersonal clusters.) This finding provides additional evidence of the heterogeneous nature of the DSM approach and helps to explain why so many patients meet the criteria for several categories.

It is also possible to place the four group roles described in Chapter 3 on the SASB space. The Sociable Role matches the characteristics of the lower-right quadrant, and the Divergent Role, those of the lower-left quadrant. These are the two roles that are most invested, positively and negatively, in the emotional transactions of the group. The Cautionary Role clearly belongs in the upper-left quadrant, and the Structural Role has many of the characteristics of the upper-right quadrant. These last two roles represent the negative and positive aspects of a more distancing connection to the group. These positionings may offer some ideas in understanding the function for the group of patients with different roles.

Interpersonal Application of SASB

The SASB system can be used to capture the essence of many of the interpersonal events common in psychotherapy. It is important that relationship connections emerging in the group not be seen in unidirectional, causal terms, because these connections describe a circular pattern. For example, persons with high levels of Self-Blame may also be more inclined to see others as acting toward them in a blaming manner. They may therefore have a habitual resentful presentation that does in fact elicit critical and negative responses from others. The SASB system also clarifies the important difference between self-assertion and anger. Self-assertion is a measure of autonomy (a Focus-on-Self statement) and is located in quite a different place than anger (a Focus-on-Other statement).

In the SASB system, complementarity, described earlier in this chapter in the application of the interpersonal circumplex, refers similarly to the conjunction of corresponding styles on the Focus on Other and Focus on Self circles. Affirmation and validation elicit confidence and disclosure (a Rogerian paradigm). Nurturing behavior elicits a trusting response (good parenting). Criticizing behavior elicits a resentful response (resulting in, for example, a passive-aggressive style). Ignoring elicits withdrawal ("Best not to get involved"). Because interactions are conceptualized as occurring in a circular, reciprocal manner, it does not matter where one begins; submitting behavior will elicit controlling from the other person, and controlling behavior will elicit submitting responses, and so on. The biting dog will elicit fear, and a fearful demeanor may elicit bites. Complementarity in the lower half of the composite circle captures the idea of the popular term *codependency*. Codependency may involve, in a superficially benign form, one partner protecting and the other trusting (lower-right quadrant) or, in a more malignant form, one partner actively blaming and the other characteristically sulking (lower-left quadrant). Usually, there is an oscillation between the two quadrants.

The expected response style for a congruent pattern between two people would be one of complementarity. Of course, it does not always work that way. Controlling behavior may elicit a response of Assert or Wall Off, which, as can be seen on the composite circle in Figure 5–5, is almost the opposite of what would be expected if one assumed the response would be complementary. How will the individual who is controlling respond to this interactional discontinuity? Perhaps initially, he will intensify the control. If there is no success, as gauged by the complementary response of submission by the other individual, then perhaps an attempt will be made to understand what is going on by shifting to an affirming position. "I can see your point; I guess I was coming on pretty strong." Such a shift in response is an example of one's disconfirming the initial interactional intent by using a response—in this case involving affirmation—that leads to a more constructive interaction (represented in upper-right quadrant of the composite circle). Controlling behavior may, of course, elicit a response of Control, in which case an escalation of tension and, often, a shift to Blame or Attack may result.

When the SASB system is being applied, occasions will arise when the individual appears to be actively using behavior from opposite sides of the circumplex, a situation analogous to Conflict Scores on the interpersonal circumplex. A common example is a Focus-on-Other statement that contains both Free-Up and Control features, referred to as a *control double-bind pattern.* "Do what you would like, but don't you think you should . . ." An elevated rating on opposites across the horizontal axis represents a love-hate combination that usually indicates major relationship problems. Such conflict patterns may suggest internalized conflicts of which the patient is unaware. These patterns may also reflect major ambivalence about a relationship. Sometimes they can be seen as the components in a wish/fear pattern. For example, "I wish to be taken care of (Submit/Trust), but I fear losing myself in the relationship (therefore, Wall Off/Separate From)." This pattern of ambivalence is commonly found in patients with marked borderline features.

The SASB patterns may help one to understand three powerful mechanisms of how we learn to be in relationships. These mechanisms provide a good example of how the language of interpersonal patterns can be used to capture the essence of psychodynamic mechanisms.

- *Identification* refers to the simple modeling of behaviors of the parent. "Father was a person who used blame a lot, and so do I." Such modeling is considered to be a powerful determinant of personality style. This is focused on patterns of others toward oneself and is the mechanism underlying identification with the aggressor.
- *Introjection,* as noted earlier in this chapter, refers to the process by which the Focus-on-Other behavior of the parent is taken on as a self-description. "Father blamed me for everything, so I am a person who must always feel guilty that I've done something wrong."
- *Recapitulation* refers to the automatic assumptions about what to expect of others. "Father was a blamer, and therefore all potentially nurturing figures are blamers too, so I have a right to be resentful toward everybody." In this way, internalized response patterns influence current relationships.

In patients from seriously dysfunctional families, all three mechanisms may be triggered at the same time in intimate relationships. "Men are cruel

(Recapitulation), but I deserve whatever I get (Introjection), so I'm going to be as critical as I can get away with in this new relationship too (Identification)." Of course, these thoughts may not be entirely on the surface, but many patients recognize such relationship patterns in their own descriptions of key relationships.

If two people interact consistently with the same interactional style, the result is likely to be an unstable relationship. For example, if both persons consistently use strongly controlling behaviors, there is an unceasing struggle to be on top. Even when both persons use highly affirming behaviors, the relationship may look artificial because both are being nice to each other but neither is utilizing reciprocal Confident and Disclose behaviors.

Finally, the SASB system provides a method for systematic consideration of how to respond to a particular behavior. *Antithesis* is defined as the complement of the opposite in the other interpersonal circle. As can be seen in Figure 5–5, for example, the antithesis of Blame is Disclose, and the antithesis of Trust is Ignore. A response that is the antithesis of the target behavior should encourage a shift in that behavior. However, this occurs mainly in less intense situations and with less disturbed individuals who are able to respond in a more flexible manner in terms of relationship adaptation. In clinical work, the therapist may apply the concept of antithesis by beginning with a response that is closer to the target behavior and then gradually shifting to responses around the circle.

For example, a patient who exhibits a high level of Blame (lower-left quadrant in Figure 5–5) will often elicit a complementary response of Sulk from others, including the therapist, who may be quite resentful at how this person is able to sidetrack the group. A calculated response would be to begin with a degree of Control: "Jim, it is important that we not say destructive things in here. I am going to ask you to put critical comments on hold for now." The response may then be gradually shifted to one of Protect: "Jim may put some of his ideas a bit bluntly, but it seems to me he often has a valid point." Eventually, but not too soon, a position of Approach and then Affirm may be adopted, and the antithesis will thus finally have been reached: "It sounds like you have been doing some important thinking about how things go for you, Jim." Hopefully, through this progression, the patient will be drawn first to agree to go along with the restriction (Submit), then to trust the therapist to some degree (Trust), and finally to develop a positive feeling about the group and so finally to feel able to talk more openly about himself (Disclose).

Introspect Application

It is easy to underestimate the power of the internalized attitudes toward self. Many patients, especially those with severe personality pathology, may clearly recognize the invalidity of their negative self-views but cannot free themselves from the effects of this constant internal voice.

Example

A 42-year-old single man had avoided any contact of an intimate nature with women because of his belief that they would find him inferior and probably disgusting. After some time in a psychotherapy group, he reported that he had had two dates with a woman who seemed attracted to him. The group responded with supportive and pleased excitement to this news. He immediately shifted to focus on how uncomfortable he felt while out with her and how he was certain that it would not take long for her to see through his facade.

A common Introject pattern, in terms of the SASB system, is a Conflict Score along the Control axis. This pattern often reflects an overcontrolled style with obsessional features coupled with a fear that if rigid control were not in place, emotional reactions or spontaneity would lead to total dyscontrol.

Patients with borderline personality disorder often demonstrate a rapid shifting of interactional positions. One common pattern is to begin with behaviors from the lower-right quadrant of excessive Trust in the therapist. As the relationship becomes closer, there may be a rebound up into behaviors from the upper-left quadrant: apparent Wall Off from therapist accompanied by Self-Neglect from the same cluster on the Introject circle. This behavior may be potentially dangerous because of self-injurious behaviors from the adjacent Self-Attack cluster. Often, there follows a further shift into Blame toward the therapist for allowing this sequence to get started. The therapist at this point will need to guard against a complementary response of Resent.

Presence of unrealistic and strongly held attitudes toward self can be taken as strong evidence that significant others have behaved toward the patient in ways characterized by the same cluster on the circumplex. In that way, the individual is constantly reliving his or her personal past. The same patterns can be expected to emerge within therapy, where a "corrective emotional experience" can occur that disconfirms *internalized* expectations.

The way in which this process is typically conceptualized may vary according to the therapeutic orientation. This process will be viewed by the cognitive-behavior therapist as learning to block negative thoughts and replace them with constructive ideas, by the interpersonal therapist as learning new ways of relating, and by the psychodynamic therapist as effecting a shift in ego structures. Underlying all of these perspectives is the same basic belief that long-standing, entrenched learned patterns must be addressed.

SASB Assessment: A Clinical Application

All clinicians are familiar with getting a sense of the nature of important relationships from different periods of a patient's life. Gaining a sense of the nature of such relationships is a standard function of an assessment interview. The SASB concepts can be woven into this process by one's keeping in mind the basic dimensions of the SASB circumplex (see Figure 5–5). Think of a patient you have recently assessed. Can that person be assessed in terms of the three circles? What is the patient's main Focus-on-Other style? How does she usually respond to others? What is her predominant Focus on Self? How did you assess her self-image using this circle? Could you do the same for a small range of the patient's key relationships, including parents and intimate partners? Does this approach help you to identify patterns across relationships? What evidence is there of the important mechanisms of identification, introjection, and recapitulation?

Another way to complement the information obtained during an interview is to have the patient complete a set of questions about each of the people on the short list of key significant others. The SASB Intrex questionnaire (see Appendix 13) consists of 32 items—8 items for each of the four parts of the interactional loop—that, when considered collectively, describe each relationship. Many patients find it quite an arousing, perhaps disturbing, process to respond to these questions. But the process gets them actively thinking about the nature of their relationships. The following example illustrates how the results from the Intrex questionnaire might be utilized in the preparation of patients for group psychotherapy.

Example

A 28-year-old male graduate student in a healthcare program was referred by his clinical supervisor because of increasing difficulties in his clinical placement. These difficulties centered on his superior attitude to permanent staff members, especially female staff members. He was opinionated and dogmatic and could tolerate no suggestions from women. He also was blunt and rude and showed no appreciation for the difficulties and stress they might be experiencing with difficult patients. These problems became particularly apparent in a community-oriented rotation where the allied healthcare staff were experienced and knowledgeable. He felt that other staff members were against him and that he had to fight to preserve his status. He was authoritarian and yet undermined the efforts of those to whom he was responsible. He also reported increasing tension in his relationship with his wife of 3 years. He was preoccupied with work issues and had little time for her interests or concerns, though he was quite devoted to his 4-month-old daughter. The workplace issues had escalated to the point that he was in immediate danger of being asked to leave the program. He reported that, contrary to the view others had of him, he experienced a despairing sense of low self-worth.

The patient's father had died in a motor vehicle accident when he was age 4. He had memories of a caring, involved relationship with his father. The accident produced severe financial strains on his mother, who put the patient in a boarding school, returned to full-time work, and began to abuse alcohol and sedatives. The patient described his mother as explosive and emotionally unavailable and noted that she frequently gave him severe physical beatings. His principal coping mechanisms lay in being passively compliant and losing himself in scholarly pursuits, at which he excelled. His mother married when he was 11. The patient described his stepfather as not abusive and "somewhat interested" but basically a peripheral figure in his life ("at least he was benign").

The patient had in his teens a small core of one or two male friends, mainly "intellectuals in the outgroup," and seldom dated. While an undergraduate he met a foreign student who encouraged him to join her in an evangelical congregation. He had not before that time been involved in an organized religion. He felt that he had found himself through her. He became very involved with their religious activities and felt that this stabilized his life and gave him some direction. They began to plan for future missionary work and became engaged. On a trip home, her parents insisted that she end the relationship because it was outside of their culture. Though torn, she followed her parents' wishes. The patient experienced a major grief reaction and came close to abandoning his studies. Two years later he met his future wife and began an exciting courtship that was particularly enhanced by the warm and loving family atmosphere in her home. On their honeymoon, he mentioned his previous love to his wife and they had a major quarrel. His sexual interest declined thereafter. He became immersed in clinical work placements and studies, and the romance quickly faded.

SASB Intrex questionnaire patterns at intake. The salient features of the intake SASB Intrex patterns are shown in Table 5–3. (Please refer to the SASB system in Figure 5–5 or on front flyleaf while reviewing this table.) These begin with self-descriptions when at his best and worst, followed by a series of relationships, each of which has four results corresponding to the interactional loop. Results described as having "No major pattern" are those in which no systematic pattern within the eight points of the circumplex emerged and thus no clear description could be made. This

Table 5–3.   SASB patterns pre- and post-treatment for 28-year-old male graduate student in clinical example discussed in text

Relationship	Pretest	Post-test
Self-at-Best	No major pattern	Active Self-Love and Self-Affirm
Self-at-Worst	Self-Attack	No major pattern
Mother to me	Attack	CONFLICT: Free Up vs. Control
I react to Mother	No major pattern	No major pattern
Me to Mother	No major pattern	Affirm
Mother reacts to me	Assert and Withdraw	Assert and Withdraw
Stepfather to me	No major pattern	Active Love and Affirm
I react to Stepfather	Accept and Disclose	Accept and Trust
Me to Stepfather	Let Go and Affirm	Affirm
Stepfather reacts	Assert and Disclose	No major pattern
Wife to me	Affirm	Affirm
I react to Wife	CONFLICT: Accept vs. Recoil From	Active Love and Affirm
Me to Wife	No major pattern	Affirm
Wife reacts to me	Affirm	Accept and Affirm
Female Co-worker	Attack	Not available
I react	Assert	Not available
Me to Female	CONFLICT: Free Up vs. Control	Not available
Female Co-worker	Assert and Withdraw	Not available

Note.   SASB = Structural Analysis of Social Behavior.

designation ensures that less-than-definite self-generated relationship patterns will not be used in the assessment.

The first indication of interpersonal issues in the patient's life arose during the process of selecting significant others to be rated. In the end, the absence of enough candidates led to the inclusion of two siblings and the only, rather distant, male friend the patient could identify from his university days.

When describing himself at his best, the patient had a diffuse picture; however, at his worst, a clear negative self-image emerged. This self-attacking type of pattern is sometimes associated with suicidal ideation, but on probing this area, the patient stated that he refused to allow these sorts of thoughts because of his religious convictions.

Among the parental ratings, the relationship with his mother stood out for its angry and distant qualities. Strong patterns did not emerge for his side of the relationship. This lack of strong patterns perhaps reflects the patient's difficulty in conceptualizing what the relationship was like, much as he experienced difficulty in trying to rate himself At Best. His description of his mother's actions toward him carried the same SASB code as his rating of himself At Worst, a result in keeping with a process of introjection of early parental actions toward him. His relationship with his stepfather was characterized by underinvolvement, although his own reaction to his stepfather had a positive quality. This rating surprised the patient somewhat, but on reflection he was able to recount a number of activities they did together. Clearly, his preoccupation with his early environment had been selectively focused on the negative images of his mother. The parental marital relationship, not shown, was seen as benign (i.e., in the upper-right area of the SASB circle).

The patient's descriptions of his relationships with his siblings, his university friend, and his first love were also positive (not shown). In his own marital relationship, he described his wife in positive terms but himself with an Affiliation Conflict Score. Affiliation Conflict Scores, which indicate a contradictory, black-and-white quality of interactions and responses, tend to reflect particularly troubling psychological tensions. No major pattern was evident in the patient's behavior toward his wife.

The patient was also asked to rate how he viewed his relationships with women at work, the focus for so much of his difficulty. His description of how his female colleagues act toward him and of their reaction to his response was identical to that of how his mother acted toward and reacted to him in childhood. His own pattern was that of Withdrawal coupled with a Control Conflict Score. This pattern seemed to match his verbal description of the situation, although he had trouble initially reconceptualizing his authoritarian stance as anything but a desire to do the best job.

At termination his view of Self had improved, as had his picture of his relationship with his stepfather, who was now seen in more positive and trusting terms. His relationship with his mother remained problematic but with less attacking. He appeared to have significantly rewritten his personal history. The Affiliation Conflict Score with his wife had disappeared, and he described greater warmth and intimacy. By interview, his relationships with women at work had greatly improved.

This extended example has been provided to demonstrate how a detailed interpersonal feedback process can be organized. It may not be to everyone's taste to actually use a questionnaire format. However, the explicitness possible with such an approach is a useful antidote to the generality that often accompanies interpersonal diagnosis. Often, therapy is most powerful when relationships with specific people and specific events are being addressed, not just general patterns. We will return to this issue later, in Section III, when we discuss therapeutic strategies. Having a clear format for the interpersonal assessment, even if such an assessment is carried out verbally as part of an interview, is helpful. The descriptions of the relationships being described can be tightened. The theoretical structure of the SASB system provides an effective vocabulary for catching the essence of a relationship in a standardized manner. The Interpersonal Work Sheet provided in Appendix 7, which is based on the SASB dimensions and can be completed by the patient, has proven useful in getting patients and clinicians to think in interpersonal terms.

For each patient, it is useful to record a short paragraph, not more than half a page, that encapsulates your understanding of the principal issues for that patient. In such a summary, ideally you would describe the immediate reasons for the patient's coming to treatment; pertinent current stress events; the patient's predominant interpersonal style; the nature and course of key relationships, including those with family of origin and other significant persons; and specific events such as deaths or episodes of abuse. The description contained in the clinical example above is a slightly longer version of a summary statement. The resultant document will pull together interpersonal patterns, major traumatic stressors, and key figures and will identify positive coping skills or circumstances. These succinct summaries can be kept together in the chart so that they can be readily reviewed following group sessions. This process, which need not be time-consuming, is a mechanism for alerting the therapist to issues that may need to be addressed or that might even be reenacted in the group process. The summary could certainly be shared with the patient as well.

These same issues can also be translated into formal Target Goals that are adapted to the nature of the patient's problem and the objectives of the group. The simple Target Goals Form in Appendix 8 is intentionally left general and provides a way for the patient to formalize his or her commitment to deal with important issues. This simple rating scale can then be used as one measure of outcome.

For interpersonal groups, it is worth considering a more detailed description of Focus Areas. These can be linked to predictable issues within the group that need to be watched for as well as to suitable changes that would be appropriate outside the group.

Examples

You describe yourself in your important relationships as being very helpful and supportive to others. At the same time, you seldom reveal much about yourself. This appears to lead to situations where you feel taken advantage of by others while not having your own legitimate needs met. Understandably, this causes you to feel resentment and then eventually to end the relationship because it is unsatisfying. It will be important in the group to be aware if these patterns are happening and to address them verbally at an early point in the cycle.

The principal pattern you describe appears to be one of remaining silent even when you have useful or important things to say because you fear that you will be rejected or ignored by others. So you find yourself living in quite an isolated state in terms of getting much satisfaction from relationships. This pattern is likely to pose a problem for you in the group as well. Perhaps it would be important to outline these patterns for the others at an early point so that you and they can work together to change them.

These Target Goals or Focus Areas can also be reviewed at intervals in a group's life to realert patients to the issues that were initially considered important. Such a review is commonly done at the halfway point of a time-limited group. Sometimes this process results in a useful discussion about how targets have shifted during the process of treatment. No matter how one chooses to spell out important issues, the underlying process of expecting that therapy will deal with specific important tasks is central to maximizing the effectiveness of group psychotherapy, particularly in a time-limited format.

CHAPTER 6

Group Composition and Pretherapy Preparation

*T*he question of group composition shifts the focus from the individual to the group system, as can be seen by the structure of the group presented schematically in Chapter 3 (Figure 3–1). No longer can the individual be seen in isolation from the group context. Indeed, the process of selecting members for a group is an important aspect of defining the nature of the group external boundary.

The process of composing a group entails two types of decisions. The clinician must first determine, based on the nature of the group objectives, what sort of group is most appropriate. The clinician must then decide who the members will be. The principles involved in making these two decisions are outlined in this chapter, and some representative examples are included. The final section of this book (Section IV: "Group Models for Service Systems") provides more detail on issues of composition for specific types of groups.

For all groups, the pretherapy preparation of the members promotes the rapid development of a cohesive group environment.

Group Composition

Group Objectives

The nature of therapy groups is defined, in large part, by the degree to which the group interactional process is a central focus for therapeutic attention. All groups are, of course, interactional by their very nature, and the group process must be skillfully managed by the therapist. The therapist is in a position to determine the degree to which the subtle nature of that interaction is scrutinized.

A simple five-step system captures the essence of this group dimension (Table 6–1). This system is meant to inform the technical decision as to how the group will be run and is in no way meant to identify more or less powerful or sophisticated psychological work. The use of supportive techniques is relatively high until the last level, the interpersonal/psychodynamic, where the therapeutic strategy shifts to a greater use of interpretive techniques and a more abstinent leadership style. All five levels require skill in managing the group environment, and all have been demonstrated to be effective for properly selected patients.

This five-level system forms a useful general background from which to make more specific composition decisions. These decisions will be influenced by the goals of the group and by the interactional capacity of the members. A clear understanding of the objectives of the group is essential when one is making composition decisions. The task of selecting types of group is discussed at length in Chapter 12, which addresses the planning and setting up of clinical group programs.

Group Characteristics

Group Format: Open or Closed

Another basic decision is whether to admit members after the group begins. Each time a change in group membership occurs, even a single member's being added or leaving, the group must renegotiate the balance of interactional forces in the system. During this process, early engagement-stage tasks must again be addressed. For a well-functioning group that is admitting a single member, the renegotiation process may be relatively brief. For

Table 6–1.   Levels of process focus in group therapy

1.   Psychoeducational
2.   Social skills
3.   Cognitive-behavioral
4.   Interpersonal-semistructured
5.   Interpersonal/psychodynamic–process-oriented

groups experiencing some struggles, however, a change in membership may result in a significant regression of group work. A group with a constant turnover of members will have great difficulty in moving into more advanced interactional work. Termination issues will be of less importance because the level of bonding between the members will be lower. This diminished emphasis on termination issues may be appropriate if the goal of the group is to stay focused on collective strategies such as learning psychoeducational material or specific skills such as assertiveness training or anger management. Cognitive-behavior therapists differ in their approach. Some prefer to keep the group at the engagement stage, whereas others are interested in making fuller use of the interactional climate. Certainly, groups planning to deal with interpersonal psychopathology will expect to move into more advanced group work.

Longer-term groups usually operate with a *slow-open* policy of filling vacancies as they occur. This approach is probably more satisfactory than discharging and admitting patients in larger blocks at intervals. If half of a group's membership turns over at once, reconsolidation is a major challenge, often accompanied by termination of continuing members who resent the disruption in the group's progress.

Time-limited groups are already facing the limitations of the established duration. Anything that can be done to simplify basic structural issues for the group is helpful. Most such groups therefore use a closed group format. Some programs modify this format slightly by allowing new members over the first two or three sessions. An advantage of this modification is that members who drop out very early in the group and thus have not really become involved in the group can be replaced. With this possible exception, time-limited groups are best kept closed. Even if the membership erodes to some extent, the price of admitting new membership is interference with the progress of the existing members.

A closed format permits the application of a group developmental model. The group as a whole moves through each stage together. When this occurs, the therapeutic potential of each stage can be fully explored and exploited. This is particularly the case with time-limited groups in which there is an effort to center attention on themes that come into focus around the final stage of termination. Time-limited groups spend most of their time getting formed and getting separated. It is not recommended that intensive time-limited group work be conducted under circumstances of constant membership change. The tasks related to doing serious psychotherapy within a specified time are challenging enough without this extra burden being added.

Some programs provide a time-limited experience with a *semi-open* group format. At the initiation of such a group, the patients make a commitment to participate in the group for a certain time period (e.g., 6 to 10 sessions). At the end of the initial commitment, the patient may be allowed to renew the contract for a similar duration. This approach works satisfactorily for relatively structured groups in which more intensive interpersonal work is not expected. However, the format is less desirable for groups that intend to use a process focus. With a semi-open format, the group must address termination issues at a relatively early point in group development and only for some members. This depletes the impact of dealing with reactions to termination. Those remaining in the group must then incorporate new members and rework engagement issues. An advantage to this format is that the continuing members will be able to impart to the new members a sense of the working atmosphere of the group—a process that can result in a rapid incorporation of the newcomers. But a common result is that over both segments, there is a significant restriction of time available for participation in more advanced group interactional work. It would be preferable to conduct two separate groups beginning at different times and consisting of 12 to 20 sessions each. Such an arrangement would result in a more integrated group experience for the members.

Groups that are conducted in the context of a day treatment program generally have weekly admissions. These changes in membership are better tolerated because of the constant integrating effects of the therapeutic milieu. Rapid turnover of membership is a fact of life on inpatient units and in outpatient crisis intervention group programs. In such settings, the group is intentionally maintained in the engagement stage, and active therapist structuring techniques are used (50). This model is perfectly acceptable for such situations and may also offer an opportunity for extended assessment of patient needs and capacity. Patients can then be referred for additional treatment when indicated. However, the nature of the format does not allow the full application of formal intensive psychotherapy techniques. Termination issues will be of lesser importance in such programs.

Group Size

The question of group size is important in any consideration of group composition. As noted in Chapter 3, as groups increase in size, the opportunity for effective interpersonal work decreases. This principle may be directly applied to the group levels described above (see Table 6–1). Because this five-level system is based on the degree to which group process will be the central therapeutic focus, it stands to reason that group size becomes more important as one moves from levels 1 to 5. In practice, there is a marked shift in therapeutic strategy between the more programmed aspects of levels 1 and 2 and the specific strategies in levels 3 to 5. A strong argument could be made for limiting group size to a maximum of 10 patients for the more intense therapeutic efforts of levels 3 through 5. Cognitive-behavioral groups in which it is planned that members will have an opportunity to review weekly journals and other behavioral records might want to be kept at a size of eight members or fewer.

Group Membership

Prediction of Problems During Member Selection

There are few absolute exclusion criteria for entering a treatment group (51). Consideration of the issues discussed in the following subsections, as well as outlined in Table 6–2, can alert the clinician to potential members who either will have difficulty using a group or are likely to present major problems in group management. It should be noted that all of these issues make individual therapy equally difficult. Paradoxically, many of these cautionary dimensions are more effectively addressed in group psychotherapy than in individual psychotherapy.

Capacity for participation. Clearly, it is necessary for a patient to be able to sit in the group room with some capacity to attend to the group process. Thus, patients with severe endogenous depression, mania, acute delirium,

---

Table 6–2.   Factors predictive of problems in group participation and/or management

---

Limited capacity for participation

Suicidal ideation

Acute stress

Emotional dyscontrol

Cluster A personality disorder features

Highly defended personality style

Antisocial and psychopathic features

Lack of focus

---

acute disorganization due to psychotic symptoms, or major dementia are unlikely to benefit from a group approach. However, even for patients with such conditions, groups may be helpful once the acute symptomatology subsides, or, in the case of dementia, before the condition progresses too far. It would be reasonable, for example, to have a manic patient attend a ward group once his symptoms had come under modest control. The patient's inclusion might be accompanied by the advice to both the patient and the group leader that the patient be asked to leave the session if he finds his mania escalating. The group environment may be experienced as quite stimulating, but it also gives the patient a realistic opportunity to test his capacity to tolerate social situations. Structured groups for patients in the early to middle range of dementia appear to be helpful in addressing goals of maintaining orientation and in providing support.

Suicidal ideation.   Suicidal ideation may surface and will need to be dealt with in any group. The acutely suicidal patient is commonly found in inpatient groups and may benefit from talking about his or her suicidal ideas. Such discussion often provides an opportunity for the patient to get some objective distance from her thoughts. In any outpatient group, it is common to find members with suicidal thoughts, but it is probably best to exclude those with active suicide plans in this setting unless the intent is to provide a more structured crisis intervention program. It is always difficult for group members to deal with acute suicide risk. Such topics, because of their critical nature, may demand a major portion of a session, which may be to the detriment of other members.

Acute stress.   Another factor in the determination of group composition is the presence of acute stress. Normally, it would be desirable to address situations of acute stress with a supportive approach in which the attempt is made to reinforce coping strategies and to help the patient gain a sense of emotional mastery over the situation. Acute grief reactions, the unexpected loss of a job, and a natural disaster are examples of situations for which such a treatment approach is desirable. Such circumstances may be effectively managed in a crisis intervention mode, either group or individual in nature. For example, bereavement groups focus in a supportive manner on the normal process of grieving and serve a preventive function regarding longer-term disability.

On the other hand, when the group is designed to provide a specific treatment approach for significant psychological problems, the presence of an acutely stressful external situation may derail the individual's capacity to address personal issues. The patient may be preoccupied with managing a difficult, perhaps catastrophic, situation.

Example

A man's entry into a cognitive-behavioral group for major depression was precipitated by marital breakdown 10 months before. At the third session, he reported that intensive litigation involving custody had begun. He found it impossible to attend to group tasks and decided to leave the group with the therapist's blessing. Individual crisis sessions were arranged, and he eventually joined another group, where he dealt effectively with the life changes resulting from the situation.

Groups for persons experiencing longer-term sequelae of personal loss are designed to focus on the problematic psychological implications of the loss. The active techniques used in these groups might in themselves be quite anxiety-producing. A usual guideline would be to delay formal psychotherapy for a period of time, perhaps 6 months as a minimum, after an acute crisis.

Emotional dyscontrol.   Poor affective control may take the form of poor anger control or of escalating emotional reactions triggered by group interaction. Patients who are highly impulsive and highly suggestible may find a group with minimal structure quite difficult to tolerate. A more structured environment in which the emphasis is on mastery of emotional control, not exploration of issues surrounding it, may be more satisfactory. These patients often have features drawn from the Cluster B categories of Axis II. There is general agreement in the literature that such patients probably do best in the short term with more mastery-focused approaches. An exploratory approach is likely to require longer-term treatment.

Cluster A personality disorder features.   Patients with personality features characteristic of the odd, eccentric cluster of personality disorders (Cluster A) do not do very well in psychotherapy. Those who have marked paranoid or schizotypal features will find group participation difficult. Their style makes it hard to engage constructively in the group process, and they tend to distance themselves and to view the efforts of other group members to involve them with a high degree of suspicion and possibly anger. This response is frustrating to the group and may impede the development of cohesion and, at the same time, is of little value to the patient. The issue of whether to include patients with Cluster A features is not typically encountered because such individuals usually avoid all possibility of group involvement.

Patients with severely schizoid personality features will derive little benefit from group involvement. As with patients with paranoid or schizotypal features, their distancing behaviors may alienate the group. However, there may be a sadness and yearning for some type of contact that may be effectively addressed in group once the patient commits himself to the idea. The clinician will want to talk to the patient at length about his reasons for wanting to join and carefully assess the motivation to participate. Are the patient's expectations realistic for the type of group being organized? This relates to the common diagnostic problem of differentiating between schizoid qualities and avoidant problems. The schizoid patient wishes to be isolated, whereas the avoidant patient wants contact but fears the implications of closeness. A detailed history of intimate relationship experiences might be of help.

Highly defended personality style.   Patients who have a highly defended personality style also will have problems utilizing a group. Often, this style is part of a controlled, obsessional picture or may occur in combination with the Cluster A features that were described above. People with a highly defended personality style tend to take judgmental positions on interpersonal situations, possibly viewing these situations in highly polarized, black-or-white dimensions. This makes it difficult for them to respond flexibly to the range of responses often found in a therapy group. Their efforts to polarize the discussion around their rigidly held positions may lead to their isolation in the group and the possibility of a negative effect. These patients have difficulty incorporating feedback in a constructive manner. At the same time, it is probably more likely that problems arising from such a highly defended style will be more effectively managed in a supportive group than in individual therapy. A group with more structure and low interpersonal demands would be a good place to start.

Antisocial and psychopathic features.   The antisocial/psychopathic dimension, addressed in some detail in the context of our discussion of assessment (Chapter 4), must be of major concern when one is composing a group. Persons with antisocial or psychopathic personality features have difficulty utilizing a general therapy group and may be actively destructive to its functioning. On the other hand, groups that are homogeneous for the problems these persons present with may have some value because the members can confront another member more effectively than can the therapist.

Lack of focus. A patient's low motivation to engage in treatment will dampen a group's working capacity. Patients who report few symptoms need to be carefully assessed, because they may also have difficulty participating in any sort of challenging processes. When a patient has great difficulty identifying a focus for treatment, the group's energy may be sapped. These patients may do better in a more structured group.

Composition Strategies

Three composition strategies might be contemplated for difficult patients.

1. One or two more difficult patients may be placed in a group to provide them with an opportunity to rise to the overall group level of functioning.
2. Patients with very similar difficult styles may be placed together and constitute the entire group. In this type of group, which will be highly homogeneous for the difficulty in question, the negative impact of the particular style can be tolerated because all the members are familiar with the style and its problems.
3. Difficult patients may be placed in more structured group approaches, where in some cases they respond better, and then may be graduated at a later phase to a more interactionally focused group.

A good general rule is to consider the overall capacity of each member in terms of interpersonal functioning. The six personality dimensions listed in Table 4–6 may be used as an informal scale. Think of each dimension as having a range from low to middle to high. Note that Emotional Reactivity is given a positive value because it acts as a motivator for involvement. If more than half of the dimensions are low, the person is not going to take to the group environment very easily and probably will need a fairly structured group such as one that involves the first two levels shown in Table 6–1 (i.e., psychoeducational or social skills). If more than half are high, unless there are some specific features of concern, it is likely that the patient will be able to handle an interactional group reasonably well. The decision would therefore focus on what kind of more intensive group experience would be most appropriate.

Those patients in a mid-range need to be carefully considered. It would be worth looking again more closely at four of our assessment dimensions. First, it should be determined whether Psychological Mindedness and Quality of Relationships have been adequately assessed. (Quality of Relationships is probably the more important of the two in this context.) Then, overall adaptation, as measured by the Global Assessment of Functioning (GAF) Scale (Appendix 1) and the Global Assessment of Relational Functioning (GARF) Scale (Appendix 2), should be assessed. The clinician should consider how these two measures of actual performance contribute to an assessment of interactional capacity.

These ratings need to be considered in relation to the course of the person's entire adult adjustment to the present, and then over the last couple of years, and then over the last 6 months. Has there been a marked drop in level of functioning in recent times? Do the problematic aspects extend back many years? This review process should alert the clinician to major long-standing problems stemming from limited overall capacity for adaptation. Some patients having problems with adaptation in the present may have had much more satisfactory functioning in the not-too-distant past.

The clinician should then decide on the optimum level of group therapy for the individual. In practical terms, the clinician chooses among the five levels of process focus listed in Table 6–1. Cognitive-behavior therapists will need to consider the extent to which they want to use process expansion for the application of the material. Therapists more comfortable with the interpersonal/psychodynamic model might view the process focus levels in terms of a shift in emphasis between using more structure and encouraging support and using less structure and more interpretive techniques.

Patients with high ratings on measures of both Psychological Mindedness and Quality of Relationships often find a highly structured group and a primary emphasis on cognitive style to be less satisfying and may resist these sorts of interventions or drop out.

Individuals are being done no favor by being placed in a situation that they are unlikely to manage. They may experience another sense of failure at seeing themselves as being less effective than the other members of the group. A serious mismatch may also act as a brake on the group. The members may either feel they always have to wait for that member to catch up or feel apprehensive about further self-disclosure in that member's presence.

Homogeneity of Membership

Clinicians almost always compose a group with some type of homogeneity in mind. The clinical setting itself often results in major preselection effects. The personality measures discussed above are automatically invoked by most therapists as they think of group composition. At the most basic level, the therapist should ask himself or herself, "Are these people likely to be able to understand one another relatively easily?" The formal measures simply help to structure that process.

As a general rule, the more constraints there are in terms of group integrity, the more homogeneity is likely to be helpful. For example, structural issues such as few sessions, more membership changes, changing therapists, and large size will make the creation of a cohesive group more difficult. These factors can be, to some extent, counterbalanced by greater homogeneity. Sometimes the nature of the interventions being utilized requires quite homogeneous membership. For example, systematic desensitization for specific phobias will result in a tightly homogeneous group based on diagnosis, as will a psychoeducational group for patients with bipolar disorder.

Homogeneity has both advantages and disadvantages (52). One advantage of a tightly homogeneous group is that the members can quickly identify with one another. As a result, the early process of cohesion is rapidly accomplished, and the group has more time to spend in interactional work. A disadvantage of homogeneity is that the lack of differences may make confrontational group tasks more difficult. In more technical terms, if most of the members utilize the same sort of defensive mechanisms, they may collude in a common resistance toward examining these mechanisms. For example, a group of dependent, dysthymic middle-age women may have great difficulty in challenging one another's passivity. On the other hand, in some situations these similarities may actually make it easier to identify what others are doing ("It takes one to know one"). This identification with others is commonly cited as an advantage in groups for persons with alcohol or substance abuse.

It is not uncommon to compose groups on the basis of age. By selecting patients who are at a common stage in their development, the therapist automatically achieves important homogeneity. The basic tasks of sequential human development have a powerful background impact that will allow members to understand one another's situations readily. This factor tends to be most relevant in earlier and later years. For example, groups for younger adolescents will be facing quite different issues than will groups for later adolescents. Patients dealing specifically with the challenges of adjusting to early adulthood also have many common themes. Such groups are often found in student counseling settings. Similarly, groups dealing with adjustment to retirement or to advancing age bring with them many common issues. Other groups may be composed to deal with the more subtle changes of adulthood such as decade markers, family status, or other middle-age transition points.

Another common method for achieving homogeneity is for groups to be composed based on gender. Historically, such groups have tended to be for women, though recent years have seen an expansion of groups for men as well. Such group formats are designed to promote a cohesive group environment with strong identification among the members. Such cohesion and identification may provide an opportunity to address issues associated with secrecy and shame. These issues often center on past or present abuse. Many of the gender-specific programs are reinforced with substantial philosophical or political orientations. Such groups clearly have been helpful for empowering many people. The perceived safety of gender-specific groups may be an important way for a person to begin the therapeutic process. At some point, liabilities may be encountered. Often, central issues in gender-specific groups, for both men and women, concern the nature of relationships with the opposite sex. A mixed group offers an opportunity to address such issues directly.

For general psychotherapy purposes, a mixed group is desirable. The usual problem is finding enough men, because most mental health programs see approximately twice as many women as men in their general assessment pool. The same consideration needs to be applied to the gender of the therapists, a topic to be discussed in more detail in Chapter 11.

A trend in recent years has been to compose groups according to quite narrow selection criteria. The intention of using such criteria is to encourage a tight focus on a specific set of circumstances. Some groups are formed based on specific diagnostic categories such as major depression or panic disorder. Others are formed according to present or past events, such as dealing with loss of an important person, having an alcoholic parent, or having been sexually abused. From a technical point of view, such composition decisions clearly promote cohesion and focus. At the same time, however, it is important to appreciate that underlying most of these conditions are common factors often relating to self-esteem and skewed relationship patterns.

There is a danger that highly homogeneous groups may reinforce the status of victim or survivor, which may subtly impede mastery over the offending circumstance. This argument may be unwelcome to some who have a vested interest in a particular set of traumatic conditions. The objective of therapy, however, would seem to be best conceptualized as a freeing from one's past, not a perpetual enmeshment in its framework. From this point of view, there are advantages to a sequential process whereby the tightly homogeneous group is used for the purpose of acknowledging, perhaps even to oneself, what has happened and to make it a public event within the group. Once this stage has been accomplished, progression to a more general group might allow more complete working through to occur. This theme will be addressed later in the book when specific group models are presented (see Chapter 13).

The subject of homogeneity in group composition is related to the question of what mix of types of groups a service system should have. This important clinical question will be addressed in detail later in this book in the discussion of the use of groups in clinical settings (see Chapter 12). To set the stage for that expanded discussion, it is worth seriously considering placing most patients in a general psychotherapy group at the interactional level to which they are most suited. General groups can accommodate patients with a wide variety of problems and facilitate moving patients quickly into treatment. The more narrow the focus of the group becomes, the more delays may be encountered in finding enough patients to fill the available slots. As implied above, highly homogeneous groups have advantages but also disadvantages. The popularization of many highly specific groups may be useful for marketing and referral purposes, but such specificity may not always allow for the best therapeutic strategies.

Mix of Members

So far, group composition has been addressed from the standpoint of the objectives of the group. The second level of decision about composition focuses on the mix of interactional styles among the members of a particular group. A general recommendation would be to strive for homogeneity in regard to level of vulnerability and interactional capacity and for maximum heterogeneity for areas of conflict. To translate this recommendation into an interpersonal framework, a reasonable theoretical position would be to strive for a mix of members within which members from all four group role categories—Sociable Role, Structural Role, Divergent Role, and

Cautionary Role—are represented. This presupposes that such social role behaviors can be accurately determined through a dyadic interview process. However, patients frequently demonstrate quite a different side of themselves once they begin the group. Later in this chapter, a pregroup preparation workshop is described that can provide an opportunity for the therapist to see patients at work in a group before final composition decisions are made.

It is worth striving at the very least to have different interpersonal styles represented in the group. Such heterogeneity of interpersonal styles provides greater opportunity for interpersonal learning. Because of homogeneous selection criteria based on diagnosis, groups may have a high degree of similarity in interpersonal style. To the extent possible, a mix of styles should be sought. The four group role categories can be a helpful guide. It is useful to try to include in any group at least a couple of members who are likely to have a more spontaneous and lively interactional style. Such members can provide important energy for the group process.

Prolonged deliberation about details of the mix of members is generally of limited value. The early sessions provide an opportunity to mold group norms and establish a working atmosphere that can override such subtle composition issues.

Potential Group Isolate

The other side of homogeneity deals with identifying group members who are likely to be isolates in the group. Isolation often centers on relatively nonspecific characteristics such as age, sex, racial origins, or socioeconomic status (e.g., a person considerably outside the age range of other members, one man in a group of women, or one member of a minority group). Isolation within the group may result from a greater depth of psychological dysfunction than in other members, such as the presence of psychotic thinking, repeated suicide attempts, or a history of extended hospitalization. The general principle would be for the therapist to try hard to find another member with whom the potential isolate could identify. It is worth scanning the prospective members of a group from this standpoint to the extent possible.

The therapist must be concerned that the isolate not experience rejection or a sense of failure because of difficulty integrating into the group. It might well be that such feared expectation is related to the patient's coming for treatment in the first place. If the composition issue cannot be corrected, then open attention to the difference, whatever it might be, is warranted in the first session. During the first few sessions, the therapist should be scanning the group to ensure that all members are becoming involved in the group interaction. Skillful handling of such issues usually allows the therapist to get around most of these sorts of situations. The issue of isolation will be discussed at greater length in the next chapter when the engagement stage is addressed.

Cotherapy

The final issue regarding group composition is the number of therapists. Because the presence of two therapists increases the complexity of the group system, the use of cotherapists is among those factors that should routinely be considered as adding more potential complications. For more structured groups, the use of cotherapists may not be a major issue. But for groups in which the intention is to make the interactional climate of the group a major component of treatment, the opportunity for problems increases markedly (53). This applies particularly to groups that operate primarily at the last three levels of process focus: many cognitive-behavioral groups and most interpersonal-semistructured and interpersonal/psychodynamic groups (see Table 6–1).

There are some circumstances in which cotherapists serve a specific purpose. For example, adolescent groups and couples groups may wish to provide a parental model. In this case, the cotherapists should be of opposite gender and be able to provide a truly functional model of communication and collaboration. In special settings, such as correctional institutions, cotherapy may be required as a safety measure.

Many training programs use cotherapy as a way to provide an opportunity for the therapist-in-training to be in a group without the expectation of total responsibility. The nature of the role would be known to the group members. With careful preparation and debriefing before and after sessions, this model can be quite effective. Usually, the trainee begins with less activity and increases the level of activity over time, often modeling on the experienced therapist. The issue of senior and junior roles can be tricky but manageable when there is a constant focus on open communication.

Cotherapy is *not* a good solution for therapist insecurity. Two therapists who are uncertain of their roles simply compound the potential for problems. They are less likely to be aware of the impact of their roles on the group. They may be unaware of covert control struggles that may stem from their mutual anxiety. Mutual avoidance of responsibility is all too common: "I was going to intervene, but I saw you were thinking the same thing, so I didn't." "Me too." In short, cotherapy is for experienced therapists. Many therapists forced by circumstances into doing a group solo come away with an exhilarated feeling of being truly responsible, with the attendant boost in professional self-confidence. Routine use of cotherapists doubles the personnel costs for treating the same number of patients, eroding much of the efficiency of the modality. Training, supervision, and program standards that assist the solo group therapist to feel secure are addressed later in this book in the discussion of service programs (see Chapter 11).

Clinical Considerations

No group is going to be composed in an ideal manner. The pressures of clinical settings work against the construction of the perfect group. Obsessive attention to composition issues is unrealistic and unnecessary. The issues raised in this chapter regarding group composition are designed to alert the clinician to situations that may cause problems. Fortunately, the generic model of group psychotherapy is based on the idea that any group that is run according to basic constructive professional principles is going to be helpful. This base of common effect will do much to soften less-than-perfect composition decisions. The therapist can assist this natural process by ensuring that composition stresses be openly discussed in the group as a normal event that needs to be resolved. In general, the earlier this is done, the better, beginning with the first session.

Pretherapy Preparation

After the group has been composed, the next task is to prepare the members for the beginning of the group. Pretherapy preparation results in fewer early dropouts and faster development of cohesion. The main purpose of such preparation is to influence the development of group cohesion. After the first six to eight sessions, the effects of preparation are washed out by the actual experiences within the group.

Preparation has two technical effects. First, it increases the likelihood that members will stay in the group long enough to have an exposure to therapeutic factors, mainly those of the "supportive" cluster. Second, it assists in the development of constructive group norms. Often, patterns that arise in the first few sessions come to establish the group's image and are difficult to change. This "primacy effect" is well recognized in the social psychology literature. Once a behavior is in place, far more effort is required to change it than was necessary to prompt it in the beginning. Some form of systematic orientation should be considered a necessary part of professional group practice (54).

The purpose of pretherapy preparation is to educate patients about what to expect in group and how to get the most out of their group experience. Such preparation provides them with some cognitive predictability, which is a major source of strength as the group begins to form. It helps to build a common set of attitudes and expectations about how to be a successful group member, a process described as "role induction."

Pretherapy material can be presented in several ways. The major choice is between carrying out pretherapy preparation in a group setting or conducting it with individual patients. Both approaches have advantages. The choice is partly dependent on service characteristics. Programs with large volumes of patients may have regular pretherapy preparation meetings for people joining several groups. Sometimes the material is covered with the incoming members of a particular group. Most settings handle the preparation task in individual sessions. No matter which approach is used, patients will be anxious about joining a group, so it is important to present the information *repeatedly*.

Patient Information Handout

The Patient Information Handout provided in Appendix 9 contains the information of most value for pretherapy preparation. This handout can be given to the patient to take home and should then be discussed in the preparation session; it should not simply be given out to be read. By spending some time with the patient going over each paragraph, the therapist has an opportunity to answer questions or clarify the information. Most critically, such careful review reinforces the importance of the issues. The final two group rules on the form in Appendix 9 regarding extragroup socializing and contact with the therapist between sessions may be modified for groups that are largely supportive in nature. However, careful thought should be given to modification of these rules because both deal with important aspects of the group frame.

Pregroup Preparation Workshops

Several programs have reported positive results from the use of a pregroup assessment and preparation workshop procedure (55). It might be argued that this is particularly relevant to the private practitioner as a method of preventing early group dropouts in time-limited groups. People who are uncertain about participating have an opportunity to leave before the group actually begins.

For the patient, it is the experiential component, the experience of "getting one's toes wet," that is the strongest recommendation for a group approach. Preparation workshops introduce the idea of group treatment in a structured manner that addresses patient anxiety and results in fewer overall dropouts. Patients can make more informed decisions about what they are getting into and therefore feel more confident about becoming engaged in the effort.

The clinician can also be better informed about which patients seem to fit comfortably together for a particular group and so can use the session to make final decisions about group composition. For this purpose, it is better to have a slightly larger number attend the workshop than will actually be in the group.

The advantage of a group approach is that it allows the material to be presented in an experiential manner. A structured series of group exercises, in addition to serving as an educational tool, permits a controlled entry into experiencing the group process. Such sessions may consist of a brief introduction about the history and theory of group psychotherapy and an opportunity for questions. Often, this introductory period is followed by a series of structured group exercises. For example, members can talk in pairs for 5 minutes and then introduce each other to the group. This exercise begins a process of self-disclosure and facilitates a level of group participation that is controlled and safe. A useful second exercise is for the therapist to ask members to identify something they would like to change or understand better in their personal relationships, or what they would most like to get out of the group experience. Through this process, central themes can begin to be focused on as a target for therapeutic work. Within the course of a pretherapy session, the material outlined in the handout in Appendix 9 can be systematically covered.

The pretherapy process should consist of no more than two sessions, to ensure that the therapeutic process does not begin before the "official" group starts. Participants are not expected to make a commitment to join the group on the spot, but instead are asked to let the leader know in a few days if they wish to join a group. Such workshops may be run with as few as 3 or 4 participants or as many as 10 or more.

A group preparation session allows the therapist to detect potential problems with over- or underinvolvement in the process, the presence of inhibiting levels of anxiety or depression, and the level at which problems are conceptualized. A patient who clearly does not fit in terms of interpersonal style may be identified as unsuitable for a particular group. Evidence of low motivation may become evident through the discussion process. A patient whose behavior poses major problems in terms of disruptions and who does not respond to guidance may be deemed not yet ready for a group experience.

The clinician conducting the pretherapy group also needs to be alert to identifying potential dropouts. Sometimes misunderstandings can arise and if not addressed may lead patients to resolve that they could never be in a group with a particular person. Such decisions may also reflect a resistance to wanting to look at issues raised during the session. These meetings may be considered "pretherapy," but for the patients they represent the beginning of the group treatment process, and some patients may be frightened off at the idea of serious work. The leader must address such reactions openly and quickly. When reactions are successfully addressed, patients are provided with a good education in dealing with process issues. If a patient decides to leave anyway, his or her leaving is probably inevitable, and it is perhaps better that it happen before the group formally begins.

Preparation of the Individual Patient

The group therapist may elect to have a few meetings with each patient individually before initiation of the group. There are several advantages to conducting such sessions. Such meetings provide an opportunity for the development of the beginning of a therapeutic alliance, which can be an important sustaining factor for the patient during the early sessions. In addition to obtaining more diagnostic data and providing information about how groups work, the therapist can be alert to concerns the patient might have about joining the group and can address these. The specific topics in the Patient Information Handout should be directly reviewed, particularly the myths and the group rules.

The danger with pretherapy individual sessions is that the patient may then become resistant to "giving up" the therapist to the group. The therapist can guard against this by continually reinforcing the preparation task of the sessions and by making regular reference to how the issues can be applied in the early stages of the group. Meeting with the patient for more than three such sessions increases the likelihood of transition problems.

In addition to obtaining more diagnostic information and providing facts about group therapy, the therapist should inquire about the fears the patient might have about being in a group. The specific topics concerning myths about groups contained in the Patient Information Handout (Appendix 9) need to be directly reviewed. The pregroup meetings can be effectively used to begin the process of establishing a therapeutic focus, which is an important priming function that facilitates the rapid emergence of a working atmosphere in the group. This objective can be specifically reinforced by suggesting to the patient that it would be useful early in the group to review such discussions with the other members. This work orientation can be the vehicle for initial self-disclosure and universality.

Group preparation material can be integrated into the two-session protocol for developing a focus outlined in the preceding chapter. The two approaches, group and individual, are not mutually exclusive. A sensible combination could begin with the two individual sessions to finalize assessment and to work toward defining a therapeutic focus. These sessions might then be followed by a single pretherapy group session in which structured exercises are used and the Patient Information Handout is reviewed. It is important for the therapist conducting the preparation to clarify that it is a warm-up session and that when the therapy begins the therapist will be less active. The first-session procedures described in the next chapter also offer an opportunity to reinforce pretherapy ideas.

Preparation for group should always be considered. In some situations, such as in an inpatient group, the preparation may be adequately handled through a brief talk with the patient rather than by a more formal procedure. In outpatient settings, the preparation material can be inserted into assessment interviews. In clinical services where the patient is referred to the group therapist after a full assessment has been completed, it might be realistic to schedule only a single pretherapy session to confirm suitability, develop some Focus Areas, and cover the pretherapy preparation material. The important point is to make sure the material is covered in one way or another.

Planning for the First Session

This subsection may seem like an exercise in the obvious. But in the rush and anxiety over beginning a group, it is not at all uncommon for mundane details to get lost.

The therapist should ensure that there is absolute clarity regarding the exact date, time, and place of the first session. This information is best written down and read over with the patient. There needs to be an unambiguous description of exactly where the patient should report, how to get there, where to park, and any other practical details. The time should be not only clearly spelled out but also reinforced with the idea that arriving a bit early for the first session would be a good idea just in case there are any transportation snags. This is also a good opportunity to double-check that the patient will not have problems attending future sessions. Similarly, the therapist should be sure that arrangements have been made for doors to be unlocked, receptionists to know whom to expect, and the room to be available a good 15 minutes before the group is to start. Consent forms are best taken care of in advance, as well as any discussion about observation or taping arrangements. Indeed, it is helpful for the patients to hold the pregroup preparation session in the group room itself and take the members through the observation room or show them how the equipment works. They may even try using the camera themselves, an exercise that helps to promote an observing perspective.

SECTION III
Implementing the Generic Group

CHAPTER 7

The Beginning: The Engagement Stage

*I*n Section II, considerable detail was provided about the assessment and preparation of patients before the group has started. Now comes the payoff for these efforts. Most of the techniques described in this chapter about the early stage of a group can be referred to in general terms as supportive strategies. They will continue to be used to some extent throughout a group's life, and especially when the group is under increased stress. Groups that begin strongly move on to deeper work quickly. Groups that get off to a shaky beginning may never achieve higher levels of cohesion or as active a working environment. The first session is a critical time. Fortunately, a desire to see the group succeed is shared by the members. They will provide most of the important input into the session. It is important that the therapist not get in the way of the developing group system.

The First Session

Careful preparation for the first session will lead to a more effective beginning. A clear and, preferably, written description of exactly when and where the group will meet should have been provided to the patients prior to the first session, as described in the preceding chapter. Nonetheless, it is not uncommon to encounter last-minute arrangements that have to be addressed. For example, perhaps all the details for the final member to be chosen for the group have not been worked out. A potential member calls 2 hours before the group begins with uncertainty about whether to attend. The therapist is feeling some anxiety and left the list of the members' names at home and is not sure that all can be remembered. It is best to anticipate that some problems will arise and not schedule the day too tightly. The major tasks of the first session are outlined in Table 7–1.

Preparing the Room

The therapist should allow time to set up the room well in advance. A room that has just been vacated by another group and is cluttered with cups and crumpled papers does not make a good impression on newly arriving patients. Chairs should be set up in a reasonably tight circle, with one chair for each member, no more and no less. If possible, long sofas that cluster members and may interfere with each member's having a clear view of all others should be avoided. In general, it is preferable not to have a table within the circle. Tables invite the depositing of cups, books, clothing, feet, and anything else that can serve as a barrier. An open space sends a clear message that the task of the group will be to talk and interact with one another. If a table is present, it must be low. The room should be well lit though not glaring. Subdued lights in a group room suggest secrecy and internal reflection, not self-disclosure and interaction. If audiovisual equipment is to be used, it should be set up, tested, and ready to go, with only the pause button waiting to be released.

Greeting Patients

It is preferable for the first session to have the group members assemble in a waiting area. They can then be called into the group room together. This avoids the tense silence that often prevails when the members go directly into the group room before the therapist is present. (In one such group, the members were sitting almost immobile, with some piece of reading

---

Table 7–1.   Tasks of the first session

1. Preparing the room
2. Greeting patients
3. Orienting to the room
4. Managing late arrivals
5. Establishing the leader's role
6. Reviewing individual goals

---

material in front of each face, like mannequins in a store window. This scene was recalled by the members with somewhat embarrassed humor during the termination process.) The therapist should join the group at the indicated start time. It is not wise for the therapist to spend time sitting with the group either before the beginning or while waiting for additional members. Doing so invites involvement in social chatter, which serves to detract from the business of the group and the role of the leader.

Often, one or more members may arrive late despite the best of planning (see discussion of late arrivals below). It may be the best strategy for the therapist simply to tell the group that an expected member has not arrived and that he or she wishes to check the waiting area one more time so that that person can be included in the beginning of the group. The therapist should relate this to the patients in a concerned, but not anxious, manner. The therapist should check only once, about 10 minutes into the session.

The therapist should rather obviously close the door, even if some group members have not arrived. This is a powerful symbolic statement regarding the external group boundary. By closing the door, the therapist avoids the situation in which the group, with expectant, perhaps pleading, glances toward the hall outside, awaits the arrival of any additional members. To latecomers, a closed door is an implicit message regarding time boundaries. To those in the room, closing the door reinforces their promptness and indicates that the group is going to work with whomever is present. These structural issues begin to create a "frame" around the therapeutic experience.

Careful adherence to these guidelines creates the impression of a well-organized and professional atmosphere in which important work is anticipated. It does not mean that pleasantness or humanness is abandoned, but that there are clear structural expectations regarding the process of group participation. Such an atmosphere allows the members to relax in the knowledge that they are in good hands. Psychoeducational and social skills groups may have a more relaxed approach to informal preliminary conversation, but the issues concerning time, attendance, and membership must not be relaxed.

Orienting to the Room

As a first priority, the members need to be oriented to the therapy room. If audiovisual equipment is being used, whether it be a simple audio recording within the room or partially hidden video cameras, it should be openly described and identified. Although it is useful to have such equipment as inconspicuous as possible, the equipment should not be hidden. It is better to directly acknowledge the presence and location of equipment to desensitize the members to any sense of mystery or secrecy regarding it. This is also an opportunity to reiterate issues of confidentiality by reviewing exactly how tapes will be handled in terms of access and erasure.

If the group is to be observed, this should also be immediately addressed. The members must be informed about the regulations and policy regarding who can observe their group. They should have the option of meeting any observers and of seeing the observation room if they wish. It is an ongoing responsibility of the leader to let the group know if there is a change in observer status. It is not acceptable practice to have random visits by any observer, whether clinical or administrative, without the group's knowledge. One may be absolutely certain that the presence of observers will be in the back of the minds of the group members throughout the session. By addressing these external boundary issues directly, the therapist is building a sense of trust in the therapeutic environment and also encouraging a common group focus to promote cohesion.

Example

In one recent group, the members met the observer briefly and expressed no specific concerns regarding his presence. During the session, no mention was made of the observation window. However, just as the session was ending, several members spontaneously waved and spoke in a humorous vein to the unseen observer behind the one-way window, wondering if he had enjoyed the session. One member took this a step further by stating that she did not think the observer could have enjoyed the session as much as the members did! Though unseen, the observer is always a participant in the minds of the members.

Managing Late Arrivals

It is not uncommon for one or two members to arrive significantly late for the first session. The late arrival may be a reflection of anxiety or the first evidence of ambivalence about the idea of psychotherapy. The therapist may feel some irritation at a member's interrupting the first session in this manner. There may be an inclination either to address the situation from an interpretive viewpoint or to come down firmly on norm expectations about not being late. Either approach would be inappropriate.

It is preferable to provide a positive example of norm establishment without invoking comments that might be taken as criticism or blame. The member might be greeted and asked to wait for a moment before introducing himself to the group. Once a natural pause occurs, such an invitation could be extended. By handling the situation in this way, the therapist acknowledges the member but does not reinforce a grand entrance with attention. Indeed, the point could be reiterated at the end of the session with a bland reminder for everybody of the importance of beginning each session with everyone present.

Example

A 30-year-old single professional woman arrived 30 minutes late for the first session. In the assessment process, she had been somewhat irritable and suspicious of the questionnaire process. She was absolute in her rejection of her parents and in her determination to never let a man take advantage of her. There was a vague hint of a disastrous early relationship, but she would not elaborate. She described having a number of good girlfriends but was feeling increasingly isolated as they became married. It was clear from this interview that she would present some management difficulties.

She entered the group room aggressively and sat down firmly in the one empty chair. The therapist nodded to her and said there would be an opportunity shortly to get introduced. The chance arose when one of the members finished a discussion of personal goals. The therapist then suggested that the group might take the opportunity of the arrival of the final group member to review names and perhaps to have those who had already spoken give a capsule summary of their goals. The late member began to visibly relax and listened carefully, commenting at the end that she wanted to apologize for arriving late. At the next session she spoke of her high level of apprehension about coming to the group and her fear that she would not be found acceptable to the members. She had hidden in the washroom before the group, trying to get up enough courage to enter. The fact that the therapist had acknowledged her and that the group had interrupted its business to include her had been a powerful experience of acceptance.

She became one of the first group members to make a significant external application of her group work. She acknowledged to herself that she had maintained a rigid view of the negative aspects of her parents since her teen years. She was beginning to see that they were not in fact as negative as she chose to see them. They had a moving reconciliation that resulted in a positive increase in self-esteem. She quickly went on to review with considerable grief a relationship in her teens that had ended abruptly when the young man began dating her friend. She had not dated since but found herself beginning to wonder about whether she might begin again.

It seemed clear that a response by the therapist in the first session that had smacked of nonacceptance or implied criticism would have resulted in an early dropout. In addition, the brief repeat during the next session helped to reinforce core themes and to succinctly extract the essence of them. For that patient, the establishment of the Therapeutic Bond was off to a good start, and her state of Self-Relatedness markedly deepened. Indeed, the experience of the first session was perhaps the most important incident in her entire time in the group.

Establishing the Leader's Role

Many members will anticipate that the group is going to be "conducted" by the therapist. This expectation is not unrealistic if they have not previously been in a therapy situation. Remember that assessment interviews are largely structured around questions, with the patient in a responding mode. Pretherapy preparation will not alter the hope and expectation that the real responsibility will continue to live with the therapist. The group members will be watching closely to see what role the therapist will take.

The activity level of the therapist will become established early in the group's life. Opinion varies considerably, however, regarding the best style for the first session. For all forms of group psychotherapy, the task of the therapist is an inherently paradoxical one: to facilitate group interaction without taking over or inhibiting group initiative. For groups with a more structured approach, an active leader style will be immediately evident. The solution for the first session is less clear-cut in groups that are designed for a greater focus on learning from the group process.

A body of evidence suggests that a modest amount of structure facilitates the development of group cohesion (56). Structure helps to lessen anxiety, which in turn makes self-disclosure easier. This promotes greater interaction among the members and, therefore, a more rapid sense of acceptance and participation. It is certainly possible to accompany early therapist activity with the message that this level of activity will not continue as the group moves on. Many therapists working from a psychodynamic orientation would argue that bad habits should not be fostered and that the members must realize from the onset that the major momentum of initiation is to come from them. However, prolonged silence or trivial conversation in the first session can be counterproductive. It is preferable that the group address its therapeutic task early, even if the therapist finds it necessary to provide some structure around which this can occur.

The decision regarding how active the therapist should be is linked to the interpersonal capacity of the members. For example, experiential training groups for clinicians are usually run with a restrained style that lays the onus on the group members to take responsibility for maintaining the group process from the beginning. A restrained style is appropriate in this context because the members are not in the group because of major psychopathology and already have some understanding of the expectations of membership. However, clinical groups are dealing with a different population. By providing some structure, the therapist can accelerate group involvement.

The following protocol provides a practical solution to beginning most psychotherapy groups. After the orientation procedures described above are carried out, the therapist suggests that members introduce themselves. "Who would care to begin?" This suggestion provides both modest structure and the opportunity for member initiation. The therapist may also suggest that personal information such as last name, area of residence, or employment is not really relevant to the task of the group. The group is to work on problems within the group room in confidentiality, and specific details about outside circumstances are unnecessary. This suggestion helps to focus the members on the task of the group. The end result of this first go-around is usually a quite brief statement from each member.

Reviewing Individual Goals

The structure is then deepened. The therapist mentions that all group members have been through the same assessment, questionnaire completion (if relevant), and feedback procedure, and so the therapist is in the unique position of having had the opportunity to get to know all members reasonably well. Perhaps a good way for the group to begin work would be for each member to discuss with the group the sorts of things that were focused on during these pregroup meetings. In particular, it would be interesting to hear of issues that were raised that were new or surprising to the patient.

It is useful around this time to acknowledge some degree of anxiety in the air and normalize the anxiety as an understandable reaction. The therapist should try to build this acknowledgment on a member's comment about feeling tense or feeling confused about what to say. Some gentle humor is not amiss. For example, with the first member to acknowledge some tension, the therapist may ask, "I suppose you must be the only anxious person here?" With the ice somewhat broken, members are then encouraged to explain in some detail what the central issues will be for them to address in the group. The therapist can immediately translate this process into an interactional format by encouraging members to ask further questions or to reflect on their own responses to issues raised.

The therapist may wish to encourage the members to state their understanding of the broader connections to their presenting problems. This process often results in quite penetrating comments about important stress issues or recurrent patterns.

Examples

One woman in an interpersonally oriented group explained that the review of important relationships during the assessment had made it clear to her that she played a major role in why her intimate partners became disenchanted and left her. It had been an unpleasant surprise for her to see that she described herself in these relationships in the same way as she saw her mother behaving toward her father. She had always been angry toward her mother for this style and blamed her for the departure of her father, whom she idealized. This realization laid the base for important future work on the implications of intimacy for her to address in the group.

A man in a structured depression group identified his angry but passive withdrawal from any situation containing the seeds of conflict. He would criticize himself for such withdrawal, and the self-criticism would trigger an intensification of his negative views of the world and of himself. The patient's addressing this issue led nicely into a discussion of the importance of addressing negative thought patterns in the group.

The challenge for the therapist is to maintain a reasonable balance between ensuring that all members have an opportunity to present themselves in some detail during the first session and, at the same time, working toward a normative expectation of interaction. The goal is to have the major issues for all members placed on the metaphorical group table by the end of the first session. This is not the time for a detailed exploration of this material, and at times the therapist may need to intervene to defer elaboration to later sessions.

The therapist can accomplish this simply by stating that the issues raised are clearly important and will need to be addressed in the group and that it was good to hear them described so clearly, but that it is necessary to keep going around the group so that everyone has the same opportunity.

This semistructured go-around procedure ensures that all members participate and that the focus is on core issues, not the weather, hospital procedures, or historical material unconnected to current problems. The members can be encouraged to translate their issues into specific goals or Focus Areas that they want to address. This straightforward approach to the first session builds on the careful assessment and preparation procedures. It almost always results in a powerful session and establishes in some detail the agenda for each member. Once such information has been put into words, it is available for recall by the therapist or other members as material related to these themes comes up later in the group.

It is very helpful near the end of the first session to elicit comments from all members concerning their reaction to the session. This process, which blends into the tasks of norm reinforcement and management of affect, can be initiated very early in the first session. The example given earlier regarding addressing entry anxiety among the members is an example of *process debriefing*, which is described in more detail later in this chapter. The modest structuring of the first session assists in a public reinforcement of the Therapeutic Contract—that is, the nature of the "helping relationship" that is emerging in the group.

New therapists should take solace from the fact that the first session of a group is almost always a success. The members are even more anxious than the therapist and will work hard to make it a productive occasion. The initial self-revelations are deeply felt and produce both relief and a sense of membership. If all is going well, the therapist may need to do very little except to stay out of the way and let these processes flow. Under more difficult circumstances, the therapist needs to be prepared to actively intervene in molding the nature of the group process in a productive manner.

Strategies for the Early Group

There are a number of strategies that will assist the group in forming and developing (Table 7–2). Most of these are not technically difficult, but, rather, consist of not getting in the way of group process and of gently shaping the nature of the group environment.

Table 7–2. Tasks of the engagement stage

1. Developing cohesion
2. Defining the external boundary
3. Promoting interaction among members
4. Reinforcing group norms
5. Using the therapeutic factors
6. Using process debriefing

Developing Cohesion

The principal goal for the therapist in the first few sessions is to foster the development of cohesion in the group. To foster group cohesion, the therapist must be continuously monitoring the overall group atmosphere. The individual members will be seen primarily from the standpoint of their participation and involvement in the group. The first few sessions are not the time for detailed individual exploration.

The process of becoming a member of the group carries with it many therapeutic ingredients. The primary marker of an effective group is the *level of cohesion.* It is essential that a sense of positive identification with the group emerge at an early point. If this does not occur, the members will become demoralized and disenchanted about the possibilities of the group's being helpful. It was noted in the discussion of the generic model of psychotherapy (see Chapter 2) that the early Therapeutic Bond is the most reliable predictor of outcome. The effects of the technical processes of therapy are mediated by the quality of the Therapeutic Bond. In the absence of positive connectedness, the most skillful techniques are likely to fall flat. Group cohesion is the analog of the Therapeutic Bond in psychotherapy groups.

The patient dimensions of the Therapeutic Bond in individual psychotherapy can also be identified in groups. Patients will appear motivated and eager to continue treatment and will have a strong sense of engagement in the process. They will show a quality of collaboration in the treatment process, as reflected by their high level of participation. The patients may express a positive affirmation of the therapist, but in groups it is more important that there is a sense of positive connection with the other group members. Likewise, the therapist dimensions of the Therapeutic Bond in group therapy are similar to those in individual psychotherapy. These include an attitude of engagement, a collaborative approach with the members, and a firm and credible presentation. The therapist will show an empathic understanding of patients' experience and will have a positive attitude toward them. The therapist should be constantly monitoring these qualities in group members and in himself or herself. The Group Cohesiveness Scale, developed by Budman and colleagues and presented in adapted form in Chapter 3 (see Table 3–4), may be used to assess group cohesion in the early sessions.

Defining the External Boundary

During the engagement stage, the external group boundary will become increasingly defined. *Boundary clarification* can be addressed in a systematic manner from several viewpoints.

The physical boundary.   The importance of beginning the first session of the group in a clear and unambiguous fashion has already been mentioned. By seating the group members in a special room, entering as the Designated Leader, and closing the door, the therapist begins the process of defining the group external boundary. These actions communicate louder than words that the group, including the therapist, are in this together and must sort out how the group as a whole is going to operate.

It is highly desirable for the therapist to have the group meet in the same room under the same conditions for each session. For example, if a group is to be observed, it should meet systematically in the observation room even if on some occasions no observers are present. Changes in the time the group meets should be considered very carefully. Shifting the time schedule to accommodate a member or the leader implies a violation of the original contract and thus weakens the external boundary.

The membership boundary.   The question of membership speaks directly to the heart of external boundary definition. Early in the group's life, the therapist must be constantly aware of the impact of changes of membership through repeated absences or premature terminations. Such issues cannot be put aside with the rationale that they will get sorted out later; they are fundamental to the definition of the group and must be addressed and resolved. A member who, for example, misses several of the first six sessions of a group must be directly confronted with the issue of membership. Confrontation does not mean that the behavior is addressed in a punitive fashion. There may be perfectly understandable reasons why the member cannot attend. For whatever reason, if a member's attendance is going to be sporadic, then it is in the best interest of the group that the member be guided into an alternative therapeutic program. This is one specific example of the therapist's acting on behalf of the group, not the individual, during the first stage.

The time boundary.   There should be no ambiguity concerning when the group sessions start and end. The clear expectation is that all members come on time and leave only at the end. As with attendance, members who cannot do this should be placed elsewhere. Groups should begin on time, even if all members are not present. They should also end on time. Only in extremely unusual situations should the ending time be extended. Such a practice invites members to delay bringing up important matters and thus to garner extra group time and attention. The group cannot substitute for real-life circumstances, and one aspect of this is the necessity of facing the "real world" on time.

An overly accommodating approach to time boundaries suggests that the interests of those who are attending regularly and on time are being sacrificed. Maintaining the time boundary is not an issue of compulsivity or punitiveness. A group can be a group only when its members are present. The absence of even one member makes a difference in how the group operates. Altering either the beginning or the ending time provides circumstances in which all members may not be able to participate.

The information boundary.   Another major process in the engagement stage involves comparing experiences in the group with those that members have had outside of the group. Through this process the group shares in an implicit recognition that there is an information boundary. The process of universalization creates a sense of what the group is about and therefore allows comparisons with other groups. This information about differences helps to consolidate a sense of groupness.

In general, members coming to psychotherapy groups have experienced adverse issues in their current or past relationships. Almost always, the early group experiences are infused with an atmosphere of positive excitement. It is therefore easy to contrast the group experience with less satisfactory outside experiences. The comparison should not be carried out by encouraging critical language that may reinforce the patient's misperceptions or distortions regarding such outside experiences. Rather, the emphasis should be on the occurrence of positive experiences within the group. For example, "You describe problems in talking openly with your wife, but it seems very constructive that you have been able to open up about these important personal issues here in the group," or "It sounds like letting some of those pent-up emotions come out in the group is a different way for you. I remember your descriptions of how you usually keep things locked up inside in your outside relationships."

Using the guideline of differences between experiences within and outside of the group, the therapist can systematically reinforce the external group boundary. Therapy is more effective when attention is devoted to the application of therapeutic experiences to outside circumstances and relationships. The presence of a clearly understood external boundary assists this process because it highlights ways in which the therapeutic experience and the "real-world" experience differ or are the same. This promotes the use of finer distinctions in how to apply what is learned in therapy to the world outside.

Once a group is well established, with a sustained cohesive atmosphere, minor lapses in maintenance of the above boundary issues can be tolerated. However, in the early sessions, setting firm boundaries constitutes an important mechanism for assisting the formation of a sense of groupness. As will be discussed in Chapter 10, many of the same principles apply during termination work.

Promoting Interaction Among Members

A simple but powerful method for enhancing cohesion is for the therapist to specifically promote member-member interaction. By members' being encouraged to talk with each other, bonds between them will be automatically created. During the early sessions of a group, the therapist should be continuously scanning the directionality of group interaction. The most common problem is a tendency for members to want to talk to or through the therapist. The leader should be comfortable in specifically redirecting comments. Initially, such redirection might be attempted by simply breaking eye contact if a member talks to the leader. Connecting phrases might be tried, such as, "Why don't you try that idea out with Helen. It sounds pretty close to what she was saying earlier," or "Henry sounds interested in what you're saying. Would you like to hear what he thinks of your situation?" Such interventions will not suggest that the leader is avoiding making a response or being too controlling if the rationale has been established during pretherapy preparation that intermember activity is to be an important component of the group therapeutic experience. Directional structuring activities make explicit the message that members are going to be of help to each other. Indeed, a simple statement during the early sessions might deal directly with the issue—for example, "As we discussed before the group started, much of the value of group therapy comes from what the members learn from each other. That's why I keep encouraging people to talk directly to each other and not just to me."

Often, more active members may begin to dominate the group interaction by talking to each other. The silent members may be relieved, because this appears to take the responsibility off their shoulders. The therapist can mold group norms by addressing such participation disparity at an early point. Simple inquiries about what a certain member is thinking may be adequate, particularly if the timing of such inquiries coincides with some sort of nonverbal reaction. But the therapist may need to make a more direct intervention—for example, "Well, Susan and Anne, it sounds like the two of you have a lot of positions in common. I'm sure we'll get back to these matters again, but I guess we need to hear from some of the other members too. Sharon, you look like some of the things they were talking about were of interest to you."

It is of particular importance that all members participate in each session. The semistructured go-around approach described earlier in this chapter to some extent ensures such participation in the first session. It is helpful if all members early on can gain experience in simply being part of the group process. The therapist should remember to scan the group after two-thirds of the session is over to be sure that no member is notably outside of the group conversation. If that is the case, then corrective moves should be considered. Again, an attitude of empathic alignment is in order, not an implied criticism. For example, "It looks like you've been quite involved in what's been going on. Any of these issues seem familiar to you?," or "Getting into the conversation is a challenge in this group isn't it? What thoughts have you been having?" All members can be encouraged to make these sorts of approaches.

Some technical aspects of the interactional climate foster the development of a strong working environment. The therapist is in a position to subtly reinforce and encourage constructive sorts of events as the group unfolds. A willingness to speak up spontaneously with ideas or reactions is helpful. Asking for clarification if one is unsure what a person means will encourage increasing self-disclosure. Listening carefully to others and monitoring one's own internal reaction to what they are saying facilitate deepening of the work. Continuously searching for specific examples rather than general comments, particularly general comments about the group, will foster interpersonal learning. For example, "Mike, you said the session was quite powerful for you. What particularly affected you the most?" or "Elaine, when you said that Jim's story was interesting, it sounded like it had some personal meaning for you. Can you speak to that?"

If group interaction proceeds satisfactorily, the group will come to assume increasing importance in the psychological life of the members. They will find themselves thinking about past sessions and about what they want to say in the next session. This reflective process should be encouraged and used as a regular part of group work. Many people find that it is helpful to keep a daily journal to record their ongoing personal work between sessions. The therapist might want to reinforce that this may be a good practice to continue after the group ends as well. The therapist can also directly underscore the idea that the work of the group goes on all week, not just in the actual sessions.

Reinforcing Group Norms

The early sessions provide an opportunity to reinforce basic group expectations and to begin molding the nature of the interactional experience. Appropriate comments can be interwoven casually throughout the session. Topics addressed through such comments would include the importance of confidentiality, of the group starting and ending on time, and of not missing sessions.

It is particularly important to address the topic of extragroup socializing through these comments. Extragroup socializing becomes an immediate possibility with the end of the first session. The rationale for the expectation that group members will not have contact with each other outside of the group should be reviewed specifically. This expectation will have more relevance for the members as they come to appreciate the sensitive topics that have been introduced in the session. Members might consider the implications for the group if some of the members were to get together after the sessions for coffee while others did not. What effect would this have on the group? The therapist restates the expectation that the group be informed of any such activities. (Note that in more highly structured skill-focused groups, extragroup contacts may actually be encouraged, though still reported back to the group.) It is also useful to remind the group that contacts with the therapist between sessions will be treated as group business and introduced back to the group at the discretion of the therapist.

With this approach, the therapist reinforces the frame of the group in a matter-of-fact fashion and, because clear rationales for the small number of group rules are provided, avoids the impression of authoritarian control. This process makes public what has already been discussed in individual pretherapy meetings.

The therapist may also weave into the group process comments about the value of self-disclosure but must also stress that each member is in control of how much to reveal at any given point in time. The importance of feedback can be reinforced, and in particular that some response is in order when any member says something having strong personal meaning. Responses from other members allow the person to know how his or her statement was received by the others. Members can also be encouraged to be actively curious about what others are saying and to feel comfortable in asking for clarification. When a member provides a response to another member or expresses understanding of what is being discussed, this can be underlined as a good way to learn through the group process. One might ask the person responded to what it was like to hear that someone seemed to appreciate what he or she was saying. This general massaging of the group interactional process is a technique that can be applied in all types of groups to maximize the therapeutic potential of the small-group experience.

This process of subtle norm reinforcement can be maintained through the early sessions until the group is routinely putting constructive interactional techniques into practice. The therapist knows that most of the constructive norms will emerge in some form in the early group. These norms can then be specifically and directly underlined. To the group members, it will appear that they are creating their own group culture and that the therapist is a participant in the process. These subtle techniques involve applying simple operant conditioning principles that most therapists draw on almost without realizing it. A low-key therapist profile allows the group members to experience at an early point that they can have a responsible role in developing their group culture.

Using the Therapeutic Factors

The therapeutic factors, particularly those from the supportive cluster, will emerge automatically as the group begins. The therapist is in a position to encourage and reinforce them.

The Supportive Cluster

The importance of fostering the development of a cohesive group atmosphere has already been discussed. The supportive cluster of therapeutic factors comprises important mechanisms that lead to group cohesion. These factors are particularly crucial during the engagement stage. The four supportive factors usually emerge together and are intertwined. The advantage of identifying each one specifically is to alert the clinician so that they can be quickly identified, promoted, and reinforced.

Universality. The most pervasive mechanism for the development of engagement in groups is *universality,* the recognition that others in the group have had experiences similar to one's own. This process forms the seed from which a sense of group identity can develop. Universality fosters an appreciation of the group as a unique entity. When members in a group first begin to interact, a process of searching for common experiences, common symptoms, and common personal reactions takes place. The use of some homogeneous criteria in group composition will now be rewarded.

The experience of universality contributes to a lowering of social anxiety, which often is accompanied by a sense of exhilaration that is sometimes close to euphoria. This process of searching for sameness typically involves uncritical acceptance of information about others, in which ambiguity and rapid assumptions go unchallenged. This forms a base from which more complex understanding can develop, a vehicle for creating a general sense of universality. It is this component that the therapist needs to reinforce. Simple bridging statements can be used, such as "It sounds to me, John, that you have had several experiences which are very parallel to those that Anne was talking about last week." Universality can be pushed further with process encouragement—for example, "You and Irene seem to have had similar experiences when your depressions were at their worst. Could the two of you explore further what that experience was like?"

The important issue for the therapist to keep in mind during the early group sessions is that it is the process of finding similarities that is of most value to the group. This is the time not for exploration into personal depth but rather for the revelation of information that will promote mutual identification. One can feel comfortable with, and have the illusion of understanding, someone who has had similar experiences.

The therapeutic technique that promotes universalization is a simple one. It consists of clarification interventions that will result in the elaboration of content themes that can be linked among the members. Although the therapist may be keeping careful track of important issues being raised by each member for future exploration. the task initially is group formation.

Acceptance.   The experience of becoming part of a group constitutes a powerful validation of the self. The sense of belonging reinforces group participation. Many individuals coming for therapy experience themselves as on the outside of "normal" society and view their need for help with shame. Once the individual is in a therapy group, the opposite is the case. The decision to seek therapy is viewed not only as a positive choice but also as an indication of strength.

Acceptance is more powerful when it is accompanied by a sense of being understood. The therapist will want to create an atmosphere in which important statements do not go unnoticed. Each sensitive or delicate issue raised requires a response from others. Highly charged statements should not be met with silence. Sometimes patients will slip in statements regarding events in their lives without any elaboration. These statements may relate to some obviously major and potentially traumatic event such as the death of a parent or a rape. If the factual information is dissociated from the affect, the members may politely let the statement pass without comment. The therapist must engineer a response if none is forthcoming. Any reasonably positive response will augment the patient's sense of acceptance and normalize the distress being described.

Many patients, in retrospect, identify the experience of acceptance as the single most important factor that allowed them to continue in the hard work of therapy. They may report that the group felt like the family they never had but always longed for. Clearly, the process of being accepted with all one's warts is a specific antidote to low self-esteem.

Altruism.   Self-disclosure early in a group places responsibility on other group members for a validating response. Members become in a sense responsible for the well-being of their peers. This experience of *altruism,* of being of help to others, is highly motivating and contributes to group cohesion. It also makes the giver feel more positive. This is a paradoxical situation in which the person coming for help experiences enhancement of self-esteem through helping others. The mechanism of altruism is seldom found in individual psychotherapy but can be specifically promoted and explored in the group context.

Hope.   The presence of this factor will have been felt from the first pre-therapy interview, actually from the first phone call to make an appointment. The experience of joining a group and being listened to and understood by others—in short, being exposed to the supportive therapeutic factors—makes the prospect of change seem possible. It is important that the therapist not take this process lightly. *Hope* is a direct counterbalance to the negative thoughts and sense of futility that bring patients for therapy. It is probably the main factor responsible for the rapid improvement in symptoms that many patients experience early in a group. Such improvement, in turn, is a strong motivating factor to participate.

The Self-Revelation Cluster

Early group sessions depend on the self-revelation factors of *self-disclosure* and *catharsis.* Pretherapy sessions will have stressed the importance of revealing internal thoughts and taking some risks in the group. The process of actually putting personally important material into words in a group is experienced as quite arousing and quite threatening. This process is a necessary precursor to universality.

The content of early disclosures is usually of a factual nature, often shaped by the goals of the group. The material is important not just for psychological understanding, but for providing an opportunity to identify with other members. The therapist therefore should not explore the significance of such self-disclosure too vigorously. The less comfortable work of the therapy is best conducted later when a base of support and a sense of safety have developed. However, the therapist can actively work to mold the nature of self-disclosure so that it is primarily centered on psychological material that will be of value for later work. Lengthy factual discourses with many specific details are less relevant than information about the meaning of experiences and nature of reactions. The therapist has to walk a delicate line between, on the one hand, shaping the material in the service of group interactional norms and, on the other hand, not shutting down participation in the process. The therapist may sometimes effectively accomplish this by referring to other members with similar problems where the relationship meanings can be seen in a more objective manner.

An important component of the self-disclosure process is to risk putting sensitive problems into words and then experiencing a response that is different from that expected. Members will be extremely alert to the reaction of others when they say something of personal importance.

The therapist must recognize the power of these experiences and the need to ensure that a constructive result emerges. The nature of the response of other members should be carefully monitored. In the great majority of cases, members will respond in an understanding and supportive fashion to the disclosure of almost anything. The therapist can ensure that these reactions are expressed clearly and that the individual hears those words. In a sense, the therapist can conduct an "instant replay" of the process with the addition of commentary. For example, "What you have just said sounds like it is an important issue for you. Did you understand what Jane was saying about it? Jane, do you want to repeat what you said to be sure that Bob understands how you feel?" This "massaging of the process" is a technique that will be used in many situations. Risking a personally important statement and experiencing a positive response from other group members can be a powerful experience. It not only indicates that the member is becoming accepted by the group but also serves as personal validation that enhances self-esteem.

The Learning-From-Others Cluster

There will be constant examples in the early group of members' providing guidance and advice. This is usually done in an attempt to be helpful and supportive. Sometimes offering guidance and advice reflects a desire to appear in a superior position as one who is more knowledgeable or in control. Generally, however, most guidance and advice giving serve to enhance cohesion and to help clarify important issues. For many patients, open discussion of the issues they perceive as problematic is a new and risky experience. It is reassuring to find that others might have suggestions. It is often thought-provoking when others are found to have a somewhat different view. To not only reveal but have to justify one's viewpoint may sow the seeds of possible change. The frequency of advice giving gradually diminishes as the group progresses.

The therapist may need to guide the advice-giving process when it becomes too directive in nature. Guidance and advice are most helpful when they are given in tentative terms, not as absolute decrees. In trying to be helpful, the group may take at face value reports of distressing situations only to find later that the matter was much more complex.

Example

A 45-year-old woman described her distress with a controlling, demanding, and unsympathetic boss in a small office. He depended on her to take care of everything. The group was most sympathetic to her situation and offered much practical advice. Only some sessions later did it become clear that the patient derived considerable satisfaction out of secretly controlling the entire office operation. She went on to describe a series of personal relationships in which her covert smothering pattern drove the other away. Indeed, this was the prime issue she wanted to work on!

Using Process Debriefing

Beginning group therapists often experience some apprehension about getting group members to talk about what the group experience is like for them. There may be the fear that members may be disappointed or critical of the therapist or that sensitive interactional material may be hard to handle. The opposite is the case. Talking about the personal meaning of the group process is the major route to a positive outcome. Therefore, the therapist should promote a constant review of what is being experienced in the group. Brief interventions are easily inserted into the ongoing group process so that they are almost unnoticed by the members. For example, "What was it like to get that off your chest?" or "It sounds like others have had experiences much like you describe. Does that surprise you?" or "John seemed to find it helpful when you kept asking him for more information so that you could understand his situation better. Is that right, John?"

Members almost always find the process of self-revelation to be a constructive experience. Encouraging them to put their reactions to the group process into words therefore reinforces group cohesion. However, the exercise may also flush out negative or ambivalent positions that need to be addressed. Usually, a lack of enthusiasm is based on untested assumptions about what will happen or misunderstanding of some aspects of the session. Opening these assumptions and misunderstandings up for discussion serves to defuse them. Such topics will also draw a response from other members as group supporters. Such supportive response reinforces members' commitment to the group and may provide an opportunity for altruistic behaviors. A brief final go-around regarding reactions to the group also allows an opportunity for some cognitive integration of the experience before leaving.

However, the focus on process debriefing has a much stronger rationale. It is clear from the generic model presented in Chapter 2 that the greatest therapeutic effects are derived from the experience of being in an interactive environment. By addressing group issues promptly, calmly, and fearlessly, the therapist is modeling a norm of learning from the group process. If this norm can be solidly established in the first session, it will become an automatic expectation that all group events will be looked upon as an important part of the treatment. Such an expectation activates the constructive development of both Therapeutic Operations and the Therapeutic Bond. It also helps to ensure that session outcomes are constructive so that a process of incremental change can begin.

Therapist Technique

The members will tend to focus on the leader during the early sessions. A positive benefit of such a focus is that it helps to define the external boundary of the group. Focusing on the leader can also be seen as one variant of universality, in which the members unite in placing their trust and hope in the therapist. This common identification is often evident in statements of exaggerated appreciation of the power and wisdom of the leader. Members are able to identify not only with one another but also as members of "Dr. So-and-So's group." It is best not to seriously challenge unrealistic assumptions early on; there will be time for that later. Personally, the clinician should bear in mind that the effusion of positive remarks is in part promoted by group necessity and therefore is best taken with a grain of salt.

The task of the leader during the engagement stage is to promote a cohesive group environment, not to undertake specific treatment of individual patients. This is not to say that members may not experience the group as therapeutic, but the technical focus for the therapist is on the whole group. The phenomena described in this chapter will emerge spontaneously from the group experience. The therapist can use his or her position of authority lightly to reinforce the most helpful aspects of the group interaction and to ignore or dampen the less useful aspects.

Therapists might think of their role as that of an operant conditioner who is molding the ongoing stream of group process skillfully. One could think of the image of riding a horse and guiding it with very light rein pressure, or of guiding a canoe through rapids by using the onward rush to subtly maneuver around rocks. Both of these images capture the idea of the therapeutic force residing within the small group—a force utilized, not created, by the leader. On the other hand, the therapist needs to be careful not to get in the way of the group process. To quote an old European saying, "It's easier to ride a horse when it's going in the right direction."

The leader can assist in the development of a group identity by making use of group-level interventions. During the engagement stage such interventions will generally focus on labeling of common group themes. Regular use of "we" will promote a common identity. A positive orientation should be maintained. For example, a state of resistance would not be labeled as such, but instead would be reframed into a more empathic format (e.g., "I appreciate that group work is sometimes difficult").

A particularly constructive technique is consistent seeking of clarification. This technique may be applied to group events or to content themes. By requesting further clarification or further elaboration, the therapist is both modeling a process that has powerful learning features and encouraging members to commit themselves with further revelations to the group. Use of this technique also provides a good model for group members to adopt to gain further information from each other. The therapist will be aware of important issues for each member. These issues are often lurking behind casual comments or brief references and thus must be listened for closely. The therapist can utilize such opportunities by becoming quite interested in just what was being referred to and what it means. For example, "You've made reference to having a temper a number of times today, Sam. Is that an area you see the need to work on?"

The early group is not a time to indulge in interpretations. It is too likely that these would be taken as implied criticisms or as a lack of understanding. If the group can achieve a good working atmosphere, there will be opportunities later for interpretive ideas to emerge from the members themselves.

The therapist should be prepared to be as active as necessary. The pretherapy preparation and opening strategies discussed earlier in this chapter usually result in an intense group process. In such cases, the therapist can only sit back and admire the astuteness of the members. In structured groups, the therapist will be more active in focusing on the target issues. In some groups, there may be a low level of interactional energy, and the therapist may need to counterbalance this with greater activity. Such activity should be focused primarily on techniques to enhance interaction and should not take the form of a succession of questions or interpretive statements. Therapist activity should generally be of an exploratory, not a directive, style.

As noted earlier, it is useful for the therapist to automatically scan the group toward the beginning of the last third of each session to check if any members have not been very active. Often such patients will leave and castigate themselves for not having been a "better" group member. The therapist has a responsibility to initiate interaction in the early sessions.

At all times, the therapist should have in mind the supportive psychotherapeutic style that is described in detail in Chapter 11. This style is rooted in a solid belief that the Therapeutic Bond and Group Cohesion are of central importance. A conversational style is appropriate. Patients are encouraged to set goals and work toward them. The therapist is responsive, a real person in a disciplined relationship with role responsibility. Emphasis is on understanding patterns. Direct measures, such as encouragement and recognition of difficult tasks addressed or mastered, may be used to enhance self-esteem. Therapy-related anxiety is addressed early, in an attempt to diminish its inhibiting effects. In general, patients are supported in their attempts to regain mastery unless the techniques used by them are clearly nonadaptive.

Above all, the therapist must appreciate that the process of simply being in an interactive small group carries with it many helpful qualities. A continuing focus on the immediate experience not only will activate these therapeutic processes but also will generally help to identify the sorts of difficulties the patient encounters in daily life. The focus on process therefore usually leads to the heart of the psychopathological difficulties.

A simple but effective technique is to inquire regularly about what members thought was going on between them. By asking such questions not in an accusing and interpretive manner but simply out of interest, the therapist can lead the group to greater comfort in exploring process events—for example, "You two just had a pretty serious exchange about things that are very important. Could you say a little bit about what it was like to talk in the group like that?" Often such seemingly benign and nonintrusive methods actually provide rapid access to emotionally loaded issues. Technically correct interpretations may run up against defensive barriers if the individual or the group is not ready for them.

As stressed earlier, therapists have as their guiding orientation in the early sessions a greater responsibility to the group than to the individual. Of course, the therapist has a professional responsibility for the welfare of each individual as well. In a way, the duty to develop the group is cloaked in interactions directed at the individual. However, on occasion, individuals do not seem to be adjusting smoothly to the group environment. There may be specific reasons for this difficulty in adjusting. The group composition may have created an isolate within the group. The stress of the group environment may inflame pathological impulsivity that is difficult to contain. Some people seem determined to turn the entire group against them despite all efforts of the therapist to mediate the process. And for some members, their ambivalence about the idea of therapy may become increasingly evident.

The therapist must be prepared to intervene if there appears to be the risk of a harmful experience. It is useful to remember that all of the members in a new group will be struggling as best they know how to survive and be accepted. They may lose sight of the effects of their actions on some members. In most cases, it is adequate for the therapist to simply draw attention to an area of concern and have the group address it. For example, "In all the enthusiasm to get started, Annette hasn't had a chance to get in yet. Annette, have you found some issues today that make sense for you?" or "Jack has been an active participant today and is sort of getting jumped on. I wonder if he's taking the heat for some concerns that others might have as well."

Sometimes it becomes clear early on that a particular member is not going to fit in the group. This situation may reflect composition issues or indicate simply that the individual is not suited to group therapy. In these sorts of situations it may be in the patient's best interest, as well as the group's, that a peaceful parting of the ways takes place. The management of such an occurrence is challenging and is reviewed later in this chapter in the discussion of premature terminations and also in the next chapter in the context of scapegoating.

The therapist should keep in mind the phrase "Trust your group." Most groups have within them surprising reserves of resourcefulness for addressing complex problems. If this creativity and energy can be mobilized, the effects are helpful for both recipient and provider. The therapist does not, and indeed should not, feel that all therapeutic effects stem from the leader's chair. If the group is hard at work, the therapist should stay out of the way and let it evolve and should intervene only to reinforce and underline events or to head off less effective or negative directions.

The Individual Member

Just as the group is dealing with becoming a cohesive entity, the individual member is in the process of making a commitment to the group. A commitment to membership is also a commitment to work. Indeed, the therapist should be sure that these two processes are regularly linked together. Agreeing to join means taking the group work seriously, but it also implies taking the self seriously. It represents a further step on the road to personal change. Beginning to address personal issues often reflects a fundamental shift in self-perception. Therapy carries an implicit statement of asserting and valuing oneself, not of being a passive recipient or victim. Although this self-assertion and self-valuation may be combined with hopes of being rescued or magically altered, the positive aspect can be identified in the early sessions and sought out and reinforced.

The experience of universality, "joining the human race," may be a powerful one. To appreciate that other people have had reactions that oneself views as extreme, shameful, or sick is a powerful first step in reconceptualizing oneself. This is another example of the parallels between group process and internal psychological states, in that the idea of being found acceptable by others, even of helping others, may be a profound experience for self.

The new member will see the challenge of the early sessions primarily as a question of how to get into the group without damage to self. Characteristic protective strategies will be fully used. Members will often comment later what a sight they must have presented in early sessions. For the therapist, this a time to observe these defensive techniques at work, not respond to them. Indeed, some members may need to be buffered somewhat lest they elicit negative responses from other members. Aligning with their anxiety and acknowledging that they probably are not the only one experiencing it may be helpful.

Example

A 35-year-old woman suffering from severe anxiety and panic symptoms along with a major depression was referred for cognitive-behavioral treatment. In the first session, she sat virtually immobile, with a visible tremor in all extremities and a blank face that was later revealed to have been related to a heavy preventive dose of anxiolytics an hour before the session. She was clearly the only member who could not participate effectively in the initial go-around. As the session wore on with good, active involvement from all other members, the therapist made several aligning comments about anxiety and the fact that people could decide for themselves when they would like to get started. Toward the end, she was able to state that she was feeling pretty nervous. At the end of the session, the therapist was careful to say good-bye and say that he was looking forward to seeing her in the next session. Over several meetings, she became more acclimatized to the group and looked back on her first session with some anxiety-relieving humor, describing herself as "being like a robot," a comment that was kindly echoed by the group.

Social Roles

The social roles described in Chapter 3 will begin to emerge early in the first session and become more evident over the next few sessions. It is useful to think of these roles as the "character armor" members use to protect vulnerable areas. The therapist can think of these patterns as further diagnostic evidence to integrate into an understanding of each member. Members in the two roles with positive valence, Sociable and Structural, will be most actIve early in the group. Members in the Divergent Role may also be active but will be less central to the group task, while those in the Cautionary Role will experience the most difficulty in adapting to the group environment.

Sociable Role

The emphasis that members in the Sociable Role place on positive interactions and the involvement of all members is invaluable during the early stages of the group. Their warmth and nonthreatening approach elicit participation from others. A trusting nature often makes it easier for them to reveal important information, thus modeling self-disclosure. These members experience the early support of the group for their activities and show early symptomatic improvement. Thus hope is reinforced for others. The therapist may feel like wanting to modestly encourage members in the Sociable Role in their social support activities. However, these very qualities will at a later point provide difficulties for them. Care must be taken that they are not identified as the ideal group participant simply because what they have to offer is of particular value early in the group's life. A safer path is to encourage generalization and modeling of the behaviors these members are using as an important group goal rather than to focus on them as the main providers of such input.

Structural Role

The members in the Structural Role, with their focus on identifying problems and establishing a work ethic, provide a useful model for the developing group. Their activity complements that of the Sociable Role members in helping to develop a positive working climate. The desire of the member in the Structural Role to understand and explain behavior, rather than just to experience it, as does the member in the Sociable Role, exerts a calming influence on the group. It addresses the fear that group emotion will get out of hand. Generally, the Structural Role members are appreciated for their efforts. If they become too active, however, their activity may be viewed as interfering with the development of the group experience. At such a point, they may need some support from the therapist and encouragement to sit back and observe rather than to try to get everything organized.

Divergent Role

Members with behaviors characteristic of the Divergent Role are welcomed for their enthusiastic engagement into the group process. However, their emphasis on differences and confrontation works against the creation of group cohesion. The therapist needs to be attentive to the input from these members and to be prepared to reframe it in terms of the engagement stage without alienating or shutting down these members. Using the language of universality and the other "supportive" factors usually accomplishes this. For example, differences expressed by a Divergent Role member may be interpreted as an important demonstration of people talking openly in the group. Support can be given for the issues raised, and reassurance that these issues will be talked about eventually can be provided.

Cautionary Role

Members in the cautionary role tend to be silent observers during early sessions. Although they need to be encouraged to participate, it should be remembered that often a small contribution from these members goes a long way. The reluctance of Cautionary Role members may be translated into the importance of taking small steps in joining the group. The therapist may be reassured that the contribution of these members, although not as important as others' early in the group when developmental issues are being addressed, will be of importance later. It is important not to align with the view that those who participate less are going to handicap the group.

Predictable Problems

Excessive Self-Disclosure

The therapist needs to monitor the depth of self-revelation to ensure that it is not too great in early sessions. Initial self-disclosure is designed for group entry, not for major psychotherapeutic work. Powerful disclosures may shut down a group if there is not yet a base of confidence among the members. The therapist should be prepared to intervene when self-disclosure begins to escalate in the early sessions. The most effective way of doing this is to acknowledge the importance of the material and provide assurance that it will be dealt with in time.

Examples

A 28-year-old man began to talk in the second session of an outpatient group about his sense of shame at promiscuous sexual activity and inability to establish an enduring relationship with a woman. He began sobbing while talking about the barrenness of his life and about how he often wondered if he could go on. The group had begun the first session with considerable apprehension expressed about how safe it would be to talk openly. They reacted to this disclosure with a fearful silence. The therapist was aware of the serious discrepancy between this highly charged material and the capacity of the group to absorb it. She intervened quickly into the silence. "I appreciate how difficult it is to talk about these very upsetting matters. It is good that you have introduced them now, and we will certainly get back to explore them further with you later. Why don't you take a moment and let things calm down a bit. I wonder if others in the group have also experienced trouble with how their relationships have gone. Maybe you could let Henry know that he's not the only one with issues in this area." The group rose to the occasion and continued the theme in part as an altruistic effort to help Henry but in the process beginning to reveal more about themselves.

In a mixed group for university students, a young woman made a veiled reference in the first session to "an incident" when she was younger. The therapist was aware that this centered on her first sexual experience at the age of 17, when she was raped while on a trip abroad. Because this was clearly not the time to get into such a disclosure, the therapist made a preemptive move by saying immediately in a low-key manner that this sounded like something that would need to be addressed in the group when the time was right. The woman took the hint and proceeded to talk about issues going on currently in her relationships. Several sessions later she returned to the rape incident as an important precursor to her present difficulties.

The problem of excessive disclosure may center on a group member who has a history of sabotaging the development of relationships by coming on too intensely or being too needy at an early point. This pattern may be replicated in the group, with the same result. Individuals who drop out of the group often report that they were carried away in the enthusiasm of the early group and blurted out sensitive information. They may have feared that they would be rejected or held in ridicule by the group members, or that they had broken some personal or family taboo for which they will eventually be blamed. One reason that it is valuable for the therapist to have a personal meeting with a patient who has dropped out of the group, as will be discussed below, is to address the patient's motivation for dropping out and his or her fears about continuing in therapy. The person may be in a critical state of decompensation and feel that there is no help available. The larger question of negative effects from psychotherapy is discussed in Chapter 11.

The leader needs to be aware that a definite move to limit a topic of discussion, even when quite appropriate, may be seen by some members as an attempt to exert undue control. In structured groups, this situation can generally be handled by giving a simple, direct explanation of the tasks to be addressed and emphasizing the need to stick with them. In interpersonally oriented groups, there are broader possibilities. An invitation for the group to discuss how they see the leader may be quite productive and, at the same time, maintains the deflection from the self-disclosing member. At the very least, the issue of leader control might be flagged for future discussion, with the group being given the message that such a topic is condoned. Control issues around therapist interventions will be a common theme in the next stage.

Rebound From Affective Intensity

The protocol outlined in this book for the preparation of patients and for a rapid start into deeper themes in the first session has proven quite useful for a range of types of groups and levels of pathology in patients. The nature of the material coming into focus varies with the intention of the selection process and the type of group. In all circumstances, however, this protocol tends to prompt the incoming member to focus on themes that have presented significant difficulty. Thus, the early sessions are preloaded with powerful affect-laden material.

This early initial focus on difficult issues has major advantages, particularly for groups with some time limitations and for groups whose members are all starting at the same time. But the therapist needs to be aware that there are some risks. The level of affect may rise quite steeply, and members may find that throughout the week between sessions they are experiencing intrusive thoughts concerning the group and the issues raised. The reality of the psychological task they have set for themselves may begin to appear overwhelming. Some patients become anxious that they will not be able to manage the tension and have to take time off, be hospitalized, or get more medications. Others fear that the group is making them worse and that they should terminate. Another possibility is that the group as a whole becomes restrained and resists continuing with the work. This resistance may go in waves, with a very active session followed by one or two quiet ones. Sporadic absences may be a telltale sign.

Simply acknowledging and accepting emotional states is helpful, particularly when these are in the direction of sadness or grief. Tears are common in the early sessions. However, if the level of intensity becomes overwhelming for the individual or frightening to the group, the therapist must be prepared to intervene. This usually means shutting down the further elaboration of the material being presented. The therapist must make it clearly known when this action is taken that the intention is to contain the moment, not to give a message that affect or the particular content behind it cannot be tolerated. Various techniques may be helpful: reference to important work for future sessions, the courage to bring such sensitive material to the group, an appreciation of how distressing the material is, and reassurance that the issues might have relevance for other members as well may all be tried. Sometimes it is best to simply acknowledge that it is very important material and therefore upsetting but suggest that the group take a break and let things cool down before getting further into the topic. Members might also be told that expressing important material in the group often results in thoughts surrounding those issues arising during the week before the next session. It is often useful to let patients know that they might try simply sitting with the affect, experiencing it, and not feeling that they have to do something immediately to address it. Journal writing can also be helpful in modulating affect.

Most of these phenomena will pass with time and are indeed found in most groups to some extent. However, they can result in the loss of members and the loss of active working sessions. The principal strategy is to directly address the concerns. The therapist should begin quite intensive debriefing exercises during and toward the end of sessions to get a full discussion of the issues raised for each member. This debriefing process can almost be a group within a group, allowing an opportunity for a process of cognitive integration to begin. By forecasting what is likely to happen, the debriefing makes it seem less intense when it occurs.

The debriefing is also an opportunity to talk about coping strategies during the week. Would it be helpful to organize some structured activities during the week to cut down on time alone? Are there close friends or relatives who could help over a particularly difficult part of the week? The therapist can suggest to the members to practice experiencing the affect in the group and sitting with it until it fades, and then to apply that technique at home. It should be emphasized that being upset is a time-limited state.

Example

A 47-year-old woman disclosed in the fourth session of the group that she had found out 10 years ago that her husband, with whom she thought she had a good relationship, had been having a homosexual affair for several years. She had insisted they separate immediately, though they continued to have considerable ongoing contact because of their son, who had no knowledge of the situation. She had never spoken of this to anyone, except briefly to the clinician who had assessed her for the group, and viewed the situation as a shameful block to her capacity to enjoy life or to have another relationship. She was filled with rage and grief about her husband's behavior that seemed undimmed in intensity despite the passage of a decade.

She was fearful of what would happen now that she had let herself open up the memories more directly. She received considerable support from the group for her courage. It was predicted that she would have an upsetting week before the next session, but it was inevitable if she was to master the situation. She planned how she would intersperse some activities and structure to some extent the time she would spend thinking through the issues she had raised.

She reported at the next session that the planning had worked well, and she was surprised at her ability to let herself think about the event and also to take breaks from that psychological work. Within several weeks she had a direct talk with her ex-husband about how destroyed she had felt at what she regarded as his treachery. She began to see him as a lonely, isolated man and converted her anger into feeling somewhat sorry for him but with no desire to establish further contact. This process freed her up to regain a sense of hopefulness about how she might develop her life further.

When the group-as-a-whole sinks into an inactive state, then once again the issues need to be activated by recalling the nature of the preceding session or the specific incident. What have members found themselves thinking about the group since then? What was it like for each member during that session? Who were you most concerned about and why? How might it have gone differently? These efforts are directed at making the resistance a natural and suitable topic for discussion and investigation.

All of these approaches give the message that what is happening is not unexpected and, indeed, is a sign that the important issues are being addressed. They also give a message of belief that the individual can cope. Such working-through activities often are recalled as the most important part of the treatment experience.

Early Conflict

Sometimes material in early sessions is laden with affect characterized by anger, resentment, or suspiciousness. The early group is not in a solid position to incorporate such material. There is a certain danger that a negative interactional tone will be established within the whole group. The most useful technique with this negative side of the affective spectrum is to align with the sense of distress that underlies the anger and simply ignore the emotional component. This strategy is usually enough to shift the theme to an emphasis on the universal distress among the members and thus facilitate group cohesion. This is an example of using group process knowledgeably to promote those aspects that will be most helpful to the early group.

The therapist needs to be alert to the emergence of themes of conflict, criticism, or rejection among the members. In general, such themes do not arise during early sessions, but when they do, they need to be skillfully handled by the therapist. Usually, drawing attention to a positive component and shifting the focus are adequate. The therapist should try to find evidence of universality that can be reinforced. At times, the therapist may need to temporarily take over control of the process and request that conflictual material be delayed until a later point in the group's life. For example, "I can understand that it must be difficult for you to understand Maureen's experience [initial alignment]. Both of you seem to have had pretty upsetting times in your marriages [universality]. As we get to know each other better in here, we will have an opportunity to get further into those things [material suitable for discussion but time not appropriate]. Let's put it on hold for now and see what others have on their minds [unambiguous control]."

The emergence of high levels of conflict in the first few sessions correlates with premature terminations and with groups that fail to progress. Patients beginning psychotherapy are generally particularly sensitive to judgmental issues, and the strength of negative comments will be amplified severalfold because of the perception that these comments reflect a general group opinion. Usually, some group members will intervene quickly if such material escalates, but the therapist has a clear responsibility to step in if the level of negative affect rises too much.

Therapists also need to be aware that they may unwittingly promote conflict. There are two common situations. Therapists may have been exposed to the highly intrusive techniques of affect stimulation such as those used in some chemical dependency programs and in some brief psychodynamic traditions. They may try using these as a way of kick-starting the group. Their style may be interpreted by the members as attacking and nonsupportive. The therapists may see themselves as being quite concerned and eager to get results, but this aspect is lost on the members. Members may simply drop out, or the confrontational style may be adopted by the members, in which case the group is likely to disintegrate before too long because of the failure to establish a supportive base of cohesion.

Therapists coming from a tradition of a highly cognitive-intrapsychic interpretation style may use these techniques at an early point in the group. The members are likely to view these techniques either as overly intrusive and shut down or as distancing and feel abandoned. Others may simply consider these techniques irrelevant and evidence of inadequate skill or understanding.

These comments do not imply that these types of technique do not have their place. However, they are clearly out of place early in a group before an adequate sense of belonging and support has developed.

Early Terminations

Most premature terminations in group therapy occur in the first six sessions. Beyond that point, unpredicted terminations are infrequent and usually result from some intense event. The therapist can be reassured that it is not a catastrophe to lose a group member at an early point, though reasonable efforts need to be extended to try to forestall this happening. The most important principle is to address directly any remarks suggesting doubt about continuing. To ignore hints about such material is to encourage the patient's leaving. Generally speaking, the source of such doubts is usually understandable but correctable. If the member does drop out, at least the matter has been addressed and is not an entirely unpredicted event. The remaining members will have some understanding of the issues, and such understanding will serve to create a rationale for the loss. Because there will be strong pressures to consolidate group integrity, this rationale will be quickly accepted. In the first few sessions, relationships between members are just forming, and the departure has its greatest importance in terms of group morale, not the loss of a specific individual.

If group efforts are not sufficient to persuade a member to remain, the therapist should have a private discussion with the particular member after the group. The task is not to dissuade the individual from the decision but, rather, to understand the basis for it and to clarify issues. This may be important for the individual. Personal material not brought up in the group may cast a different light on the circumstances, and an alternative referral might be helpful. In addition, a negative therapeutic experience may block future efforts at seeking help, so efforts to defuse separation tension may be of value. Care should be taken that a critical tone is not adopted.

When a member does decide to leave a group at an early stage, some therapists insist that the person come back to a final session to "say good-bye" or to "clear up unfinished business." Such efforts are usually futile because the person has been backing out of the group for several sessions and is not really committed to it. Thus, the question of group relationships is not a highly charged one. For the other group members, the major concern is the survival of the group. If the individual does return, a perfunctory explanation is made, this is accepted by the group, and everyone sits around in uneasy apprehension waiting for the actual separation to occur. It is important that the departure not get in the way of ongoing group cohesion.

An exception to not insisting on the patient's attending a final session is when the decision to leave is directly related to a specific group event. Some opportunity to clarify the intent or meaning of the experience may be useful both for the one departing and for the other group participants. A common reaction at an unexpected termination is for other group members, or perhaps the therapist, to feel that the circumstances were mishandled and that someone must bear responsibility for the loss. In fact, such situations almost always are complex and stem from powerful interactional processes. The group needs an opportunity for a thorough discussion of the circumstances with or without the departing member.

It is useful to bear in mind that the decision to terminate therapy might be in the best interests of the individual. Individuals who drop out may correctly sense that they are getting into dangerous territory that they will not be able to handle. They may be concerned that to continue would risk negative or unsuccessful experiences that might reinforce doubts about self-effectiveness. In short, early terminations are not uncommon and are not necessarily damaging to the individual or to the group. What is important is that the issues are openly discussed in the group so that misconceptions and individual reactions can be clarified.

In the next chapter we discuss the idea of the scapegoated group member who is in fact acting out group tension. The issues surrounding dropping out in this case are entirely different from those related to the early dropping out of a patient who is not yet fully committed to the group.

Completion of the Engagement Stage

By the end of the engagement process, group membership issues should have been resolved. If the group is to lose members, it has usually occurred by this time. A general consensus of how the group operates, as well as a reasonable sense of the group task, should have been reached. The therapist can consider the task of engagement to be nearing completion when all members are comfortable in participating and all have made some self-revealing statements, both of which indicate a basic trust in the group process.

For a weekly outpatient psychotherapy group, the first stage is usually accomplished in three to six sessions. Some groups get off the ground more quickly than others, but a group that is still having difficulty with general positive participation after six sessions is showing developmental strains. When these strains emerge, the therapist needs to carefully review the group's life up to that point with a view to identifying the issues that seem to be interfering with progress and to carefully consider strategies for addressing those issues.

It is very important to understand that the first stage is not lacking in therapeutic effectiveness. The group process is being utilized in a preliminary fashion, but the experience for the individual member can be powerful. The "supportive" factors that are mobilized address the demoralized state in a specific fashion. A positive shift in self-esteem results in a spiraling sense of self-confidence and self-efficacy that allows the individual to regain a sense of control. Once initiated, this building of self-confidence may become a self-reinforcing process that allows continuing progress with or without the group (57).

It is possible for groups to become stuck in the engagement stage. This may reflect problems with composition decisions or a mismatch between therapist's expectations and the capacity of the members. It may represent leadership difficulties about addressing issues of conflict or difference. Membership problems regarding attendance or terminations may thrust the group back to basic engagement tasks. Some groups leave the support and encouragement of early sessions, try to address more conflictual matters, retreat from this attempt with a drop in cohesion, and then oscillate between the two stages. The material in this chapter and the next may offer some insights into how such a situation might be handled.

Just as the positive developments of the first stage are coming to fruition, the challenging tasks of the differentiation stage emerge. As a group moves through the engagement stage, the sense of group cohesion and commitment steadily increases. Once the stage tasks are achieved, the intensity may lessen and a sense of vagueness or lack of direction may develop. The contributions of the Divergent Role members are often stimulated by this situation. The leader needs to be sensitive to an emerging sense of disillusionment or irritation. Once convinced that the group is together in mastering engagement tasks, the therapist can begin to promote the expression of more negative themes. Nurturing therapists are alarmed at these developments, whereas confronting therapists cannot wait to get on with the action. The result is entry into the second stage of group development, the differentiation phase, to which we turn in the next chapter.

CHAPTER 8

Dealing With Conflict: The Differentiation Stage

*T*he second stage of group development, referred to as the *differentiation stage,* is often referred to in the literature as the stage of conflict because it is characterized by an atmosphere of dissatisfaction and confrontation. The term *differentiation* describes the primary functional task of the stage for group development. The preoccupation with criticism and justification serves the purpose of developing a greater awareness of the individual in the group, which is a counterbalance to the assumptions of universality, uncritical acceptance, and similarities developed in the engagement stage.

The central task for the group in the differentiation stage is to develop a cooperative approach to conflict resolution. This must begin with recognition by the group members that they do not all see the world the same way. The presence of different points of view threatens the sense of universality that initially allowed the members to get closer. The work in this stage focuses on the ability to tolerate differences and learn from them in a collaborative fashion. It also offers an opportunity for patients to behave more assertively.

Characteristics of the Differentiation Stage

Hints that the transition from engagement to differentiation has begun often take the form of minor complaints or dissatisfactions. Such complaints may initially center on issues outside of the group. Discontent with referral sources such as family doctors or with previous groups or therapists is a common theme. Normally punctual members may start arriving late, and there may be some unpredicted absences. There may be a mounting sense of frustration or irritation and an edgy confronting tone to the discussion, first between members and eventually toward the leader. A direct breakthrough of anger or criticism is a good sign that the work of the differentiation stage is progressing. In response to criticism, members make self-justifying assertions, often of an exaggerated nature. The therapist may find that the sessions do not seem as enjoyable, may feel a sense of irritation, may feel a desire to get people back into line, and/or may experience physiological arousal, such as toes curling up or increased sweating. Several features of this group climate are worth identifying.

Assertiveness

The members begin to seem more comfortable with a higher level of self-assertion. There may be a sense that members are energized by, or almost reckless in, daring to speak up more firmly. The group seems to enjoy the secret challenge of acting up.

Expression of Negative Affect

Firmly, perhaps vigorously, stated opinions, challenges, criticisms, and misunderstandings may seem to contribute to an unproductive atmosphere. However, in this way the members become more self-disclosing, often by blurting out ideas or reactions that must then be defended. This process forces an increased appreciation of the uniqueness of each member and breaks down some of the unrealistic sense of commonality of the engagement stage. The amount of information available about each individual increases as a result. For these reasons, the members sense that the work is important, although some may not enjoy it as much as they did in the engagement atmosphere.

Identification of Differences

Opinions tend to be stated in terms of stereotypic descriptions that reflect a global judgment, not an individualized reaction. Opinions expressed in this way should not be seen simply as the ventilation of negative affect but rather as self-definition. It is typical of adolescents that they set up straw men to tilt at with strongly held opinions. This process promotes the development of a greater sense of autonomy and a clearer idea of self. The atmosphere during the differentiation stage of a group often has such an adolescent quality. The importance for the individual member lies not so much in the actual content of the discussion, but in the process of self-assertion. By adopting this perspective, the therapist is able to intervene effectively by promoting and encouraging the exploration of the tension among the members. This will defuse the affect constructively and permit the members to understand that they can continue to interact effectively even though they do not always agree.

Leadership Challenge

Another feature that is central to the differentiation stage relates to the role of the therapist. Just as members identify differences between themselves, so the membership as a whole may identify differences between the group and the therapist. Criticism of the therapist frequently focuses on a perceived failure to care or provide enough—for example, "You just get paid to do this and can't really know what we are experiencing" or "If you gave us more direction, the group would be more helpful." Such a focus can be seen in one sense as the members' needing to differentiate themselves from the control of the authority figure. At a deeper level, it reflects disillusionment with the idea that the perfect solution is going to be provided by the therapist. In the engagement stage, the group was able to bask in the untested assumption that if everybody got along a healing process would occur without further work. In the differentiation stage, the members now begin to realize that the process will be more challenging.

Conflict Resolution

A further major task during this stage is the development of a group approach to conflict resolution. If an approach to conflict resolution cannot be achieved, then the group becomes bottled up in unproductive criticism or self-justifying defensive rhetoric that may lead to a serious drop in group cohesion and member commitment. The approach to be fostered is one of exploring differences so that individual positions can be tolerated as being neither right nor wrong but different. Unresolvable competition can be replaced with a sense of cooperation, although not necessarily agreement.

The danger is that if this cognitive exploratory work does not take place, either the group will disintegrate or the tensions will go underground. The latter result may lead to a situation in which the group oscillates between the relatively superficial style of the engagement stage and bursts of negative affect from repressed differentiation-stage material.

Reassessment of Group Norms

The therapist's role in setting group norms in early sessions was clearly identified in preceding chapters. Now these ideas about how the group should operate must be critically examined. The importance of this process is that the members achieve a personal stake in how the group should function. This results in an increased identification with, and responsibility for, the group. At the same time, the influence of the therapist is somewhat tempered. Underlying this process is a strengthening of normative expectations about the group. Usually, the norms that emerge from this process are not greatly different from those at the beginning, but the process of challenging helps to make them more explicit. Here again there is a parallel to the necessary challenges of parental values and control that are characteristic of adolescence.

Group rules are usually tested in the differentiation stage. Some members unconcernedly barge into sessions a few minutes late. There are whispered leaks about how the group assembled for coffee after the preceding session. These events should be seen as minor transgressions in the service of a greater goal: the forging of a group consensus. For example, after several late arrivals the group may have a serious discussion about how difficult it is to begin when members are late. Group pressure will be brought to bear on the tardy members in a much more effective manner than is possible from the therapist. After all, the members now feel, it is "our" group now, not "yours."

Dominance Hierarchy

The phenomena of the differentiation stage may also be conceptualized as the enactment of the formation of a dominance hierarchy. This ranking process is part of our primate heritage. One of the first things to happen when a new group is formed is that judgments are made as to who has more influence. There is usually considerable agreement in the members' conclusions about this. These evaluations, though initially made early in the group's life, are tested in the differentiation stage. Much of the competitive jockeying at this time can be understood in this light (58).

Challenge of leadership tests the top rung of the hierarchy, which, in the case of group therapy, is the therapist. One important way to describe a social system is by the *gradient* of the dominance hierarchy. For example, in military groups the level of control is absolutely prescribed. Therapy groups may vary considerably in the degree of therapist control. In general, greater member participation is achieved with a middle level of control. This level of control reassures the members that someone is in a position of responsibility but still accommodates member initiative. This idea is developed more completely in Chapter 11 in the discussion of therapist style.

Development of the Group Structure

Boundary Focus

It will be clear from the foregoing descriptions of group characteristics that the boundary that now comes into focus is that of the individual member. In the engagement stage, it was important to identify information regarding differences between the group and outside experiences. In the differentiation stage, it is important to focus on the public expression of internal information in the form of beliefs and reactions. Through this process, the individual begins to emerge as a more rounded and fully developed personality. Boundaries can be viewed as opening and closing. The typical process of expression during the differentiation stage is the statement of a strongly held opinion followed by justification of that opinion. This process represents a sequence of openness followed by closedness—an affect-driven self-disclosure followed by cognitive justification.

Another boundary of importance is that between the therapist and the group members. On the group schematic presented in Chapter 3 (see Figure 3–1), the leadership subsystem boundary was identified. The work of the differentiation stage inevitably deals with issues across this boundary. Initially, questions about leadership may be raised between a particular member(s) and the leader. But commonly, a collective group stance about leadership develops that polarizes most of the group against the leader. This stance creates an illusion of unanimity in the service of the differentiation task. It is important for cotherapists to discuss the tensions they may be experiencing during this stage. One component of differentiation may be pressure to split the leaders into divergent positions. Given time and patience, the conflict resolution processes will allow the group to work through such issues.

Therapeutic Factors

It is important that the tasks of the differentiation stage be addressed on the foundation of solid group cohesion developed during the engagement stage. Groups that begin with high levels of conflict generally do not fare well because they do not have the positive cohesive "glue" to keep them together during the disintegrating effects of conflict resolution. It is for this reason that the therapist needs to dampen and divert conflictual themes during the engagement stage.

At first glance, it may appear that all those carefully nurtured "supportive" factors operating during the engagement stage have disappeared. Although not as visible, they are still very much present. The laughter and reconsolidation that occur after a heated interchange, for example, may reveal their presence. It is as if the members are saying, "We can get away with this heavy stuff, because we know we won't let each other down." The therapist may usefully remind the members from time to time that they do have a positive past together.

The confrontational process results in further self-revelation. Indeed, the amount of personalized information available about each member often increases markedly through the second stage. The interactional process of the differentiation stage lays the groundwork for the psychological work factors of insight and interpersonal learning in later stages.

Therapist Technique

The general comments about therapist behavior during the engagement stage in the preceding chapter continue to apply in the differentiation stage. The therapist should remain as a predictable and sustaining force in the group. However, the change in group atmosphere does increase the pressure on the therapist. For the beginning therapist, it is useful to understand that differentiation-stage phenomena are basically constructive in nature. The process of therapist challenge is normal and inevitable. A defensive or apologetic response from the leader deprives the group of the opportunity to learn from the experience and may drive it back into an unsatisfying engagement-stage condition. The following suggestions are intended to be superimposed on engagement techniques, not to replace them.

Keeping Calm

The most important thing the therapist can do during this stage is to remain calm. This sends a powerful message to the members that nothing catastrophic is going to happen. Further, the therapist's calmness acknowledges the legitimacy of the issues raised, even if they may have been somewhat overstated. The therapist needs to be careful not to intervene too early in the group process, lest this be interpreted as an indirect message of concern, disapproval, or defensiveness.

There is a danger that the therapist may be driven by anxiety to actively collude in the avoidance of the conflict of the differentiation stage. The therapist may fear that the anger will get out of control or that members will drop out and the group will dwindle away. If the therapist can tolerate differentiation issues with equanimity, then the group has a chance to master them as well. It is a time for the therapist to take a few deep breaths and reassure himself that this too shall pass. Some therapists will find it very difficult to tolerate an atmosphere of tension. Such concerns need to be addressed through supervision, because they will get in the way of the group's reaching its potential.

Exploring Differences

The main technical task for the therapist in learning to manage the conflict of the differentiation stage is to accurately label the central mechanism. The expression of negative affect is not the main mechanism. A more powerful underlying mechanism is the exploration of different points of view. It is this dynamic that underlies the conflict and the sense of dissatisfaction characteristic of the stage.

The climate of differentiation typically is characterized by the expression of polarized points of view. Members may express their points of view with an exaggerated tone of self-justification or outrage, often stereotyping people into less-than-desirable pigeonholes. This process may give the impression of quite unrealistic assessments and perceptions. Whereas in the engagement stage there is uncritical acceptance of self-revelations in the service of universality and engagement, in the differentiation stage there is unrealistic exaggeration of differences, still with a tendency toward distortion.

The process of confrontation increases the level of affect, and this increase in affect results in pressure to disclose firmly held opinions or reveal negative and painful experiences. Such information may be blurted out in a burst of self-revelation. Once out, it must then be justified or defended, and this leads to some of the polarized and stereotypic statements. The need to defend one's position requires the revelation of strongly held beliefs or reactions that cut deeper into interpersonal issues. The result of this process is that the amount of personalized information available concerning each member, especially regarding interpersonal style, is greatly increased.

The therapist must develop a sense of timing regarding the point of optimum intervention. The affective climate should be allowed to reach a reasonable degree of intensity. This ensures that real interpersonal process tension is present. This feeling of encounter makes the work productive. At an appropriate opportunity, the therapist can begin to shift the interchanges to a focus on the fact that members clearly are seeing things differently and to encourage them to clarify their perception of the issues under discussion. Such a focus helps to validate each member's ideas and defines the process, not in terms of right or wrong, but in terms of varying viewpoints. The group can thus be led toward a mechanism for tension reduction based on cooperation.

In structured groups and to some extent in cognitive groups, the management of tension during the differentiation stage may be more indirect. The more assertive style has an important function for the members, but it may not be explored to the same extent as in interpersonal groups. Simply accepting that it is all right for members to express their frustration may be adequate. Often, the negative material can be transposed into a discussion about negative thought patterns and how these might not always reflect the total situation. For example, "I heard your concerns about how the group is being run, and I guess there is room for some difference of perspectives. But I wonder if, to some extent, you are also experiencing in here negative thought patterns that apply outside the group as well. Would it help to explore these patterns and test for yourself what they are based on?"

An optimum result is that the members can agree to disagree but continue working on the issues. This approach lays the base for greater tolerance in perceptions of others and the possibility of empathizing with people even in the face of disagreements—qualities that will be very important for later group work. For example, as the group progresses, much discussion can be expected to center on misinterpretations concerning aspects of close relationships, including the contributions of various members. It is important that members can challenge such phenomena without their opinions being rejected outright. Differentiation-stage experiences lay the base for such work.

Managing Leader Challenge

The group during the engagement stage operates under the guidelines laid down by the therapist in pretherapy preparation and the first few sessions. One of these normative expectations is that members should speak up about issues they are concerned about. This expectation of truthful openness about internal thoughts is central to all forms of therapy. It is somewhat of a paradox, therefore, that to obey this normative expectation means to challenge the very leader who stressed it in the first place.

This process of group challenge to the therapist plays an important part of the work of this stage. It reveals a deeper commitment by the individual to the group process and a higher investment in the resulting normative shift. Not surprisingly, this process often has a somewhat adolescent quality to it. It is as if the members know that some of the issues they are raising are of less than central importance, yet they are bound to vigorously make their points. Just as adolescents establish close peer relationships, so the group during this phase may at times band together as "co-rebels" determined to alter the system. There is minimal danger that nontherapeutic norms will eventually prevail. What is critical is that a leader has been challenged and everyone has survived.

The response of the leader to the challenging process will help or hinder the mastery of the stage tasks. The therapist must not respond with an intensification of rules or authoritarian or judgmental statements. Nor should the issues be trivialized by the therapist's ignoring them or shutting down discussions of them. A few deep breaths to recognize the inevitability of the process are useful, and a parental perspective of "this too shall pass" is a great asset. If the group believes that therapist challenge is not permissible or not safe, it may revert back to the safety of the engagement stage or may seek an alternative outlet by identifying a group member as a scapegoat on whom the negative attitudes deflected from the leader will be projected.

Addressing the Fear of the Individual

A common fear of members as they engage in differentiation-stage work is that the interpersonal challenges will be destructive. This fear may take the form of concern that other members will not be able to tolerate criticism and may be driven from the group. An associated fear is that oneself will be found unacceptable for uttering critical or angry words. Fears such as these will be universally present. It is useful therefore for the therapist to put them into words and to review with the members how they are reacting to the process. In most cases, members are able to say that they may not be comfortable with the process but can manage.

Preventing Harmful Interactions

The therapist must be alert to overpowering messages of blame or rejection between members that may prove damaging. Attacks that are mean-spirited and meant to humiliate or shame another member are not acceptable. The therapist must mediate situations in which such attacks occur. Usually, simply drawing attention to what is happening and asking the group how it sees the situation are enough to begin a reparative process. Often, the excessive negativity is driven more by anxiety than by maliciousness. If this approach does not work, the therapist may need to become more active. (I liken it to putting on my hockey referee's sweater and blowing the whistle.) The norm about no destructive attacks is restated, and the main protagonists may need to be asked to sit quietly until they become more settled. On rare occasions, a member may have to be asked to stay for a discussion afterward with the leader.

The therapist has a clear responsibility to monitor the confrontational process and to ensure that no one is harmed, and must be prepared to intervene if there appears to be some danger of that happening. Toward the end of a hectic session, it is always useful to have a go-around to check members' reactions to group events to forestall members' leaving upset. Further techniques are discussed below in the section on scapegoating and also in Chapter 11 in the discussion of negative effects.

The Individual Member

The challenge for the individual member during the differentiation stage is to tolerate a negative group atmosphere, with its dimensions of hostility, conflict, and confrontation. Patients presenting for psychotherapy often have difficulty in either over- or underexpression of anger. Therefore, the work of this stage is generally relevant to many members. The therapist needs to carefully monitor this work to ensure that it is proceeding in a constructive fashion and that the affective issues are being mastered through the cognitive mechanisms described in the previous subsection. During the differentiation stage, the individual must arrive at a comfortable position regarding acceptance of social norms versus continuation in a challenging position. Although part of the group task is to throw the question of normative expectations up in the air, the resolution is to come down with a general agreement concerning them.

While the group challenging is going on, a parallel process is found within the individual. Just as individual members are challenged within the group, so components of self-image and self-perception are raised for consideration. Material tentatively raised during the engagement stage must come under greater scrutiny. During the differentiation stage, the individual is more likely to become aware of parts of self that are in an uneasy alliance or frankly contradictory. Split-off or isolated interpersonal components may come to the fore and may be the source of intense reactions of guilt and shame. The general sense of anxiety, confrontation, and disgruntlement in the air may be seen in part as a projection from these internal dimensions.

Example

In the sixth session of a weekly outpatient group, the atmosphere was beginning to heat up with, for the most part, constructive interpersonal challenge. Members were addressing a woman who was stuck in a protracted separation process and seemed unable to take firm action. She acknowledged that there were two sides in her role: part of her wanted to make everything right and avoid conflict, and the other part knew she was being treated unfairly and felt angry about it. A man in the group came in with a passionate plea to see the positive side of things—to just keep thinking that things will turn out for the best. This caricature of cognitive therapy was actively challenged by several members who felt that difficult situations had to be confronted. The "pacifist" acknowledged in a debriefing go-around before the session ended that he always avoided confrontation and that this had been a real challenging session for him. But it had got him thinking about the difficulty he experiences in standing up for his rights in his relationships. He was encouraged to pursue this issue in the next session both for himself and in conjunction with the woman who began the sequence.

The therapist needs to look for evidence of introspective work and encourage exploration of the themes involved. Statements such as "It seems as if you can behave in two different ways with different people; with Mary you seem to be always attentive and accepting, while with Joan you need to find fault with everything she does" or "You seem to be describing two quite different ways of seeing things, either in all positive or all negative terms, like we talked about as dichotomous thinking." The therapist has a powerful tool available in identifying parallel processes within the individual and the group. The group application functions like a projection of internal issues onto the persons in the group. What is difficult to discern in the smaller image of the person becomes evident when it is projected onto the larger screen of the group.

The pressure during this stage to justify and defend oneself provides an informal experience in assertiveness training. Indeed, the therapist may want to incorporate some aspects of this modality into the management technique. An important by-product of this process is the opportunity to create a more complex self definition, one built on the "focus on self as an object of concern" that characterized the engagement process. It may be an important occasion for a member to truly take the self seriously as an object of inquiry.

Social Roles

The social role most in focus during the differentiation stage is the Divergent Role, the "scapegoat" in the group. Members in this role eagerly express contrary viewpoints. They are intuitively aware of process events, particularly that aspect of process dealing with evasive or defensive behavior. They are ready to dive in and identify avoidant behaviors and label the issues. They often do so in a blunt and relatively tactless fashion. With these activities, the Divergent Role members are contributing a vital ingredient to the task of addressing differentiation issues. Groups without such members will experience difficulty in coming to terms with conflictual themes.

Therapists must learn to value and acknowledge members in the Divergent Role who are being scapegoated. Without these members, the task will be much harder. The therapist must be careful not to align with the other members in attacking the scapegoated member. People in this role often lay themselves open for abuse and seem to relish the process even though they may be hurting inside. Their vigorous and extraverted methods may obscure the pain they experience at perceiving themselves once again on the outside. The therapist may need to offer support to the scapegoated member not only in terms of role behavior but also in regard to self-esteem. The therapist can do this by acknowledging the contribution that that person is making to the work of the group and reinforcing this importance by acknowledging the validity of the issues being raised. Members who are strong on the Divergent Role will, hopefully, emerge from this period with their need to challenge authority under somewhat greater cognitive control. They will be able to use this constructive quality in a functional, not a dysfunctional, fashion. This may be a central therapeutic accomplishment for such individuals.

Example

A 47-year-old separated woman in a semistructured interpersonal group eagerly applied herself to early group tasks and homework. About the sixth session her tone shifted and she developed a sharp tongue. She roundly criticized other group members for not trying harder and the leader for not following the plan of the sessions. In her personal life, she felt she was the butt of her family's criticism—that the children all blamed her for splitting up the household, though it was noteworthy that they kept in constant contact with her, although she interpreted their doing so as their wanting to cast blame. The leader, with some effort, maintained an aligning stance and supported to some extent the validity of her rage. Her attacks on the leader were accepted without response except that it was important for her to talk about her perception of the group even if others saw it differently. At one point in the ninth session, it was clear that she was near tears, though seemingly angry. It was possible to slip in a quiet comment about the sadness of the course her life seemed to be taking. This resulted in her sobbing heavily and expressing her belief that she was destined always to turn people off with her anger. Other members revealed that they too had trouble with anger, but in the opposite direction. They could never feel worthy enough to express it. By the end of the session, there had been a major resurgence of cohesion. The work in this session was a major turning point both for this patient and for the group. As others were able to become more assertive with negative affect, she could relax. With time, she was able to see a parallel dynamic in her own family, where she felt responsible for all and became overly controlling and irritable.

During the differentiation stage, the functions of the Sociable Role and Structural Role leaders continue to be important. Members in these roles are the culture bearers of cohesive engagement. The Sociable Role members in particular will be appalled to see their "nice group" apparently unraveling around them. They will need some reassurance that group cohesion will be able to survive the confrontational process. This stage may be particularly useful to these members as the more confronting behaviors of other members serve as models. Structural Role members are more comfortable bridging the changing climate because of the stress they place on task accomplishment. They also can understand the importance of individual perceptions and opinions. They are helpful in the group's working through differentiation issues.

Cautionary Role members, who may have come to a grudging acceptance of the group system during the engagement stage, will find in the tumult of differentiation the confirmation of their worst fears about group participation. Attention will be required from the therapist to ensure that they continue to be motivated. They may be able to offer constructive thoughts about the importance of the individual. Such comments may be presented in an angry or critical manner that aligns these members with those in the Divergent Role position.

Predictable Problems

Projective Mechanisms

During the differentiation stage, projective defense mechanisms are in evidence. Projection refers to the unconscious attribution to another person of thoughts or feelings that are one's own. This process is understood as a way of managing self-evaluations that are considered unacceptable or dangerous. Such phenomena are a regular feature of psychotherapy groups, perhaps more so than in individual therapy, making groups a particularly advantageous place to observe projective mechanisms at work. Generally, the group phenomena of displacement to and projection onto a given member can be handled through an exploration of the differences in viewpoint, as discussed earlier in this chapter, with an emphasis on the internal state of the active member.

Remember that the scapegoat role is developed as a manifestation of the group's need to contain unacceptable negative affect. That affect needs to be contained and managed in some fashion. In more structured groups, it is best to accept the ideas being expressed and tacitly acknowledge that it is permissible for the group to have periods of tension. In groups designed to have a more introspective component, this stage offers the opportunity for members to explore the nature of the reactions they are experiencing with a view to understanding and tolerating the negative affect.

Projective Identification and Splitting

Projective identification and splitting are frequently found together and may lead to serious distortions in interpersonal perceptions (59). Internal perceptions of the self both as good and as bad exist as if in separate compartments. Individuals may fluctuate from one state to another, seeing themselves at one time as special and entitled and at another time as evil and destructive. These internal perspectives are then projected onto separate people. In this splitting process, some group members come to be viewed in unrealistically positive terms, and others are viewed in totally negative terms. If stress develops in one of these relationships, there may be a sudden shift from positive to negative in how that relationship is seen.

This more extreme form of the projection mechanism is seen particularly in patients with difficulties in basic object relations, such as those typically found in borderline personality disorder. Such patients have difficulty in clearly defining themselves, and they tend to fuse their perception of self into that of the other. Therefore, both positive and negative relationships become highly charged. The individual sees herself as having justifiable reactions to the other person. This often elicits from the other the very behaviors that are anticipated, and this reaction by the other confirms and consolidates the projective identification process. Patients with this tendency are likely to use any movement toward group scapegoating as a vehicle for an extension of their personal projections. They may lead the group in this direction and carry the negative process beyond levels where it can be easily addressed. The intensity of psychopathology of such patients makes it difficult for them to utilize cognitive meditating mechanisms. It is for this reason that such characteristics are noted as cautionary signs when making group composition decisions. Can the patient tolerate an intensive group? How many members with such potential can be included in the group? The use of homogeneous groups for patients with more severe personality psychopathology may be considered. These groups can move at a slower pace and can give careful and systematic attention to the distorting mechanisms. Projective identification may arise in any group when tension levels increase.

The Scapegoat

The metaphor of the scapegoat originates in the Old Testament, as part of the ritual associated with the annual Day of Atonement:

> And Aaron shall lay both his hands upon the head of the live goat, and confess over him all the iniquities of the children of Israel, and all their transgressions in all their sins, putting them upon the head of the goat, and shall send him away by the hand of a fit man into the wilderness: And the goat shall bear upon him all their iniquities unto a land not inhabited: and he shall let go the goat in the wilderness. (Leviticus 16:21–22 *The Holy Bible* [Authorized Version])

The designation of a scapegoat demonstrates the projective mechanism at work in the social system. A group consensus forms that if a particular member were no longer in the group, everyone else could get along satisfactorily. This allows the other group members to become unified and still deal with themes involving negative affect, though with the wrong target.

The displacement process of scapegoating can be seen as a group mechanism for dealing with the conflict inherent in the differentiation work. This process effects an unstable compromise, however, because the collaborating members are at the same time denying that other differences exist among them. If the chosen "scapegoat" leaves the group, then the process must be repeated to maintain the defensive position. Groups may go through several members in this fashion.

A variant on this process is for the group to agree on an external source of the problem. This may be a collective agreement in a group of women that "men" are the problem, or in a group of men that "militant feminism" is the problem. This group-level mechanism reflects in the collectivity of the group the same sort of projective process as may occur in the individual. This type of group displacement process is discussed further in Chapter 9 when the ideas of Bion are introduced.

The therapist must be ready to intervene if the scapegoating process becomes overly active. Patients who become group casualties report being the victim of this process and of suffering humiliation and severe damage to their self-esteem. The therapist has several possible approaches to consider.

Clarify differences. The therapist may need to become more active in structuring a discussion on the roots of the tension. Often, the discussion will come to include associated material concerning issues for the main protagonists in their lives outside of group. In this way, the group interaction is made more understandable and, therefore, is more easily channeled. Group members who are less involved in the controversy may be very helpful in this process.

Identify the source of conflict. The presence of a scapegoating pattern reflects some underlying issue with which the group is trying to grapple. If this pattern can be identified and dealt with, then the need for a scapegoat vanishes. Often the real target is the therapist, who may have been giving mixed messages about the acceptability of leader challenges. When the negative atmosphere seems to be getting locked up in unproductive, inhibited, and unexpressed resistance, therapists need to take a good look at their role in the group. It may be necessary to directly address this possibility. "There seems to be a lot of dissatisfaction in the air the last two or three sessions. I was wondering if some of that might have to do with how you are seeing my role in the group." This message may need to be repeated in various forms more than once.

Support the scapegoat. Others in the group may share some of the opinions being promoted by the identified scapegoat. If these members can join the scapegoat, then there is less danger. The therapist may need to align himself or herself with the scapegoat. This alignment, when necessary, is done most smoothly at an early point in the process. "I hear everybody getting on Bob's back about these things, but it seems to me that he has a valid point." Sometimes simply letting the scapegoated member know that his or her role is appreciated provides enough support.

Halt the process. When all else fails, the therapist may need to specifically call a halt to the process. "I think this has gone on long enough and everybody has things out of perspective. Let's put the subject on hold for tonight and see how it looks next week."

Completion of the Differentiation Stage

The successful outcome of differentiation entails an undertaking to cooperate, not necessarily to agree, as was the case in the engagement stage. Failure to master this process has one of two predictable outcomes. The group may grind on in a chronically dissatisfied competitive fashion with ebbing morale and gradual loss of members. Or the group may bounce back into the less critical atmosphere of engagement. This will soon become boring or dissatisfying, so that the group will likely keep testing conflictual issues, only to rebound each time. This pattern may continue for extended periods of time, with the therapist recognizing that something is not working but not quite being able to identify the problem. The differentiation stage contributes to the normative development of the group. Through the process of leader challenge, the group gains a more consolidated view of its nature and functions. Through this process, individual members become more recognizable in terms of greater information and interactional activity. The therapist carries a responsibility to ensure that no member is hurt by the negative atmosphere.

It is common for the work in the differentiation stage to build in intensity and then rather suddenly settle. The therapist may leave one session wondering where the group is headed, only to begin the next with the group settled into a determined stance of collaborative work. As in all stages, it is important that each member participate in the work of the stage.

Summary of Group Development Through the Differentiation Stage

The first two stages of group development—engagement and differentiation—lay the groundwork for more complex interpersonal functioning and the capacity for more sensitive levels of empathy. Groups that have mastered these tasks are equipped to be engaged and supporting and, at the same time, are able to deal with differences and confrontation. The members have experienced a sense of being understood and accepted. They may have committed themselves to increasing depths of self-revelation. They have also experienced assertion, tolerated anger, and challenged authority.

The therapeutic work during the two early stages can be represented in terms of Structural Analysis of Social Behavior interpersonal space as interaction focused on, in the engagement stage, the Protect/Trust quadrant and, in the differentiation stage, the Blame/Sulk quadrant. The focus in both of these stages suggests a high degree of enmeshment in the group atmosphere, with alternating positive and negative valence.

Many groups may purposefully be maintained in an engagement-stage atmosphere. If the group does move into differentiation tasks, it is important that there be an opportunity to work through issues related to these tasks so that the group can move into the interpersonal work mode. Groups that end while still in conflict may be viewed by the members as having been unsatisfactory, and gains achieved in the early part of the group experience may be lost.

CHAPTER 9

Interpersonal Work

*T*his chapter addresses a number of topics related to understanding and dealing with interpersonal events in the more mature group. Addressing these topics as if they were separate from the early stages of group development represents a somewhat artificial division, because during the earlier stages of the group a multitude of interpersonal situations will have arisen that required skillful management. However, there is some logic to delaying discussion of this material until this point. In a pragmatic sense, the goal of the early group is to help the individual through the process of joining the group and experiencing the supportive group therapeutic factors. The principal task for the member has been to make an initial presentation of self and to experience acceptance into an increasingly cohesive group. In the differentiation stage, the focus was on more rigorous testing of the interactional environment. As a result, members became more comfortable with assertion and with tolerating disagreement and anger.

The purpose of group interventions has been to augment this process of group formation. The individual member will have many therapeutic experiences during this period, but the focus for the therapist is on creating and maintaining the group environment. Now, the therapist can shift the focus to promoting more specific understanding of interpersonal issues as they are enacted within the group (60). For the general weekly outpatient group, this transition can be expected to occur around the sixth to eighth session.

If a group meets for long enough and is allowed to create an interactional climate, it will move into a more intimate style. This shift will occur not only in interpersonal/psychodynamic groups but also in structured behavioral or cognitive groups. Groups designed for simple support functions will also experience group development. In fact, with less emphasis on formal treatment, the group as an informal social vehicle may move quite rapidly into greater intimacy. Therefore, the information presented in this chapter is not just for clinicians running groups that have a defined interpersonal focus. Clinicians who maintain that they simply use the group format to deliver specific material are likely ignoring, at their peril, the ongoing group process. They are also losing the opportunity to maximize the impact of their treatment through intentional use of the power of the group.

This chapter was written with the generic model of group psychotherapy in mind. Several formats for understanding and tracking the interactional process are presented. These formats are based on the interpersonal descriptive literature but are relatively free of theoretical emphasis in terms of traditional treatment approaches. They help the clinician to make sense of the group interaction and provide guidelines about how to manage it. If the group interaction can be managed successfully, then the group will be able to stay on track with its goals. In some groups the challenge will be to learn to focus on negative thoughts and to challenge them; in others it will involve looking intensively at personal motivations and reactions. But in either case, the work is carried out through an increasingly personalized interactional process. An attempt is made to couch this material in terms of group dynamics, not intrapersonal dynamics. The purpose is to develop an approach to the therapeutic use of the group modality that can be applied in all types of group situations. Different theoretical models, different patient populations, and different circumstances will result in specialized techniques. However, the clinician needs to be sure that consideration of these variables does not get in the way of the basic interactional strategies that underlie all effective psychotherapies. The chapters in the last section of this book, on group models for service systems, will address modifications of this material for specific types of groups.

Interpersonal Learning

The point at which the group moves beyond the confrontational style of the differentiation stage marks a critical shift in the group atmosphere. The members are now prepared to engage in more introspective work and have the interactional experience to do so in a collaborative manner. For the therapist, this transition implies that the group system is well in place and that more attention can be paid to the individual members and the nature of their interactions. In terms of the group structure diagrammed in Figure 3–1 (see Chapter 3), the focus shifts to the interpersonal boundaries between members and to internal issues. The major themes that will now come into view reflect the members' more comfortable approach to introspection and lower resistance to psychological exploration. This group environment may be used for various purposes. In cognitive-behavioral groups, the group interactions may be used as examples and as an opportunity for practicing new skills. In interpersonal/psychodynamic groups, the psychological meanings will be emphasized.

The point when the group moves beyond the work of differentiation can be described in terms of the generic model presented in Chapter 2. At this point, the Therapeutic Contract is now firmly in place. The interactional loop of Therapeutic Operations has been well established, with a particular emphasis on increased patient self-presentation and patient cooperation. The group atmosphere is able to provide considerable reinforcement for these aspects. Up to now the therapist has concentrated primarily on understanding the events at the group level and reinforcing them. Now the focus shifts to the individual, and the group process takes on more of the characteristics of individual therapy. This shift, of course, applies to the members' understanding and interventions as well as the therapist's.

The Therapeutic Bond to the leader and the sense of group cohesion should also be well in place. The group environment is particularly helpful in addressing problems with Self-Relatedness. The individual who is stuck in a defensive and closed state receives both support and encouragement to join the group from the other members, who also provide a model of greater openness. The therapist is often wise to stay out of this process. A direct approach by the leader in many cases only increases the resistance.

The generic model would suggest that the stage is now set for important In-Session Impact experiences, to be described later in this chapter in the discussion of *Focal Incidents.*

Three major dimensions will be in continuous interplay as the level of intimacy increases. These dimensions are usefully conceptualized with Structural Analysis of Social Behavior (SASB) terminology:

a. Learning to tolerate increasing levels of intimacy (a preponderance of positive warm relationships as opposed to negative, angry ones)
b. Managing the degree of interdependent involvement (a balance between excessive distancing autonomy and excessive overinvolvement and enmeshment)
c. Managing issues of power (a balance between excessive control and excessive submission)

As the interactional climate deepens, members will automatically begin to think about themselves in more complex ways in regard to the actual relationships that are forming in the group. This process will serve to "turn on" old response patterns stemming from early relationships in the family of origin as augmented by the nature of adult intimate relationships. Because, by definition, patients coming for psychotherapy often experience difficulty in their relationships, critical dysfunctional patterns may become evident. Therefore, by focusing on current group events, the members are at the same time addressing early learned patterns. These patterns are often heavily imbued with negative interpersonal implications. This process leads to an increased focus on self definition and self-concept, which triggers quite deep feelings about personal meaning.

Groups provide a range of close-to-real-life experiences that serve both to elicit interpersonal behaviors and to provide the context for members to examine them. The group approach stands in contrast to individual psychotherapy, in which there is only one relationship, and that one characterized by an imbalance of role status. In the generic model of psychotherapy, experiential enactment stands out as an important component in the process. The group can be seen as developing through a deepening spiral of interpersonal meaning. The issues first seen during the engagement process return now with more specificity around the theme of intimacy. The relative turmoil of the differentiation process reappears when issues of personal autonomy within the group are addressed.

Groups will, of course, regress to earlier interactional styles when subjected to pressures. Any change in group membership necessitates a reworking of engagement issues, even if only quite briefly. When the intensity around difficult issues rises, the group may experience a regression back to earlier styles to recoup. A Focal Incident involving much anger or rejection will often trigger regression. All groups tend to cycle through the three basic dimensions outlined above with deepening appreciation of their implications and increasing attention to the application of this material to their personal lives.

Groups provide a rich environment for interpersonal learning. This is certainly not to deny that internal, or intrapsychic, events are not occurring. These internal processes will provide the motivating factors that are then enacted in the group. However, there are some advantages to focusing primarily on interpersonal concepts. These concepts are more accessible and thus easier to describe, and therefore more understandable to the patients. There is also likely to be greater agreement about what happened in the group between members than about what is going on inside a given member. Interpersonal language can be used for internal material as well— for example, "It sounds as if you are hearing right here in the group your father's voice telling you how inadequate you are as a daughter and as a person."

Interpersonal learning forms the basic rationale for group psychotherapy. Such learning is also implied in the "corrective emotional experience" of individual psychotherapy (61). In the group context, the nature of the learning process is rather different. The peer interaction of a group does not entail the influence and power of the professional role. Instead, it offers the reality of interacting with people who are also experiencing problems, which gives the interchanges a quality of genuineness that adds to the therapeutic effect. One of the major strengths of therapy in a group is the manner in which group members can get at important issues or penetrate defensive style because they are peers. Insightful comments from another group member cannot be easily dismissed as coming from someone who "doesn't understand my situation" or discounted as not applying to the realities of life outside the group.

The majority of therapist activity is directed at ensuring that the group stays focused on its task. The therapist may find it necessary to bring the group back to reconsider a statement just made, or to probe for further reactions or to elicit responses from a greater number of group members. The therapist may be able to compare and contrast some of the responses, thus revealing important differences in how members react to the same events. The overall result is an intensification of the group interactive process. The therapist can be thought of as promoting the here-and-now process by stimulating action across a diversity of boundaries. A group that has developed therapeutic interactional norms will, with some assistance from the therapist, be able to carry much of the work of interpersonal learning. It is therapeutic for the members to experience a greater sense of self-responsibility for maintaining the working atmosphere.

The mechanisms of interpersonal learning discussed in this chapter are described primarily in cognitive terms to help the therapist to identify the processes clearly. It must be kept in mind that for the patient, interpersonal learning is an absorbing and powerful total experience. The therapist can deepen the impact by exploring the emotional reactions of the participants. Typical questions might be "What was it like to speak of these matters that you have always kept as a secret?" "The experience of telling him what you disliked about his answer sounds like you took a risk in the group. How was it?" "What sort of reactions are getting stirred up by their comments to you?" "Have others had the same sort of experience as Ken is describing?"

Intense emotional expression is only a part of the total corrective emotional experience, not an end in itself. Indeed, members who have critical experiences that are solely emotional tend to have less satisfactory outcomes. Integration of the meaning of the experience through cognitive understanding assists the process of internalization and application and also serves to bind the affective component to specific issues, rather than its being spread inappropriately over all situations. For example, it is one thing to be mad at all men, another to be mad at all controlling men, and different still to be mad at a specific controlling man. Note that the word "feelings" was not used in the examples in the preceding paragraph. This is intentional. Often, the question "What are you feeling?" elicits a simple answer—for example, "Upset" or "Confused" or "Angry." The exploration of affect is only the starting point. Once the affect is mobilized, an understanding of its meaning provides an opportunity for applied learning (62). Interventions like "How are you reacting?" "What are you experiencing right now?" or, even more simply, "What's going on?" promote a more in-depth response.

The Johari Window

One way of conceptualizing how learning can occur in a group is the Johari Window (63), which was included as part of the Patient Information Handout used in pretherapy preparation (Appendix 9). In a straightforward fashion this diagram encapsulates the idea of psychological processes that may interfere with interpersonal functioning. It takes into account the existence of material either purposefully hidden or not available to the individual because of unconscious mechanisms. It acknowledges the importance of learning from what others tell one about oneself, as well as through an introspective process. The format of the Johari Window is easily grasped by patients and can be used to explain how learning takes place in psychotherapy.

The Johari Window format can also guide the therapist in tracking group process. The goal of therapy may, in one sense, be described as increasing the amount of "public knowledge." This may be accomplished through self-disclosures by the patient, through which information is transferred from the "hidden" box to the "public" box. Similarly, feedback to the individual from others transfers information known to others into the "public" box, where it can be understood by the patient as well. The process of personal insight is reflected in movement across the unknown/known-to-self boundary. In practice, all of these events may occur simultaneously. However, by considering these events as specific components of the learning situation, the therapist can identify and reinforce them. Conceptualizing interactions in terms of the Johari Window provides another boundary-managing technique.

In Chapter 3, a somewhat similar 2×2 matrix was used to conceptualize the role of group norms (Figure 3–2). In that context, the goal was to increase behaviors under "positive normative control" by encouraging "risky" behaviors and having them validated. Norms are the social-system equivalent to personal criteria for appropriate behavior and reflect internal values or fears. Such attitudes take their shape from early experiences. As the members strive to clarify the relationships within the group, they must apply the issues raised to their own situation.

The Johari Window and the norm matrix provide parallel information structures that are helpful in clarifying process events. For example, the "risky" box from the norm matrix in Figure 3–2 corresponds to the "self-disclosure" box in the Johari Window in Appendix 9.

Self-Disclosure

Self-disclosure is a mechanism by which information from the category of "personal secrets" moves to that of "public knowledge." In terms of the generic model in Chapter 2, it represents the enactment of Patient Presentation in Therapeutic Operations. In early group sessions, self-disclosure tends to be mainly factual and increases in levels of personal sensitivity with time. At a pragmatic level, it is obvious that people must say something about themselves if they are to address personal problems.

The decision of whether to allow the transfer of personal secrets to public knowledge has some interesting implications. The withholding of information is a component of interpersonal deceit and is a perfectly normal process. We choose to tell things about ourselves when we judge the situation to be safe. To tell too little is to be interpersonally overly cautious; to tell too much is to be interpersonally naive. Self-disclosure therefore has a direct relationship to levels of trust and, in groups, to cohesion. That is one reason why so much stress has been laid on preparing patients for groups. By facilitating a rapid sense of groupness, the therapist is at the same time creating the conditions for increased self-disclosure. It is also appropriate to warn patients that behavior that is productive in a therapy group may not be indicated at the workplace or in casual social situations.

As the group develops, it is to be expected that the nature of self-disclosure will shift into more introspective areas of personal feelings and also into interactional areas of giving feedback to others by revealing personal reactions to what others say. In addition, if the therapeutic process is advancing satisfactorily, the individual member will begin to have access to more material from the "unknown" area. An emerging sense of internal conflicts or of contradictory and split-off parts within the self may force the individual to make critical decisions about self-disclosure. Often, this sort of material is accompanied by deep feelings of shame or incompetence. It may involve behaviors that have been kept hidden or feelings and reactions about significant others that have never been shared. To acknowledge these behaviors or feelings publicly to the group may have a powerful therapeutic effect; to keep them hidden may lead to disengagement. The therapeutic factor of catharsis lends much of the power to this experience.

Example

A 27-year-old single secretary became increasingly tense during a discussion of intimate relationships by several members. After a brief recognition of her distress by the therapist, she stated forcefully that she had to deal with an important issue. This involved a rape at age 19 after meeting a stranger in a bar. She had never discussed this with anyone and was consumed with guilt because she felt she was responsible. She had not dated since that event. This self-disclosure broke the taboo about this imprinting event so that it could be put into reasonable perspective through sharing and feedback from other members.

Interpersonal Feedback

Interpersonal feedback is complementary to self-disclosure. It is represented in the generic model by Therapist Understanding and Therapist Intervention, which in groups involve all members as well. One way or another, the individual is provided with information about the impact of his or her thoughts, feelings, or behavior on others. If received and acknowledged, this information may stimulate an introspective process. Feedback may involve, for example, a supportive or understanding reaction to some quality in or information about the other. Through feedback, one can identify a discrepancy between nonverbal behavior and verbal content. Feedback often involves alternative viewpoints about perspectives or attitudes. In general, feedback enhances the ability to understand the real effect one has on others.

As noted earlier, the group context offers some advantages over individual therapy in terms of feedback. Interpretive or confrontational messages are frequently more easily accepted from other group members than from the therapist—a phenomenon that may be related to the dimension of control or power. At the same time, the members offering such statements are often participating in an altruistic process of helping others. Others may benefit vicariously by watching and thinking about the exchanges. A well-developed working atmosphere can be a potent vehicle for introspective work.

The process of feedback has a theoretical base in operant conditioning. *Positive feedback* is that which increases the targeted behavior, whereas *negative feedback* is that which decreases it. Most systems operate primarily on the principles of negative feedback. In the group psychotherapy setting, both positive and negative feedback loops may be desirable. For example, for the withdrawn patient who has difficulty in assertion and self-presentation, positive feedback of encouragement and support may be effective in increasing these behaviors. For a person with impulse-control difficulties, negative feedback is appropriate to decrease such episodes.

Note, however, that positive and negative as used above do not necessarily imply positive and negative emotional tone. For example, a strong reaction of anger or criticism to an impulsive gesture may actually provide positive reinforcement for that gesture. One of the technical challenges of working in groups is how to effectively set limits and provide corrective negative feedback. Simple lack of response or diversion to another topic is a common negative feedback technique. But in general, learning is augmented when the process is more explicit.

Several guidelines are available for maximizing the use of feedback. These mechanisms are simple, at first glance seemingly beneath the dignity of a graduated professional, but are frequently ignored. They should be purposefully nurtured in the group so that members can become comfortable with this important interpersonal skill of providing feedback. When these principles are attended to, the infrastructure of the change induction process can be carefully constructed (64).

Begin with the positive. A positive emphasis establishes a receptive atmosphere that promotes a collaborative response. The therapist should search for some positive features to the situation—evidence of some strength or determination—that can be reinforced. The idea is for the therapist to support the individual even though some of the patient's behavior is excessive or dysfunctional. Providing such support enables one to avoid an implied condemnation of the whole person.

Identify the target.   The specific issue to be addressed needs to be identified. This sequence can increase motivation for change and, at the same time, provide specific information about what to work on. The focus may be on overt behavior or internal thought processes.

Be rational.   The therapist is in a position to model an approach that emphasizes understanding before judgment. In particular, strong expression of therapist anger or criticism reflects a loss of the "therapeutic attitude" of aligning with the patient against problematic behaviors. Such therapist actions are commonly cited as reasons for negative effects.

Be consistent.   Once a particular issue has been identified, the therapist should ensure that the issue is discussed by the group. At the same time, the therapist should reinforce changes in adaptation. Often, therapeutic effect is seen first in subtle shifts in behavior that reflect a reordering of internal priorities or attitudes.

Use the group.   The goal is to train the group members to be of help to each other. The impact of feedback is greater if all the members can apply the feedback skillfully.

● ● ● ●

Feedback is a technical term that may be misused in its therapeutic application. In fact, it is recommended that therapists not even use this word in clinical work, because the term almost always evokes an image of negative criticism—"Now it's our turn to get him"—and feedback may be transformed into verbal flagellation. Alternative terminology might be "How do people understand what's just been going on between Don and Marianne?" or, even more simply, "What does the group make of this? Any reflections?"

It is easy for the therapist who is experienced in the process of therapy to forget just how important comments from the leader or members can be. One major advantage of group therapy is the power of the group to induce change. However, this same power can be destructive. The therapist must assume responsibility for monitoring the nature of this loop and actively intervene to modulate negative criticism. In particular, any evidence of a malicious intent to harm or reject must be addressed promptly.

Strongly expressed negative criticism is commonly fueled by the personal issues of the person delivering it. Exploration of both sides of the process is therefore warranted. The therapist may need to provide support to the recipient, not necessarily by denying or dismissing the issues being raised, but by assisting the individual to use the issues raised in a constructive fashion. At the same time, the personal issues of the member who is delivering the criticism may need to be explored. Introspective work may carry with it a threat to the individual's sense of self-esteem. The support derived from a cohesive group environment usually addresses this adequately, but the therapist must ensure that the individual member can tolerate the process. Feedback, both from the therapist and from the members, is most effective if it originates from the "therapeutic attitude" that is directed at aspects of the person's behavior, not the whole person.

The learning cycle of self-disclosure and interpersonal feedback may move in both directions. Self-disclosure will stimulate responses from others, and feedback may trigger self-disclosure. Both mechanisms result in a clarification of issues about the individual and about the impact that the individual makes on others. These basic processes are at the heart of therapeutic change. The content will vary according to the goals of the group, but the process greatly augments the learning experience.

Introspection

By its very nature, introspective work deals with material that is hidden to the individual, is highly charged with affect, and may involve significant distortions in how the individual sees his or her interpersonal world. These attitudes and perceptions are then revealed indirectly through the group interactional process. Actions of others trigger sensitive internal issues, and this results in responses to the others that in turn evoke further elaboration. The therapist can assist the group in introspective work by continually translating material of an intrapsychic nature into its interpersonal application. For example, if a patient is experiencing guilt, it might be useful to find out who within or outside of the group does the patient feel has the most critical attitude toward his story or behavior. What negative distortions are being introduced into this process of giving personal meaning to the situation? By using such techniques, the therapist can promote the enactment of the interpersonal behavior that will identify and open up important issues. This approach moves away from intrapsychic language and yet still implements a psychodynamically informed perspective.

Because of the opportunity in groups for many different types of relationships to emerge, a broad panorama is available on which the individual can display the types of relationships that are adaptive or problematic. To state this more formally, there is the opportunity for multiple transferences to occur within a group in a manner that is quite different from that in individual therapy. The introspective process can be accelerated by utilizing these various relationships to focus on those that are more functional and to contrast these with others that reveal dysfunction.

The therapist can expedite the learning process with the systematic use of *clarification*—clarification about what the individual knows about herself and what she can express to the others, about what the others find in each individual's presentation and can clarify back to the individual, and about how these negative cognitions get generated. Whenever a member makes a personally important statement, the primary task of the therapist is not to offer interpretations, but rather to elicit the response of other group members. Usually, a rich network of reactions and ideas, often of a quite sophisticated nature, is produced.

Another way of describing the process of interpersonal learning is through the language of *personal construct theory* (65). The focus of this theory is on the manner in which individuals construe and therefore create their interpersonal world. For example, the depressed person systematically picks out the most negative interpretations to apply to current events and to those of the past and the future. At a more complex level, these "personal construct" ideas may be applied to an understanding of the dimensions used by people to explain their relationships. An idiosyncratic view of the interpersonal world is actively manufactured through the application of unique sets of ideas about people. This process has been described as an attempt to provide a sense of regularity to one's experiences. George Kelly defined a psychological disorder as a "personal construction" that is used repeatedly in spite of consistent invalidation. For example, a common pattern in neurotic men is a strong link between the constructs of love and weakness. Thus, the idea of being in an intimate relationship automatically calls up an association with being weak and passive. This personal-construct orientation is relevant to the idea of defining a characteristic theme of interpersonal tension as the focus for therapeutic attention.

Described in this way, introspection is not restricted to interpersonal or psychodynamic techniques. Indeed, it is every bit as relevant to cognitive therapy and to the thoughts that interfere with carrying through on behavioral techniques. The goal is for the individual to recognize patterns of thoughts or behaviors and to test the way in which these distort and disrupt relationships and attitudes toward oneself. The experience of receiving both support and challenge in a cohesive group provides an opportunity to see the self in a different way. This shift into a more vulnerable state allows the individual to take the risk of trying out new responses, which can then be confirmed by the interactional responses they generate from others.

Example

A 45-year-old accountant was referred with symptoms of depression and a stated desire to learn that it was socially acceptable to be a bachelor. As the group progressed, he became increasingly open concerning his ambivalent relationships with women. He had several quite close women friends, one of whom he thought might, after having been friends for many years, have romantic ideas. He did not see how he could broach this subject without feeling foolish and destroying the relationship altogether, yet felt very anxious when with her lest she make advances. It also came to light that he felt quite attracted to another woman in a romantic way but feared asking her out on a date. The women in the group over a period of several sessions provided him with important feedback about his progress in asserting himself in the group and the unrealistic nature of his fears. The men acknowledged that they had experienced similar apprehensions. These responses freed him up to review in more depth painful experiences in his teens that lay behind his fears. He resolved his feelings of being blocked by undertaking to address these issues and report back to the group. This resolve triggered a marked shift in self-esteem and led to a successful resolution of the impasse.

Focal Incidents

One way of organizing and conceptualizing group events is to consider a session as a series of *Focal Incidents*. This orientation is useful at any point in a group's life. It is described in detail here because the notion of specific learning episodes is particularly important once the group is equipped for more challenging work. Focal Incidents not only are important as a way of tracking group events as they occur but also are useful in reporting what transpires in groups for purposes of supervision. A number of intervention strategies are mentioned in this chapter, and further ideas about leader strategies are presented in Chapter 11.

Conceiving of a session as consisting of Focal Incidents is only one way of considering group interactions, one selection from a continuum of time frames. Sometimes it is useful to think of the entire group experience, from start to finish, as a unit. This perspective can be useful, for example, when one is comparing the features of a group for anorexic patients and a group for schizophrenic patients. Another perspective, and one already used in this book, is to consider the group in terms of a series of developmental stages, each lasting a number of sessions. Yet another perspective, one representing a tighter time frame, is to view each full session as a unit, as reflected in studies using group climate reports in which the members are asked to describe the group as a whole during a single session. Viewing each session as a series of Focal Incidents, our concern in this section, divides the action up into segments lasting a number of minutes. Many research studies using videotape or transcript analysis focus on even shorter time segments: a single utterance as the unit of attention. Each of these time frames has its own value and focuses on different aspects of groupness.

Viewing each session as a series of Focal Incidents involves the identification of short segments with interactional punch that center on a relationship theme. Within any given group session, several such events might take place. If the number of Focal Incidents grows beyond six to eight, the therapist should use less detail and look for larger thematic segments. A Focal Incident is defined as having a common theme, a common emotional tone, and often a subset of active group members involved. It is sometimes possible to identify the specific action that initiated the Focal Incident and then to track the swell of attention around that particular focus as it peaks and then begins to diminish. Experienced therapists probably think this way intuitively. They are able to align with the current thematic material at an early point and thus are able to ensure a continuing focus on the implications it has for the members. They then sense when that theme is beginning to lose its intensity and the time is ripe for "processing" it. A *critical learning event* has been succinctly described by Yalom as an event characterized by elevated affect that leads to an attempt at new and risky behavior, a realization that the feared catastrophic result of the behavior did not occur, and, finally, an opportunity to work through the entire situation from a reality orientation (66).

A Focal Incident is a useful time unit for the therapist to use in applying many of the ideas in this book. It can also be used as a framework for keeping notes in terms of the succession of important themes running through a session. Each incident can be viewed from many perspectives, as follows.

Group structure. An incident can be scanned in terms of a group structural diagram, with the focus on each boundary in turn and with consideration of the four levels of the system hierarchy: the group system, subgroups, interactions between members, and internal issues. What boundary focus best captures the essence of the process? It is helpful to actually plot these patterns out with paper and pencil after the group. Arrows can be drawn between the main actors in the scenario, and an "involvement boundary" can be drawn around all of the key participants. Would it be useful to compare and contrast opinions and reactions of those participants inside the Focal Incident boundary with those of members functioning as observers? Often, the therapist may be aware of other group members who have issues directly connected to those being addressed and can quietly recruit their involvement if they have not already become active—for example, "This sounds like some of the concerns you have been dealing with, Mary" or "Can anyone else identify with what Ken has been saying?"—with a glance in the right direction.

Agazarian has described a technique that focuses on identification of members as part of subgroups (67). This focus serves to contain the individual member within a subgroup and prevents the development of a stereotypic role figure. Members within each subgroup begin to realize that they have differences, and members across subgroups see that they have similarities. Such a boundary-managing technique can be a powerful way to mobilize issues and enhance the reality of the here-and-now process experience. Members can see their issues being enacted by other members of the subgroup. The deliberate splitting maneuver avoids members' feeling paralyzed with indecision as to how to resolve both sides of the issue and the ambivalence that such a feeling engenders. A way of managing conflict by working through the issues is modeled.

Cohesion. The therapist should rate the Focal Incident as to its impact on group cohesion. Has the incident increased or decreased the sense of group involvement? The support of the group is an important sustaining factor for members when dealing with Focal Incidents. Activation of the supportive cluster of therapeutic factors may be indicated, or at least acknowledgment that difficult but important matters are being discussed.

Precipitating event.   The therapist should review the incident and try to identify exactly when it began and what was going on at the time. The use of videotapes is helpful in reviewing such an incident. The initiating circumstances not only set the tone for the incident but also may reveal why it is important. Focal Incidents often begin with a personal story by one of the members that is thematically echoed by others. Sometimes an incident will begin with an interchange between two members that has a strong, perhaps overdetermined emotional surge behind it.

Affective tone.   The therapist should consider the principal emotional quality to the incident and try to describe it in terms of the major affect states: happiness, sadness, anger, fear, surprise, interest, and disgust (68). Is there a mixture of emotional dimensions? Are contradictory or incompatible dimensions present? Is there a quality of guilt or shame that is hanging in the air but not expressed? What is the intensity level? Emotional arousal enhances learning. It is often useful to simply label the affective state for the group—for example, "I have the sense that a lot of people are resonating to Anne's disappointment and irritation at the lack of support from her partner." Members can get caught up in the details of a story and respond to the concrete issues while neglecting the emotional interpersonal meaning of the event. Their neglect of the emotional interpersonal meaning may be in the service of avoiding similar experiences of their own. Group consolidation around an affective theme often provides an opportunity to break through such denial.

Interpersonal focus.   The therapist should identify the central interpersonal theme underlying the Focal Incident. By identifying the emotional tone and the content, the therapist can frame the Focal Incident in terms of the SASB interactional space. What is the interpersonal style of the main participants, as represented on the composite circle in Figure 5–5? This process may lead to helpful speculations about what interventions would be most therapeutic.

Developmental stage.   The therapist should compare the interactional climate and thematic focus with the group's developmental stage. Are they at an appropriate level for that developmental stage? Has the group moved into a regressed position? Or is the group testing new behavior?

Social role.   The therapist should consider the behaviors of the major participants in the segment in the context of role ideas. Are the roles exhibited by the participants their customary roles in the group, or are they trying out new ones? Role behavior may be strongly reinforced by the group and can come to shape the individual's inner sense of self. This reinforcement may bring a sense of order, but it can also have a restricting effect. In the process of identifying what social role is leading the action, the therapist often comes to recognize that that person is in fact speaking to common issues for the whole group. Labeling this process may open up the material to broader participation. It also serves to divert attention from the thematic leader and allows that person to begin to reflect on the issues.

The leader.   Focal Incidents may be centered on activities of the leader, in which case they offer opportunities for particularly powerful learning. A general theme in this book has been that therapy is conducted through the group process; a leader-centered group process is *not* encouraged. However, the role of the leader is of particular significance to the group members and can be used effectively to stimulate important issues, especially around themes of authority or parental roles. These techniques are more likely to be used in intensive interpersonal/psychodynamic groups and, to a lesser extent, in more structured groups. The therapist must be comfortable in tolerating group attention and avoid shifting into a defensive position. An attitude of great interest in what people are experiencing in regard to ideas about the leader is appropriate. If questions or challenges are occurring, it is helpful to try to explore the rationale behind them and the associated needs or fears. This does not mean that specific questions might not be eventually answered; but a prompt answer will only stimulate more questions and leave the matter unexplored. Because many emotionally loaded themes have connections to earlier parental patterns, to avoid exploration of leader-centered material is to deprive the group of an important opportunity to work on such issues. It is usually helpful to end a session in which such leader-centered material has been addressed with a debriefing discussion around the impact it has had on members.

Examples

A male leader in an eating disorders group composed entirely of females was challenged by the members, who felt that it would not be possible for them to deal with the interpersonal aspects of their disorder in his presence. There were demands that the administration take action to replace him. The members' demands were met by a quiet statement by the therapist that a change would not be possible but that he appreciated the importance of the issues being raised. Could he learn more about the nature of their concerns? This resulted in a major exploration of sensitive material around previous rejecting or abusive males both in the family of origin and in subsequent relationships.

A man in his early 30s described a pattern in schooling, in jobs, and in relationships of initial success followed by self-sabotaged breakups. In the group, he had been an active and constructive member until the group moved into its differentiation stage. His style shifted into one of criticism of both others and self delivered in a manner of black humor and provocative taunts. At one point, the leader responded somewhat sharply to one of these. The man lapsed into a sulking silence. In a postgroup review, the therapist became more aware of how he had spontaneously complemented the member's interactional style (Criticism responded to by Resentment) and re-created the conditions of the past. The member continued his silence into the next session. The therapist acknowledged the man's dissatisfaction and admitted that his response in the preceding session had not been helpful. Indeed, on reflection, he realized that he had not responded to the distress underlying the member's black humor. The member experienced an immediate shift to a somber state that led to tears about his inability to sustain a relationship. This marked a turning point in his treatment.

Once the therapist is familiar with a system for applying each of the perspectives discussed above, she can quickly work through a Focal Incident as it evolves. As a training experience, going over videotapes is invaluable in learning the process of identifying and understanding Focal Incidents. It is easy to get caught up in the action of a specific member and lose sight of the importance for the group system. The therapist has a responsibility to monitor group dynamics as well as individual psychodynamic themes.

By striving to understand the interpersonal dimension that lies behind or within a particular Focal Incident, the therapist is forced to examine group events over a brief time frame. It is easy to become fascinated by content and avoid the process. By asking the question "What are these people doing to or with each other?" the actual enactment in the group of historically derived interpersonal meanings can be examined. Analysis of Focal Incidents provides in the group a parallel opportunity to the "corrective emotional experience" extensively discussed in the individual therapy literature.

One result of applying this approach to understanding a Focal Incident is the necessity of using the language of interactional process. Consider the difference between saying to oneself in a group, on the one hand, "Joe is using denial" and, on the other hand, "Joe is refusing to acknowledge what Patricia just said to him." With the first statement, one is led toward an introspective search for the internal processes responsible for the block. With the second statement, one might be led to say, "Tell him again, Patricia. It didn't seem to penetrate. Try looking him in the eye when you say it." The latter statement "massages" the interpersonal boundary between the two members and increases the affective tension that contributes to a "corrective emotional experience."

A member will frequently raise an issue of concern using the language of "there and then" outside-of-group experiences. By translating the external story into interpersonal language, the therapist is in a better position to detect similar qualities in the group interaction. This "here and now" within-group focus intensifies the experience, makes it more real, and facilitates the working-through process of desensitization and understanding. The original external context can then be reviewed in the light of the group experience. This may result in a "rewriting" of personal history in terms of how early events are understood. It may also result in new ways of approaching current situations or the development of a different view of self.

Focal Incidents are another way of describing what the generic model terms In-Session Impact events. It is useful to think specifically as a Focal Incident ends whether or not the important reactions stimulated by the event have been adequately brought to closure. The therapist may wish to prolong the event somewhat to be sure that there has been a debriefing process about its essentials. Similarly, it is wise at the end of a session to consider if there might be important reactions left hanging and again to provide a debriefing opportunity. This end-of-session review often sets the stage for the members involved to think constructively about the experience before the next session. This enhances the likelihood of a personalized In-Session Impact from the event and a positive Post-Session Outcome.

The therapist activity described here is essentially of a focusing nature and is intended to wring the most therapeutic potential from the group interaction. Consequently, the overall level of therapist activity may in fact increase during the interpersonal work stage compared with that in earlier stages. The nature of the language used to reflect on the Focal Incidents will vary depending on the nature of the therapy, but the concept of episodes of group interaction that encapsulate important clues related to dysfunctional adaptation can be used in all groups.

Focusing on themes related to the group-as-a-whole can help to maintain a sense of group work and indirectly reinforce the group external boundary, both of which will help to support the group when it is addressing difficult tasks. For example, "This has been an important session. It sounds like people are finding that they are getting more involved with each other in here, more intimate, and that is creating some pretty powerful reactions. But the process seems to be a very central one for a lot of you. Maybe at times a little scary. We'll keep at it next week."

Predictable Problems

Intense Emotional Atmosphere

At times, the level of emotional intensity may increase to the point where the therapist has concerns about how the members will manage when they leave the session. This situation may occur when new affect-laden material is introduced such as awareness of past abusive episodes, or when there is a strong surge of common group experiences. In such situations, the therapist might utilize the final 5 to 10 minutes of the session for a systematic review. The systematic debriefing could include a review of the experience, including the sensitive areas with which it connected, and what it meant to each member. Bringing such reactions out into the open in a cognitive manner helps to contain the affect. If one member is particularly upset, then it is useful to deal specifically with how the individual will manage. The group members are generally of great help, both in normalizing the experience the person is having and in offering ideas about how to cope. This ending discussion should specifically avoid intensifying the affective material; instead, it should focus on understanding it and gaining some degree of cognitive mastery.

Sometimes patients find it helpful in such circumstances to go home and write out in detail the experience. Describing the experience in writing slows down the processing of the event and encourages an observing position. Certainly, the upset member can be encouraged to make use of available resources within his or her family or with friends for support. The messages of containment, however, should also emphasize the importance of the material and the fact that it is bound to be upsetting but that the task embarked on is an important one. Very often, predicting that a distraught state will ensue will help to modify it. Suggestions that the member attempt to simply sit with the emotion without feeling that he needs to do something immediately about it can also be helpful. Above all, the member may be encouraged to renew the discussion at the next session. The group will usually make sure this happens immediately.

A variant on this scenario is when a member is experiencing acute suicidal thoughts. Once again, direct ventilation of these thoughts in the session is often helpful. The therapist will need to assess on the basis of this information whether or not additional safeguards are required. Such assessment may entail meeting with the patient after the session to review resources and, if necessary, to address further diagnostic questions. Such a check also demonstrates to the other members that the therapist is willing to assume professional responsibility in such circumstances. The problem, of course, is with the patient who has a history of multiple parasuicidal gestures and for whom the talk of suicide has become an important interpersonal currency. For these patients, the better approach is not to focus on the question of suicide but to address other interactional aspects of the situation. This approach may require a degree of therapeutic courage. However, to reinforce talk of suicide by being overly attentive to the physical details of the suicidal actions themselves is only to make the matter worse. This subject is discussed in more detail in Chapter 13 in the context of the Personality Problems Group.

The therapist also needs to be alert to situations in which many negative comments are being exchanged between members, particularly when the comments have a vindictive or demeaning quality. Such events undermine the sense of safety in the group and must be addressed promptly. At the same time, the message must not be that having disagreements is forbidden. In these activities the therapist is acting to make sure that no one is harmed by the group experience. At the same time, the material being presented may be of considerable importance to all of the members involved in the exchange. The goal would be to return to the discussion again at a later point to deal further with the issues.

Expressions of threatened violence are not acceptable in a group and must be dealt with immediately. This may require a time-out followed by an attempt to understand the issues that have been mobilized. Sometimes it is best to put the matter on hold until the next session. Above all, the therapist must make it absolutely clear that any physical action is prohibited and will be dealt with as an illegal assault. Such situations are more common in groups for the treatment of severe personality disorders.

Group Resistance

Group resistance may be shown in many ways. Uneasy silence, anxious laughter, and preoccupation with trivial topics from outside the group all suggest some difficulty in addressing the group task. There may be avoidance of a clearly relevant topic or situation. All these indicators will alert the therapist to the fact that constructive work seems to have ground to a halt. Any issue that threatens the integrity of the group (i.e., that alters events across the external boundary), such as lateness, absenteeism, or extragroup socializing, may be an indicator of resistance.

Bion has described a group as existing in two modes: a "working" state and a "basic assumption" state (69). In a working state, the group has a clear idea of its tasks and is able to address them in a rational and collaborative manner. In a basic assumption state, the group behaves "as if" it were driven by some unseen force, often accompanied by a sense of confusion, high energy, or strong affect. Bion describes three such states.

1. *Basic assumption "dependency."* A previously well functioning group may move into a state in which it behaves as if everyone were helpless. There is a vague search for someone to provide direction or answers, especially the leader. This state is common early in a group's life.
2. *Basic assumption "fight/flight."* At other times, the group may seem preoccupied with unrealistic fears about external situations or what might happen within the group. This preoccupation may alternate with equally unrealistic anger about minor issues. Often, this pattern is rooted in a reluctance to address conflict, especially with the group leader. Sometimes there is a sullen, resentful, stuck quality to the flow of the group, as if everyone were mad about something. This state is characteristic of the differentiation stage.
3. *Basic assumption "pairing."* At still other times, the group may become quite preoccupied with what is happening between two members or a small subsystem as if everyone would benefit if only those two or three members could resolve their issues. Frequently, this outlook is reflected in a hopeful and optimistic tone to which the group contributes.

All of these patterns may reflect a process of displacement, that is, of projected group affect. Although these patterns are to some extent characteristic of group stages, they may arise whenever the group is addressing a difficult task. These group-level states may be quite powerful, and therapists may find themselves getting caught up in the group version of what is going on. This commonly occurs, in particular, with the negative angry affect that may go along with the scapegoating process described in Chapter 8. Bion also described how some group member or members would rise to lead each of the states, while other members would be more or less involved. This idea of the group as an amplifier of emotion under the leadership of selected members is a useful way of thinking about group-as-a-whole phenomena. You might see in these "basic assumption" states echoes of the group developmental stages and social roles described in Chapter 3.

Therapists often speak of resistance as if it were a bad thing. There may be slightly demeaning comments about the "resistant patient" or the "stuck group." Inherent in these comments may be the secret hope that if a particular patient or patients were not in the group, then everything would be fine. Sometimes therapists find themselves in a battle of wills between their desire to have a working atmosphere and the group's stubborn resistance to every attempt by the therapist to get things going. In such situations, therapist frustration and anxiety may mount and result in impulsive attempts to break through the apparent logjam. These attempts usually make things worse.

It needs to be made very clear that resistance is the gold coin of therapy. If a group experiences no evidence of resistance, then surely it must be avoiding core issues. Evidence of resistance is a sure sign that you are on target. Remember the idea from the Therapeutic Alliance literature that the essence of effective psychotherapy is constant attention to threatened breeches of that alliance.

Rather than getting into a position of opposing resistance, the therapist is far wiser to align with the resistance. Think of the fable of the Sun and the Wind looking down on the Traveler and wagering who could get him to remove his coat. The Wind blew and blew with no effect except that the Traveler wrapped his coat even more tightly around himself. The Sun then shone benignly on the Traveler and soon the coat was off.

So the therapist can be calmly and persistently interested in what appears to be happening. Perhaps some leading comments to test out hypotheses might be in order. An attitude of puzzlement may be helpful. Above all, from the therapist side, the air should be free of frustration, annoyance, or anxiety. The group, knowing it is in firm hands, can then feel more comfortable in returning to important matters.

Example

In the third session of a time-limited outpatient group with university students, two members began expressing concerns about where the group was going—a theme commonly encountered in the early stages of a group therapy—and a third was nodding in agreement. Was it going to be just sitting around discussing? When were they going to get some concrete advice from the therapists? The therapist showed interest in these comments, mentioned that it sounded like an important issue, and wondered how others saw it. Another member said that he was finding the group a useful opportunity to think about things. Indeed, he had been stimulated to consider after the last session the growing imbalances in his relationship with his wife. A young woman commented that for her it was important to be able to put into words long-standing issues around her sense of low self-esteem. She was beginning to wonder if she had imagined her parents' expectations of her to be much higher than they actually were. The therapist reflected that there seemed to be quite a variety of opinions about how the group should work. Shortly thereafter, the topic of intimate relationship issues developed, with some quite important breakthroughs occurring into deeper levels of self-disclosure, with much of what was disclosed being of a shameful nature.

By the simple technique of aligning with the resistance and encouraging a group exploration of it, the therapist helped the group to move beyond the sticky point. The therapist's approach is also an example of "trusting your group." The group had the resources readily available to deal with resistance.

Extragroup Socializing

During pretherapy preparation, members are made aware that contact outside the sessions is not recommended and that if it occurs it is to be brought back into the group for discussion. It needs to be made clear that this restriction has nothing to do with members who do so being bad or irresponsible. It is simply because such outside-of-group connections make it much harder to use the group effectively. This restriction may not apply to groups that have primarily a social support function. In fact, in such groups, members may be encouraged to do things together. However, for most formal psychotherapy groups, the restriction applies.

Some contact between members outside of the group is inevitable. There is almost always casual chatter between members as they leave the group room, and going for coffee may seem like a logical and benign extension. The therapist is wise to keep a sharp ear for such developments. Often, important issues underlie such events, especially evidence of anxiety or resistance to group work. Remember that the issue is not that of breaking group rules, although in some contexts this may play a role. More important is the orientation that such events are a way for members to unknowingly sabotage the treatment process.

The most helpful approach to extragroup socializing is one of persistent curiosity. When did this contact take place? Who initiated it? What sorts of things were talked about? What was it like experiencing this time of greater intimacy? How is it that the members involved did not think to bring this up in the group directly? Are more contacts planned? Do they have any ideas about what brought the two of them together? Any recognizable patterns there? Usually, being in such a seemingly benign spotlight results in a useful exploration of important issues and the subgrouping disappears.

Occasionally, two group members will find themselves entering into a romantic relationship. This may or may not be wise, but there is little that the therapist can directly do about it except to explore the issues. If a definite relationship exists outside of the group, then it is generally better that one of the participants find alternative treatment resources. This approach underlines for all concerned that the purpose of treatment is to help people change and that situations that might interfere with that goal will be directly addressed.

Lateness and Absenteeism

Lateness and absenteeism are violations of the external boundary of the group. As such, every incident warrants careful consideration. The first episode may go without comment if the circumstances appear to be not too unreasonable. However, at any hint of a pattern developing, it is essential that the issues be addressed promptly. More often than not, such occurrences represent a "leakage" of anxiety or resistance. By definition, therefore, the focus should be on these elements. The challenge for the leader is to draw attention to the tardiness without alienating the patient and increasing the level of defensiveness. It is important for the therapist to give some thought about how best to introduce the topic. In particular, a tone of accusation, verbal or nonverbal, is best avoided. The goal is to increase understanding, not administer discipline. "I know the group is important for you, and I wondered what it was like missing a session?" or "The group was discussing issues that would have been of interest to you last week. They wondered where you were, and I had to report that I received no phone call" or "I know that the last session you were at was a difficult one. I wondered if that had anything to do with your absence last week" or "This is the second time you have arrived late, John. Has there been some change in your thoughts about the group?"

When the group is well into the interpersonal work stage, such references often suffice to elicit either a working response from the individual or a process of more rigorous inquiry from the group. If either does not occur, the therapist needs to be prepared to maintain a focus on the situation. Such interventions may eventually result in a more charged atmosphere, but such a result only reflects the importance of the issue. Seldom does such an approach fail to yield important working material. The therapist may have some pretty good hunches about what the issues are and can feel free to introduce such topics if they do not emerge spontaneously.

As an end result of such a process, worthwhile material is usually flushed out or a lack of motivation to attend becomes apparent. Bringing things to a head is therefore in the service of both the individual and the group. A member who is just along for the ride may have an inhibiting effect on the rest of the group, who may sense that member's indecision and try to avoid such a touchy subject. Other members may be prompted to move into a discussion of habitual patterns of avoiding situations so that they sabotage their efforts at accomplishing goals they have set for themselves.

A clear indication of trouble is when several group members are experiencing problems with lateness or absenteeism. Once again, the therapist must address such phenomena directly and nondefensively and must not cease doing so until the issues are clear. In such a situation, there is usually something going on at the group level, above and beyond issues for an individual. It may be the stultifying effects of one or two members, perhaps unhappiness with the leader, or simply that the group is moving into deeper material and the members find this disturbing. In any and all of these eventualities, bringing the issues into the open can only be helpful.

Phone Calls and Individual Sessions

Group members are informed at the beginning of treatment that it would be greatly appreciated if they would let the leader know in advance if they are unable to attend a session or if they will be arriving late. Generally, such phone calls pose no problems in themselves. Sometimes patients assume that because they gave forewarning, their absence will not be challenged.

Of course, recurrent absences or late arrivals are always important to consider. Therapists may also receive between-session phone calls regarding emergency situations or for discussion of some aspect of treatment or the possibility of alternative or additional treatment. Such calls need to be managed with care because they are a breach of the external boundary of the group. Members will hopefully already have been told that such calls will be considered part of the group frame and will be reported back to the group at the therapist's discretion. When such a call does occur, the patient should be encouraged to bring this material back to the group and also told that the therapist may make reference to it as well. Recurrent phone calls need to be addressed at greater length in the group and must not be allowed to continue. Stringency around these guidelines often has important therapeutic effects, because quite central issues of wanting special attention, feeling that one is not getting enough, or wishing for greater dependency are involved.

Requests for individual sessions must be treated with even more caution. Once again, the guidelines of referring the patient back to the group and of informing the group of the request could be followed. If there is a true crisis situation that has arisen outside of the group, then the occasional individual session might be considered. Usually, however, such requests are quite closely connected with the patient's perception of issues within the group, in which case the requests are accepted only at the therapist's peril. They are the start of erosion of the frame of therapy. They will detract from the involved member's need to use the group and will raise doubts, jealousy, and uncertainty in the minds of other members. The question of concurrent therapy is discussed in Chapter 11.

Removal of a Patient From Group

On rare occasions, it may be necessary to contemplate the removal of a patient from a well-established group. The issue of removal usually centers on negative interactions between the group and the patient. The therapist finds himself in a difficult situation. It may be clear that the patient has been put in the scapegoat role and is serving in some ways to bind negative feelings for the group. The therapist should consider this possibility first and address this issue with the group. For example, "Everybody seems to be getting on Sam's back, but I wonder if he is just an outlet for thoughts others are having. I recall that there has been some general discontent recently about the way the group has been going and my role in that." This approach has the advantage of drawing the negativity onto the leader and away from the targeted member. In general, such attempts to work with the negative phenomena eventually pay off, often to the mutual advantage of the "bad" member as well as the rest. Bear in mind that if the negative focus is indeed reflecting general group tension, then removing the involved member will inevitably lead to the group's focus shifting to another.

Sometimes the involved member demonstrates a persistent and profound defensiveness about exploring any of the issues raised. If this goes on too long, it may sap the energy of the group and lead to a general disenchantment with the process of therapy. Such a situation may reflect a significant error of composition, with the identified member having less capacity to use the interactional forum of the group.

A similar situation may arise when a given group member has been showing no progress for some time in an otherwise hardworking group. At some point, the question needs to be asked if this particular group environment is likely to be of benefit to the patient. Keeping a stuck member in a progressing group for too long discourages the group in their attempts to involve the member and may reinforce low self-esteem in that member. In such situations, it is worth considering alternative treatment approaches.

Removal of a member is always a delicate situation because one does not wish to re-create a situation of perceived failure or rejection. However, the therapist has a responsibility to both the individual and the group, especially in a time-limited format, where every session is precious. Although there may be a temptation to align with the group opinion, the therapist needs to attempt to align with the member's situation. A private meeting with the individual may be in order. Often the involved member is relieved to hear that a graceful exit could be arranged. An offer may be made to find alternative therapeutic resources if requested.

A proper termination sequence is to be encouraged, but only when the decision to remove the patient has already been made. The group itself should not be burdened with the responsibility of making such a decision. If the situation has gotten to the point of requiring a member to leave, the entire group will be aware of the circumstances. Encouraging as constructive a tone as possible during the member's final session is important.

Relapse Prevention

There is a substantial literature on relapse prevention that is seldom mentioned in group psychotherapy publications (70). Much of this literature is centered on criminal recidivism rates or substance abuse relapse. Many of the ideas, however, can be usefully transferred to a more general group psychotherapy context. The principal strategies address two main areas: general lifestyle patterns and self-mastery, and high-risk situations. This material may be introduced early and kept as a background theme throughout the group's life, with the expectation of applied efforts to change patterns. It can be returned to with more emphasis again toward the end of the group.

One of the two main areas of work in relapse prevention involves general lifestyle patterns that may contribute to negative experiences or preclude positive experiences. This cognitive work can be introduced in parallel to consideration of interpersonal matters and, indeed, can complement that process. Patterns under consideration might include inadequate exercise, lack of sleep or relaxation opportunities, dieting or eating patterns that are getting out of control, increasing alcohol or drug use, avoidance of socializing opportunities, and self-isolation from intimate friends or family—in short, how to take care of oneself. A daily journal is one way of keeping such matters under attention.

The other main area of work in relapse prevention is identification of high-risk situations that lead to anxiety or depressive symptoms that may initiate a vicious downward cycle. These situations often center on negative internal states such as anger, frustration, or boredom about which the patient feels guilty but that the patient is unable to express openly. Interpersonal conflict involving anger, confrontation, or lack of understanding from others often triggers negative states. Trying to live up to real or fantasized expectations of others may lead to a sense of futility. Circumstances involving loss or perceived loss are particularly potent triggers. Patients can be encouraged to identify such situations at an early point and begin to address the predictable effects before they become too intense. These themes are commonly encountered in all psychotherapeutic work. The group, with the assistance of the leader, may create a climate in which members are expected to address such situations directly in their outside life as in the group itself and report back on the experience.

This relapse prevention strategy can be layered on top of other group events. For example, a member complains about having too full a schedule to find time to think about personal issues before the next session. The discussion obviously may focus on the difficulty being experienced about addressing issues raised in the preceding session. But there could also be a focus on how to prevent this sort of situation from happening again.

What practical techniques can be used to prevent avoidance of situations that need to be resolved? For example, it might be helpful for the patient to structure adequate time into his schedule to think about the issues raised in the group, just as the patient needs private time to think about issues raised in his life. These topics are introduced in the spirit of helping the patient seriously learn new skills, not simply as giving advice. Such interventions are quite compatible with, and indeed promote, psychodynamic work about the same topic.

CHAPTER 10

Termination

*T*he question of termination brings us back to some of the time-related issues raised in Chapter 1. Utilization data indicate that the great majority of patients do not attend therapy for more than a few months. Much of the group psychotherapy literature assumes that everyone is in an open-ended group for years. This is probably one of the reasons that the technical aspects of managing termination have received relatively little theoretical or research attention. This chapter addresses the management of termination as a central component of the treatment process.

Time and Psychotherapy

Brief treatment was common in the early period of psychoanalysis. However, the length of treatment was gradually extended, and, eventually, shorter treatments were dogmatically criticized. Some early practitioners recognized the importance of separation issues in therapy (71). They recommended setting a termination date at the beginning of treatment and warned of the dangers of inducing excessive dependency through frequent sessions and prolonged duration of therapy. However, the subsequent brief dynamic psychotherapy literature dealt primarily with techniques for defining and maintaining a focus for interpretive interventions, while termination was given relatively cursory consideration (72). More recently, there has been greater emphasis on the termination process as an opportunity to address fundamental issues related to the process of individuation from parental figures and how this process has shaped subsequent relationship patterns (73).

James Mann was an early advocate of utilizing termination as a pivotal component of psychotherapy. When therapy was strictly limited to 12 sessions, a focus on termination became a central feature of the treatment process. Termination is seen as a means to activate core themes of self-responsibility and maturation. The approach to termination in this book has been heavily influenced by Mann's ideas. As Mann notes,

> With its specific time limit and the concept of the central issue, time-limited psychotherapy brings to the forefront of the treatment process the major psychological plague all human beings suffer, namely the wish to be close, to be as one with another, to be intimate, the fulfillment of which demands learning how to tolerate separation and loss without undue damage to our feelings about the self. (74)

Budman and Gurman devote considerable attention to the termination process for both individual and group psychotherapy (75). They espouse a "family practice" of psychotherapy, anticipating that most patients will have recurrent episodes of treatment. With this model, a wait of several months before seeking more treatment is recommended to allow a consolidation of gains. Service statistics indicate that well over half of all patients receiving psychotherapy will return for more. This applies to those receiving quite brief therapy as well as those completing lengthy and intensive psychoanalytic treatment. These authors suggest that the practice of psychotherapy in North America, even in settings in which long-term treatment is practiced, could be termed "unplanned brief therapy by default" (76). They cite the unrealistic goals of therapists who expect "total resolution" of all psychological issues and the demeaning terms applied to those who seek more treatment, such as "relapser," "recidivist," or "treatment failures."

Three methods may be used for setting the time limit (77). In the *procrustean* alternative (i.e., one size fits all), the termination date is set at the outset as in the Mann 12-session model. In the *sporting* alternative, the finish line is marked by establishing a final date, but the pace is varied by decreasing the frequency of later sessions. In the *elastic* alternative, the number of sessions is not predetermined, but there is constant attention to time; therapy will be as brief as required, and in any case not too long. The elastic alternative is probably the most common form of individual time-limited psychotherapy. Most time-limited group psychotherapy follows the procrustean alternative.

The group literature makes reference to termination themes, but most authors have focused primarily on how the decision is made to have someone terminate in an ongoing group. This focus reflects the fact that formal time-limited group psychotherapy using a closed group model has a relatively short history.

The Meaning of Time

In preparation for dealing with termination, it is helpful for the clinician to consider thoughtfully the importance of time in human existence. This philosophical orientation makes the work of managing termination more exciting and relevant. We all chronicle our personal history and the history of those dear to us on the basis of biological time. Time is the basis for determining if we are "on track" in mastering developmental tasks. Often, patients seeking therapy are dealing with major and long-standing blocks to normal developmental challenges. "At what age were you aware that things were not progressing as predicted?" Who can forget the excitement and tumult of hormonal changes in early adolescence? Think of the significance of the "biological clock" for the working professional in her 30s. Which "big zero" are you approaching: 40? 50? 60? Is retirement a safe haven or a threat of emptiness? Many people seek therapy at critical transition points in their lives. Conceptualizing adulthood in terms of developmental tasks is one of the most powerful ways of understanding the context of current psychological distress. This perspective often involves the individual's perception that expectable life achievements have or have not been accomplished.

Frequently, issues surrounding loss are given additional power when the loss occurs in an untimely manner. For example, the early death of a parent may produce an enduring sense of deprivation and of opportunities forever lost. The premature death of a spouse strikes to the heart of the bonding process. The early death of a child is one of humankind's most severe catastrophes, one that is forever actively present in memory. Man is the one animal that predicts the future. The theme of death runs through all great creativity—"To be or not to be."

Group termination has the power to stimulate these basic considerations of time. Fully acknowledging the reality of death and the inevitability of loss equips the therapist to address termination issues in a direct manner. Such acknowledgment also helps as a corrective to ideas that one always has to do more, with the attendant guilt over not providing enough. The strategies developed in this chapter strive to turn the limitation of time into an opportunity to explore basic developmental themes. This approach will have its greatest impact in time-limited formats, especially if the entire group ends together. Questions concerning the essential aloneness of the individual and the necessity of managing for oneself lie at the heart of this task. The process of maturation is compressed into the time frame of the group. In short, the ending of the group is analogous to an existential crisis (78). For that reason, the question of time must be kept continually before the members.

Time and the Therapist

The therapist, like the members, will experience a mix of reactions to termination. All therapists feel a sense of loss at the departure of a group. Group work is intensely involving, and the therapist comes to know the members well. It is impossible not to feel some sense of satisfaction at progress achieved or concern about work yet to be done. At the same time, a major time commitment has been removed, and there is the opportunity for a new beginning.

Therapists may seek to prolong treatment or to avoid termination for more personal reasons. A recurrent pattern of forgetting to address termination in a timely manner is a warning sign that topics related to termination are worthy of personal consideration. Some clinicians become anxious that all details have not been addressed. A desire to achieve closure on every issue may be revealed in a continual postponement of setting a date for ending the group. Of course, life being complex, such an expectation of total cure cannot be fulfilled. Other therapists may find themselves quite emotionally upset over termination themes and experience acute sensitivity to loss. Helping professionals are at risk of suffering from the need to help too much and may find it hard to give up that role, perhaps because in part they derive considerable personal satisfaction from their participation in sustaining the members. This need may lead to patterns of overinvolvement with patients and the taking on of undue responsibility. These activities may in fact impede patient progress toward autonomy, the opposite of what is desired. Any of these patterns may be accompanied by guilt at not doing enough or of not being an adequately skillful therapist. Remember the goal is to be a "good enough" therapist, not a miracle worker. It is always helpful to make sure there are opportunities to talk with colleagues about the stresses of termination and to use this interchange to keep a reasonable perspective on the circumstances.

Strategies for Managing Termination

A number of technical strategies serve to keep termination issues clearly in focus for the therapist and for the group. Systematically implementing these techniques will provide a therapeutic frame within which termination can be effectively used as a major component of the time-limited experience. There has been increasing interest in the development of practice guidelines that outline basic therapeutic strategies. The format presented in this section can be seen in that light, as a protocol for the management of issues related to termination. Using a format such as this one ensures that termination is not avoided.

Termination is not, of course, a separate component divorced from the preceding group work. In truth, the ending provides an opportunity to pull together the entire therapeutic experience. To be effective, the therapist must address the termination process as a serious task, not a trivial saying of good-byes and a hug. Above all, an empathic attunement with the deeper levels of distress that may be elicited during termination is important. The issues inherent in the termination task address universal human fears and challenges directly connected to a sense of personal responsibility and competency.

In groups, unlike in individual therapy, termination can occur in two ways: the ending of the entire group at once or the termination of an individual member within an ongoing group. These two situations call for different strategies and will therefore be discussed separately, though many themes are common to both.

Termination of the Entire Group

The most common setting for entire-group termination is with closed time-limited groups. In such groups the question of termination is determined in advance. The entire group experience is therefore conducted with the knowledge of exactly how much time remains. Time-limited group psychotherapy utilizes many techniques in common with group psychotherapy in general. Its uniqueness lies in the purposeful use of time to accelerate and concentrate the therapeutic process. Members have the opportunity of pacing their psychological work within this time frame. The group process can be concentrated on fundamental themes elicited by the knowledge that the duration of therapy is finite. The group format provides an opportunity for the members to address such termination issues collectively. The key sequence of management strategies is presented in Table 10–1. (Note that the first three strategies begin before the group starts.)

Considering Selection and Composition Issues

Members are chosen for their capacity to use the time format selected. In practice, this means identifying those patients who clearly require longer-term treatment, usually on the basis of major dysfunctional personality problems or a chronic clinical course. Others are best managed in a time-limited group format.

Using a Closed-Group Format

Setting the termination date in advance has the major advantage of ensuring that time is available to deal with the issues involved in endings. The closed-group format is the simplest way of structuring time boundaries. Because the whole group goes through the process together, the termination focus is intensified. This increased attention to termination builds in the opportunity to use termination themes to maximum therapeutic advantage. Therapists who shrink from making a hard decision about termination might consider the roots of their resistance. The psychotherapy dose-response

---

Table 10–1.   Termination strategies

---

1. Considering selection and composition issues
2. Using a closed-group format
3. Clarifying time boundaries
4. Reinforcing the time frame
5. Focusing activity by therapist
6. Predicting premature termination
7. Addressing termination themes
   Deprivation
   Resentment and anger
   Rejection
   Grief and loss
   Responsibility for self
8. Managing the final session
9. Scheduling the follow-up visit

---

relationship graphically represented in Figure 1–1 (see Chapter 1) clearly demonstrates that the great majority of patients benefit adequately from a few months of treatment. Those who need more can be referred for longer-term work after a time-limited group experience. The time-limited group serves as an opportunity for the therapist and patient to assess whether more treatment is required.

Clarifying Time Boundaries

The time frame of the group is specifically and clearly addressed during the assessment and preparation process, preferably with a written description of the group format that contains the date of the first session, the total number of sessions, the exact duration time of each session, and the date of the final session. Members also are informed that a follow-up meeting will be scheduled approximately 4 to 6 months after the final session and are encouraged to refrain from seeking further treatment during that time period. This attention to detail might seem at first glance to be excessive. However, it is important that there be no ambiguity regarding the dimension of time.

Sometimes longer-term groups with a gradual turnover of membership suffer gradual attrition and sort of fade away until there are not enough members to make it worthwhile to continue. This process should be forestalled whenever possible. This might entail initiating a detailed discussion about termination when the membership begins to shrink. For example, a group of eight members may face the prospect of the loss of two members, plus some questioning comments from another one or two about when they also should end their treatment. This would be an appropriate time to have a serious discussion about where members stand in relationship to the issues that brought them to group and what their sense is of how much more time would be required to address these issues. It could be mentioned that if several members do decide to leave there will be a major shift in the group as new people are introduced. The members should be given the opportunity to consider the option of everyone ending the group together, rather than facing the disruption of incorporating new members.

Such a discussion might crystallize a decision to end together, or at the very least stimulate some serious thought about the progress of treatment to date. If the decision is to proceed, then there would be some advantages of clustering the departures onto a specific target date. That way, the group could deal in a systematic way with the issues raised. When the time comes to end the entire group, it is useful to establish the date 2 or 3 months in advance. This provides the opportunity to deal effectively with termination issues.

Reinforcing the Time Frame

Most time-limited groups run for 3 to 6 months. No specific mention is made of the time line during the first half of the group's life, because this would interfere unnecessarily with the development of group engagement. At the halfway point, say session 8 of a 16-session group, the therapist makes a clear statement that the group has reached the midpoint and that 8 sessions remain, with the therapist specifying the date of the last session. The therapist reminds the group of this clearly and firmly and suggests that the group members take the opportunity of this middle session to review the course of their personal work to date. They are encouraged to describe their present sense of where they stand on issues that were initially considered important. Often, members use the session to recalibrate their therapeutic goals in view of their original objectives and what has transpired since the group began. If written goals or focus areas were developed during the assessment, they can be redistributed at this session. A review of these might fill the entire session. This task reinforces the realization that the clock is ticking.

Following the midpoint time marker, an opportunity is found at each succeeding session to make reference to the session number, the number of sessions remaining, or the date of the last session. Often, this will be done by the members themselves. Thus, a clear focus on impending termination is established from the midpoint onward. Time-limited groups therefore spend the first half of their time becoming a working group and the last half with the implications of termination always present. This provides a sense of urgency and immediacy to the therapeutic process.

For longer-term groups, once the termination date has been set, the same policy of regular reference to the date should be followed at each session during the last 2 or 3 months.

Focusing Activity by Therapist

Throughout the course of group psychotherapy, active application of group work to outside circumstances is encouraged. This comes even more directly into focus in the later sessions, when therapist activity may actually increase somewhat. The real-life application process may be enhanced by reviewing ideas from the relapse prevention literature discussed in the preceding chapter concerning lifestyle issues and high-risk situations. It is important that the group have an opportunity for specific discussion of how members imagine they will manage without the group.

Another ongoing component of the termination process is for the therapist to encourage internalization of the therapy experience. The intention is to fix group learning experiences clearly in memory as reference points to use in postgroup situations. This can be done through reference to specific critical incidents, particularly emotionally laden situations, and how they were resolved. Much of the work of historical integration of the group experience is likely to be done by the group, with the therapist being prepared to underline and punctuate the material. Members are actively encouraged to think of what the group would say when they find themselves in a critical situation. These statements often involve attending to relationship dimensions such as assertiveness, clarifying their own emotional state, or simply participating in open discussion to clarify issues.

Every group will experience attempts to avoid termination. During the later sessions, and increasingly during the last four sessions, the therapist should be alert to subtle evidence of termination anxiety. Such anxiety may be lurking under the surface in discussions about managing without important others or about dealing with loss or separation. A major therapeutic task is to ensure that the group deals directly with such material. Consequently, the therapist needs to be prepared to be relatively active if necessary. If the group is proceeding on its own to address these matters, then the therapist is able to sit back and let the group accomplish the termination tasks. In most circumstances, modest therapist activity is indicated. This does not mean, however, that the therapist controls the group process. The function is one of maintaining a thematic focus and encouraging broad participation toward this focus from all group members. Much of this work can be done by simple reinforcement or minor encouragement.

It is common for therapists to resist an open discussion of termination. There may be apprehension about how members will react. Will they be demoralized? angry? blaming? Will they demand more? An insecure clinician is open to such perceived threats. Often, the idea of termination activates guilt that more is not being provided, that the therapist is somehow failing in the task. The therapist may have a vulnerable area regarding endings. This vulnerability may be the other side of a pressing need to provide ever more for the patients. If termination routinely brings anxiety or is repetitively avoided, the personal issues of the clinician may need to be addressed.

It is a major therapeutic error not to address termination material. Any tendency to collude with patient resistance must be carefully avoided. Therefore, the therapist must be comfortable with wading into powerful and evocative areas. Such exploration, though inevitably inviting criticism and evoking anger toward the therapist, is an important part of working through the issues raised. It is for this reason that the therapist needs a positive attitudinal posture toward the implications of time. The therapist may hesitate somewhat about delving into powerful new material at a late point in the group's life. However, the awareness of time and existential pressures may elicit important work from members who have become stuck. This evidence of hard work may tempt the therapist to extend the number of sessions, but this temptation must absolutely be resisted. Important work may continue up to the last minute of the last session, but not longer.

Predicting Premature Termination

At the fourth session from the end, the therapist introduces the idea of premature termination in a straightforward manner as follows. Reference is made to the date of termination. The rationale is presented that dealing openly and directly with the forthcoming end of the group may be uncomfortable or difficult. Sometimes the thought arises that it would be easier to simply stop before the final sessions. This impulse is seen as understandable. However, the group started together, has worked together, and it is important that it end together. "Has anybody indeed considered premature termination?" Bringing the topic directly into the open in this way is a useful preventive strategy. Most groups have some members who have wondered about this way of avoiding the end. The ensuing discussion usually results in a constructive review concerning termination matters and clearly marks the beginning of the final phase of the termination process. The group can be encouraged to take time to discuss such material. This simple strategy of formally predicting premature termination also ensures that the therapist does not avoid the impending end of the group. The remaining sessions are viewed primarily through the lens of termination.

Addressing Termination Themes

The most important task of termination involves the exploration of several strategically important termination themes. These themes will arise in most termination circumstances but are particularly powerful when a cohesive interactive group environment has been created. Note that this material will be found, and should be addressed, in both supportive and exploratory groups. The therapist should assume that such material will be implicit in the members' reactions to the impending termination, even if not put directly into words. The therapist's task is to ensure that all of the themes are verbalized and confronted, and therefore the therapist must be prepared to be active in directing attention to them.

Deprivation.   Early termination work often centers on the belief that not enough time is available and that the members have not gotten as much as they would like from the treatment program. This theme of deprivation is often introduced with an affect of sadness or hopelessness. It can be helpful to label this affect as *sadness*, not depression, to emphasize the understandable connections to ending. The group may move into strong universalization mechanisms with this material, a temporary regression in level of group functioning. This group-level regression may take the form of requests for additional sessions or private interviews or advice about finding other therapists. It is useful to promote this resurgence of group cohesiveness as a counterbalance to the disintegrating forces of termination. In this way, the group is presented with the paradoxical situation of becoming closer as they discuss separation.

The theme of deprivation may have important historical connections for members. This theme often entails the belief that they received inadequate or damaging parenting. The process of becoming a full member of a cohesive group provides a symbolic replacement for this sense of inadequacy of nurturing figures. The ending of the group is seen as the therapist's replicating the experience of deprivation. This situation may activate themes of abandonment, and the member may experience the ending with a deep sense of disappointment, and even despair, at again not getting enough nurturance. "How can I be whole now, since I received so little then?" Patients may find themselves sobbing deeply when the therapist comments on "appreciating the sense of not having gotten enough of what one wished for as a child." Tolerating this affective experience in the understanding environment of the group can be an important step in mastering the nihilistic personal expectations that may accompany it.

Resentment and anger.   The theme of deprivation brings with it undercurrents of resentment and anger. For example, "If they didn't have these strict rules about service limits . . ." or "I suppose you always herd patients through these groups so quickly" or "I have been thinking about finding an individual therapist this week." The therapist needs to be attentive to the theme and feel confident in bringing it into a discussion of *the present* group and *the present* therapist. Once again, the principal therapeutic guideline is to tolerate, accept, and encourage such ideas. The angry underside of the theme of deprivation brings with it energy and constructive possibilities, which almost inevitably lead to a more balanced view of the importance of continuing after termination the personal work begun in the group. The therapist may indeed be quite explicit that such is anticipated and that most patients routinely continue the work.

Rejection.   Within the deprivation material, there may also be an important subtheme of rejection. Often, this sense of rejection is directed at a core sense of unworthiness. "I am always rejected [in friendships, marriage, work, social organizations] because of the sort of person I am." This powerful core belief may have a major role in distorting all aspects of interpersonal adaptation. It is important that the sense of rejection be clearly expressed in the group and that responses from others be solicited. Such statements should never be allowed to go without a response before the session ends. Often, connections can be made to the issues identified at the beginning of the group as being important goals. For example, difficulty with low self-esteem and a pattern of being exploited in relationships may be connected to the childhood fear of total abandonment if any word of disagreement or complaint were uttered.

The most effective therapeutic strategy for dealing with concerns about inadequate time is simply to accept that the members are experiencing difficult reactions to the impending end of the group. A simple, matter-of-fact reconfirmation about the duration of the group may be made. It may also be useful to draw the analogy between the sense of not having gotten enough out of the group and one's living with the idea of not having gotten enough out of life. Such statements addressed to the whole group may assist in building the momentum to address such themes. The philosophical attitude toward the importance of time described earlier in this chapter may be of value to the therapist at this point. It is important that the therapist not demonstrate, verbally or nonverbally, any sense of guilt or apology that more time is not available. A steady course is best that reaffirms that the group is talking about important experiences even though relatively little time remains.

Grief and loss.   Another powerful theme inherent in the termination process is that of loss. The ending of the group may be experienced as analogous to earlier loss and grief, and it is common for distant losses to again come into awareness. When this occurs, areas of unresolved grieving may open. It is an opportunity to speak unspoken last words that often contain the same ambivalent mixture of sadness and resentment that is being experienced in the group itself. At first, one might be reluctant to address new material of this nature with only a small number of sessions remaining. However, the force of the group atmosphere encourages discussion of such material, which in some cases is being openly expressed for the first time. The opportunity of expressing this grief in the public arena of the group and of receiving an understanding and encouraging response helps to facilitate a sense of personal mastery over the historic situation.

Example

A 16-session intensive interpersonal group was near termination. One member, a 45-year-old woman, had done important work on issues relating to self-esteem and the impact of this on her relationships with men. Three sessions from the end she reported having had a powerful and unsettling dream about her mother. Her mother had died when the patient was 16, and her death left the patient feeling undefended to manage with an alcoholic and abusive father. The patient saw her mother in an idealized manner, and since her mother's death she had lived with the idea that she could never really cope—an image personified in the use of a little girl's voice and mannerisms. The topic of her mother's death had never been openly discussed with anyone even though it was an almost daily thought. Over the next two sessions, the patient became aware of her ambivalence at her mother's inability to provide a more secure environment and her insistence on staying with her husband even though there was constant turmoil around his drinking. The patient had never dared to think such thoughts because it might mean having to give up her positive image of her mother, which was a major support whenever she became depressed. Before the last session, she went to her mother's grave, at the urging of the group, and spent a couple of hours talking to her mother. This experience was a powerful one, and she reported that a great weight had been lifted. At 4-month follow-up, she reported that her chronic sense of depression was gone and that the grieving process of the last few sessions had been the most important aspect of the group experience for her. The therapist's opinion was that involvement in a cohesive and understanding group had made it possible for her finally to address the maternal issues.

Responsibility for self.   A final common theme of termination centers on the necessity of managing for oneself, which constitutes a powerful existential message (78). The therapist may reinforce this experience by actively pursuing what it will be like not to have the group to attend in future weeks. This approach dovetails nicely with the material on relapse prevention discussed earlier in this chapter ("How I can become my own therapist"). The therapist might inform the group that most patients find that they make further gains during the months after the group ends. However, the therapist should not attempt to palliate termination themes by repeatedly referring to the planned follow-up session.

It will be clear at this point that all of these themes have a direct connection with self-esteem. By forcing an open discussion of this material, the therapist also forces an examination of attitudes toward self. These connections need to be reinforced by the therapist if they are not expressed directly and clearly. The intent of this focusing strategy is to promote an increased sense of self-efficacy. The time limit of the group provides an opportunity to directly challenge negative beliefs. The implicit message is that the therapist and the group anticipate that the members will manage and will continue to accomplish further self-improvement goals.

Managing the Final Session

The last session always seems to begin with new and important material. The therapist must avoid the temptation to pursue this material. Making a virtue out of necessity, one might say, for example, "It sounds like you are beginning to focus on some important issues to work on over the next few months." The final session returns to a modest degree of structure. This might be outlined in the next-to-final session so the members can give it some thought. The format of the last session is similar to that of the first session, in which members were asked to make an extended opening statement regarding the issues that emerged as critical for them during the assessment process. The impact of the ending will be strongest for groups that have achieved higher levels of interaction and cohesion. The following format may be abbreviated for groups that have had a less interactive focus. However, remember that it is easy to underestimate how much the group experience means to people, so it is important to be sure to test the depth of these responses.

Most of the final session is devoted to a systematic go-around in which each member speaks directly to each other member. For a group of eight members, this usually requires at the very least 45 to 50 minutes. The therapist always feels in a bind in regard to timing. One needs to make sure that there is sufficient time to accomplish the go-around. On the other hand, it is helpful not to finish the task with too much time remaining in the session. In general, allowing a good 5 minutes for each member seems about right. If the process ends up taking longer than anticipated, this is one occasion when the time boundary may be slightly extended.

Members are encouraged to view the go-around as an opportunity to say things they would like to have said to each other but had not had the opportunity to say. Identifying specific critical events between themselves and another member is common. Specific use of the word or phrases "good-bye," "the end," and "it's over," as well as statements such as "I shall miss seeing you" and "Next Wednesday will seem empty," is encouraged. This process is clearly analogous to expressing final words to a deceased loved one.

The group process for this final go-around focuses on one member at a time. The sequence of participation is left up to the members. The members are encouraged to view the go-around as a serious opportunity to deal with the process of separation and to bring to a firm conclusion the various relationships that have been developed in the group. This exercise virtually always results in powerful reinforcement of the importance of the group and functions as a support for self-esteem. At the same time, the structure helps to contain and channel the level of expressed affect.

The members' comments often pertain to how another member served as an important model or an inspiration to try something new. Often, advice that was helpful is recalled—a reminder that therapy groups are filled with ideas, suggestions, and advice whether or not the therapist thinks this is a good idea. In many cases, specific critical incidents in the group's life are reviewed. The review may center on an experience of confrontation or anger that was worked through. The members may refer to powerful bonding experiences that took place early in the group. Members often talk of their hope for other members' progress when there is mention of issues yet to be addressed. This reinforces effectively the idea of continuing personal psychological work after the group ends.

Generally, the therapist is included in these comments. The therapist here experiences the same sense of mild apprehension and careful listening that each member has experienced when specifically addressed by the others. As a general practice, it is best for the therapist to avoid making specific comments to each member. Doing so would invite highly sensitive comparative evaluations that are unnecessary. The therapist would be better advised to make general supportive and empathic comments to the whole group. It is useful to be sure to position oneself so that a final good-bye can be given to each member as he or she departs. A handshake or a hug is a social symbol of termination.

It is common during the last few sessions for members to talk of reunions. Often, phone numbers are exchanged and tentative plans put in place. In general, such efforts do not come to fruition. Because the therapist has no power, or right, to restrict what happens after the group ends, such plans are best treated with benign neglect. "I have no opinion on the subject." A discussion of the possible pros and cons might be helpful. The focus continues on addressing termination issues in the belief that if these are adequately worked through, the need for maintaining the illusion of the group will automatically subside. During the follow-up meeting described below, an effort is made to determine what contacts have actually taken place. These contacts are usually restricted to a few phone conversations or a single dinner together that lacked much enthusiasm.

At the very end of the final session, the members are reminded that they will be contacted for an individual follow-up visit in about 4 months. They are encouraged to use the intervening time to continue their work begun in the group and not seek further active treatment. The follow-up visit is described simply as an opportunity to see how things are going and to check if anything further is required. Although not specifically put into words, one purpose of this visit clearly is to provide an inducement for members to continue working on issues raised in the group so that the therapist can appreciate their capacity to achieve further progress.

Scheduling the Follow-Up Visit

The decision to conduct the follow-up visit 4 months after termination is based on the outcome literature, which indicates that improvement following psychotherapy continues at a substantial rate for several months. The 4-month visit is designed to catch this process at its peak. Some programs utilize a group format for this follow-up contact. However, an individual visit avoids fostering the idea of the continued existence of the group that might undermine the termination message.

The follow-up visit is not defined as, or conducted as, a formal therapy session. The visit begins with a general discussion of how the patient has been managing in the 4 months since the group ended. This material is reviewed in terms of the issues raised as objectives before therapy began and in the light of learning experiences during the group. The visit is also an opportunity to repeat any questionnaires that were administered at the beginning of therapy. A generally cognitive stance is maintained. It is useful to reinforce those areas of accomplishment that the patient may underplay. Often, the therapist will be able to note shifts in self-esteem or relationship dimensions that the patient has not quite appreciated. Areas that continue to be problematic can be reviewed in a brief fashion to clarify what they entail. The general approach is to foster an attitude of self-sufficiency. On occasion, significant difficulties require referral for further formal treatment, though further treatment is not commonly needed. It is more likely that the patient will return 1 or 2 years later, often with quite a new set of issues to address.

Termination of an Individual Member

Planned Terminations

The termination of a single member from an ongoing group has quite different dynamics. The ideal circumstances for termination of an individual member would be a considered decision that goals have been accomplished, with adequate forewarning of the decision, and the opportunity to deal with termination themes over at least a minimum of four sessions (79). With this scenario, the protocol for entire-group termination can be more or less followed. The number of remaining sessions should be monitored and not allowed to go unnoticed. Issues involved in application of group learning to outside life, including life without the group, would be relevant. Themes of grief and responsibility for self are likely to have the highest profile. It is important that the individual who is leaving directly address the process of saying good-bye. Prediction of the temptation to end prematurely should be mentioned. For many patients with attachment difficulties, the termination process constitutes a consolidation of mastery over the fears concerning individuation. A final go-around with the terminating member—both to and from each member—would be appropriate. A general goal is to imbue the termination process with energy and affect, not to let it slip quietly by.

The next few sessions of the continuing members are often haunted by the ghost of the departed member(s). There may be themes of envy about the "successful" one who "graduated." Some members will experience guilt that they had not said something or that they had done something they regret regarding the departed member. Members may experience elements of shame that either oneself, or the group, has not been more effective in reaching the goals of recovery. Previous intragroup tensions may again surface as the group adapts to the change. The next few sessions should therefore continue to be viewed through the lens of termination adjustment. It is useful to wait for three or four sessions before refilling the empty chair to provide time for an exploration of such topics.

Unpredicted Terminations

Many terminations do not occur under the ideal circumstances described above. Sometimes patients in longer-term groups will simply announce, often near the end of a session, that they have been thinking of ending for some time and that this will be their last session. This usually reflects the activation of some important issue for them, often reflecting larger group issues. The emergency strategy is to buy time to allow further exploration. One useful approach is for the therapist to make it clear to the patient that her decision to end is indeed entirely up to her and that the therapist will accept the patient's final conclusion. However, if the individual has been a member for some time, a statement like the following would be appropriate: "It is important to talk about termination and for the other group members to have a chance to participate in this. Remember the struggles to become part of the group. It's just as important to give equal effort to leaving it. Could this be a major agenda item for the next session?" If the member has truly been a participating member of the group, it is reasonable to use as much pressure as one can to engineer at least a good-bye session. Note, however, that patients who drop out without notice early in the group usually do not fit this requirement and are probably best left to go their way with some mediating rationale from the therapist, as discussed in Chapter 7.

A member may decide to leave because of some specific negative event in the group. The reason to leave in these circumstances usually centers on anger or confrontation or may involve a sense of not being heard or accepted. Such situations need to be addressed immediately and vigorously because they predict negative or damaging effects for the individual and a possible drop in cohesion for the group.

The thought of losing a member will activate fears in other members regarding the instability of the group, and of life, and often results in important group work.

The most common themes behind an impulsive decision to leave are the threat of increasing intimacy in the group, the challenge of dealing with a more confrontational group atmosphere, and apprehension about directly confronting termination. Better to simply leave and not court the risk of being left by others. Not uncommonly, the member talking of leaving is in fact voicing a common group resistance to such themes. The therapist's goal is to promote a general exploration of members' reactions. Such exploration may represent a critical juncture in the group and result in more intense work. Usually, group members can mount more telling arguments to discourage termination than can the therapist. This process may result in a surge of cohesion in the group. If the member does indeed decide to terminate, if at all possible, a final session could be selected in a few weeks, which enables the member and group to deal with issues of termination. Often, these last few sessions are filled with important work driven by the impending termination point.

There is some merit to having periodic reviews within the group (e.g., every 6 months in longer-term therapy) concerning where people see themselves in their therapeutic course. Such reviews can be introduced as a routine checkpoint for refocusing and, it should be stressed to patients, do not imply that termination is warranted or expected. Inevitably, some patients will find themselves experiencing a shift in the balance toward primarily supportive reasons for staying in the group and away from change-inducing personal work. This review procedure can be helpful in keeping the group work vital and relevant.

Much of the group literature regarding termination has focused primarily on how to make a decision to terminate an individual patient in an ongoing therapy group. Foulkes suggests that therapists tend to err on the side of too-much rather than too-little therapy (80). He describes critical points at which termination for an individual in a group may be appropriate: often first occurring at about the 6-month point, then a year later, and then at increasingly longer intervals. This pattern, by the way, corresponds fairly closely with the psychotherapy dose-response relationship depicted graphically in Figure 1–1 (see Chapter 1).

The general goal would be to seek to achieve maximum improvement from therapy, although this could be reframed as maximum improvement *given the capacity of the patient to change*. Criteria for determining the timing of termination involve achievement of the original goals (as defined by the patient) and accomplishment of theoretical tasks such as "attainment of object constancy" (as defined by the therapist). On both sides, there is room for considerable ambiguity regarding when such achievements have been met.

There is some value in carefully considering outcome status in terms of how well the individual is managing outside of the group by considering the following five levels of functioning:

1. *Social functioning.* At the most general level, is the patient able to manage basic social tasks such as attending school or work, participating in usual social activities such as shopping and traveling, and being a functional member of the community?
2. *General relationships.* Is the patient able to adequately manage general social relationships with friends and acquaintances?
3. *Intimate relationships.* Is the patient able to tolerate and maintain intimate relationships without enmeshed overinvolvement or excessive distancing? Has the patient developed the capacity to resolve differences or disagreements and to tolerate closeness without high levels of control or submission? Can the patient experience and demonstrate an empathic response to others? Is the patient able to be affectively open and not excessively defensive, allowing himself to be moderately vulnerable in close relationships? Can a range of responses to others, with both positive and negative components, be tolerated?
4. *Self.* Can the patient demonstrate reasonable control over emotional responses and mediate them from a rational perspective? Can a basically positive attitude toward self be maintained, including a sense of a coherent self-image and nonintrusive levels of dissociation or denial?
5. *Symptoms.* Are specific symptoms such as anxiety or depression reduced? To what extent do they interfere with desired activities or accomplishments?

CHAPTER 11

Therapist Style and Technique

*T*his chapter provides an integration of ideas concerning effective therapeutic style and technique. Also addressed is the role of the leader. Many of the examples provided elsewhere in the book have applied parts of this material.

The Supportive-Interpretive Continuum

An approach to psychotherapy can be conceptualized as lying on a continuum extending from highly supportive to highly interpretive, though these terms are not entirely accurate (81). It is important that therapists understand where on this continuum to position themselves in terms of the needs of the patient population being treated. It would be more realistic to reframe this as what mix of supportive and interpretive strategies is best used at a particular point in time. The tasks of the generic model can be addressed with any combination of strategies. The difference in the mix would be identified by the nature of Therapist Intervention in Therapeutic Operations. In the generic model, it is specified only that the interventions must be of a nature to elicit a response of patient cooperation and foster a positive Therapeutic Bond.

There is a common misunderstanding that supportive therapy is only for the severely dysfunctional patient. Nothing could be further from the truth. Indeed, there has been increasing interest in a supportive model for individual psychotherapy. Some have argued that the "default" mode should be that of well-informed supportive techniques and that the use of an abstinent therapist stance and intrapsychic interpretations should be restricted to those patients for whom it is specifically indicated (82). Certainly, when dealing with patient populations that have lower interpersonal capacity, the use of supportive techniques is essential as a starting point. Because this is such a central concept in determining therapeutic positioning, the principal features by which the supportive model and the interpretive model can be compared are listed below. It should be noted that both models apply an interpersonal/psychodynamic understanding of the patient. The difference between the two models lies in how this perspective is utilized. These points of comparison also highlight the fact that the very terms "supportive" and "interpretive" do not really capture the essence of the two approaches.

1.   *The Therapeutic Bond.* The Therapeutic Bond is of central importance in both the supportive model and the interpretive model.
2.   *Degree of neutrality.* In the supportive model, the therapist is no more neutral than is necessary, feeling free to express acceptance, liking, and respect for the patient. In the interpretive model, the therapist gives up only as much neutrality as is necessary to maintain the Therapeutic Bond.
3.   *Therapist style.* A conversational style is utilized in the supportive model. The therapist is responsive in a professional manner, but a real relationship is acknowledged. Therapy is not a casual conversation, but silence and nonresponse do not occur. In the interpretive model, the therapist maintains a restrained position to the extent possible.
4.   *Goal-directedness.* In the supportive model, the conversation is goal-directed. In the interpretive model, the free flow of associative material is encouraged, and no preset message is delivered.
5.   *Therapeutic focus.* In the supportive model, there is a focus on identifying and describing patterns at a behavioral, cognitive, or interpersonal level so that they can be modified. In the interpretive model, greater emphasis is placed on affective experience and interpretations linking internal conflict between wishes and fears with current anxiety and early experiences.
6.   *Approach to self-esteem.* In the supportive model, direct efforts are made to enhance self-esteem. Encouragement, recognition of progress, instilling of hope, and praise might be used. In the interpretive model, self-esteem is expected to improve as a by-product of better functioning and symptom reduction.

7. *Approach to anxiety.* In the supportive model, therapy-related anxiety is avoided and addressed immediately if it emerges as a by-product of psychological work. In the interpretive model, the more abstinent stance is expected to increase therapy-related anxiety, which will be directly treated only if it becomes disruptive.

8. *Approach to defenses.* In the supportive model, defenses are supported unless they are distinctly maladaptive. In the interpretive model, gaining an understanding of defenses and of the need for them is a central task.

9. *Therapist techniques.* Focusing, reframing, clarifying, and challenging are used in *both* models. In the supportive model, the therapist supports strengths and tries to maximize autonomy. Use may be made of suggestions, environmental interventions, and reassurance. In the interpretive model, such techniques are not used.

10. *Transference.* In the supportive model, negative transference is examined if it is interfering with progress, but positive transference is not discussed. In the interpretive model, all aspects of transference are actively explored.

These 10 distinguishing features can be applied to group psychotherapy as well. However, some interesting differences between group and individual psychotherapy emerge with respect to these key features. For most of the items, groups provide a healthy dose of the supportive model whether or not the therapist desires it. The Therapeutic Bond, as reflected in group cohesion, is a central feature of groups (no. 1). Members are certainly not neutral toward each other (no. 2). A conversational model and real relationships are inevitable (no. 3). Conversation tends to be quite goal-directed as members strive to help each other (no. 4). The nature of the therapeutic focus (no. 5) is a technical dimension under greater therapist control. Efforts to enhance self-esteem are in constant evidence (no. 6). Therapy-related anxiety (no. 7) and challenge of defenses (no. 8) are prevalent in group interaction but can be dampened by the leader if desired. There are usually strong efforts to support strengths (no. 9). The management of transference (no. 10), like the nature of the therapeutic focus, is a technical dimension under greater therapist control.

So an interactional group, no matter what the theoretical stance of the leader, is bound to be heavily loaded with supportive qualities. The leader using interpretive techniques may need to be careful not to interfere with the supportive elements and shut down the group process. The therapist must be particularly careful not to do this during the engagement stage, when the supportive cluster of therapeutic factors is an essential feature.

Treatment Manuals

The term *protocol* has been used a number of times in this book, particularly in chapters dealing with assessment, establishment of a treatment focus, and initiation and termination of the group. This is in keeping with the increasing use of treatment manuals for training purposes (83). Clinicians trained in behavioral and cognitive treatment will be familiar with this approach. Manuals are also available for some kinds of interpersonal psychotherapy and for several models of short-term dynamic psychotherapy. Fewer manuals are available for group treatments (84). The best known is that developed by Piper for patients experiencing a prolonged maladaptive reaction to person loss. Piper's manual is based on psychodynamic principles and emphasizes group-as-a-whole interventions.

Many people picture a treatment manual as being a cookbook compilation of specific do's and don't's. This is not the case. Effective manuals lay out treatment strategies in general terms. Most, in fact, read like a good, though succinct, textbook. The manuals identify important issues to be systematically addressed. Most leave the clinician plenty of scope for individualizing the technical application.

There is a perfectly valid reason for the development of manuals. A clinician's theoretical orientation does not predict what that person actually does in a treatment context. Treatment outcome is predicted not by theoretical orientation, but by actual clinical behavior. Therapists who have been trained according to manuals achieve higher levels of technical proficiency and predictability. They are able to provide more consistent structure, explicitness, and organization to their therapeutic work.

The downside of the use of manuals is that there is a risk that the guidelines may be applied rigidly without allowance for unique problems with a specific patient and perhaps with some loss of spontaneity. Some reports have suggested that the use of manuals interferes with a need to establish a good working relationship. In most cases, these potential problems represent poor application of clinical judgment, not necessarily the effects of manuals per se.

Characteristics of Leader Style

A number of general therapist characteristics and techniques have been well described in the individual psychotherapy literature and apply equally well to group psychotherapy (85).

Caring and Support

One of the most critical therapist attributes is a basic attitude of positive regard and concern toward patients. This theme has consistently been identified since early on in the psychotherapy literature as a necessary condition for effective therapy. It is directly connected to the development of the Therapeutic Bond described in Chapter 2 as well as to most other aspects of therapist involvement in the generic model. This basic relationship attitude does not imply giving in to all patient demands or approving of all patient behavior. It does embody a central ethic of the helping professions that their function is to support mastery, not judge deficiencies.

Carl Rogers considered several components to be both necessary and sufficient for effective therapy (86). Contemporary research has confirmed that these therapist ingredients are very important in establishing a working environment, but also has found that additional factors of technique need to be considered. The basic components for effective therapy identified by Rogers are

1. *Nonpossessive warmth.* The therapist maintains a caring attitude that is not controlling. It is somewhat paradoxical that the caricature of the Rogerian therapist is one who exudes a "taking care of" attitude.
2. *Accurate empathy.* The therapist attempts to understand how the patient sees his personal and interpersonal world so that the therapist is able to predict how the patient is likely to view events. Accurate empathy is an important part of the Therapeutic Operations loop. The term does not imply agreement, or even a feeling of kinship. Such responses would be better termed sympathy.
3. *Genuineness.* The therapist acts as a real person responding in a personal fashion with some degree of spontaneity. This quality is connected with therapist Self-Relatedness. It does not preclude the therapist's using clinical judgment to filter the strength of responses.
4. *Unconditional positive regard.* The therapist maintains an attitude that the patient is attempting to cope as well as she can and that the patient's efforts therefore should be seen as adaptive even if misguided. The therapist is seen as aligning with the patient against the psychopathology.

Cognitive Understanding

Another broad area of therapist responsibility is to promote an understanding of the problematic behavior in the patient. This refers to a general quality of understanding the rationale for difficulties and for the methods proposed to deal with them. Conveying such an understanding is important in all types of therapy as part of the Therapeutic Operations. Some studies suggest that the content of the proposed rationale is less important than the fact that there is one. A framework for understanding permits a sense of cognitive mastery over the situation.

This focus on the cognitive dimension of therapy is an important and pervasive therapist activity that has been found to correlate with positive outcome. Much of the material in Chapter 9 on interpersonal work deals with ways of establishing a focus for addressing a cognitive understanding of patients' issues, as does the discussion of supportive psychotherapy in this chapter.

Process Control

The optimal degree of leader control over the group process will vary according to the goals of the group, the stage of group development, and the capabilities of the members. The most common problem is when the therapist either slips into a style of leadership that involves a greater degree of management than necessary or provides less control than is required to keep the group focused on its tasks. The challenge for the leader is to select the optimum amount of control of the group process for a particular group at a particular time.

Clinicians who adopt behavioral, cognitive, and other "action-oriented" perspectives see the therapist in the role of teacher or guide and use a lot of the supportive features discussed earlier in this chapter. Those using interpersonal/psychodynamic approaches tend to adopt a less active but more evocative and interpretive role, though there may be considerable variation, with greater use of supportive features on occasion. Clinical experience suggests that patients who are rated higher on the personality dimensions outlined in Chapter 4 (emotional reactivity [neuroticism]; conscientiousness [compulsivity]; openness, including psychological mindedness; quality of relationships; extraversion; agreeableness) do better with less leader control and that those who score lower do best with more control.

The role of the therapist in group psychotherapy is quite different from that in individual psychotherapy. In a group the therapist is not the main source of influence. Many more responses come from the members than from the leader. It is worth remembering that an interpretation is a move of power, implying "I know what you are thinking or experiencing." In groups the interpersonal process is less influenced by dominance issues from the leader and more influenced by group norms. The therapist can influence the nature of the therapeutic experience by promoting helpful interactions. By having faith in the resources of the group members, the therapist can promote intensive applied psychological learning.

Control may be exerted in many ways in psychotherapy groups. The most obvious way the therapist exerts control is by structuring group activities. For example, a specific task may be prescribed, such as a go-around of responses, role playing, psychodrama, or gestalt techniques. The use of homework tasks would also function as such a structuring activity. Less obvious control may be exerted by the therapist through a subtle molding of process events. For example, some therapists establish a style in which most patient statements are directed to the therapist and are answered by him or her. Thus, group communication channels are restricted. Control may also be exerted by the use of interpretive statements that serve to bring closure to an issue. Through the use of summarizing or absolute conclusions, the therapist may "put the lid on" further discussion.

All of these interventions may be quite correct in terms of the content expressed. However, the interpersonal process message is that the leader is in charge (and therefore the members are not). An overly active and controlling therapist produces passivity and submissiveness in group members. Members in this position not only are more likely to have lower levels of initiation in the group but also will approach their own personal problem resolution with a greater degree of passivity, expecting answers from the therapist. As a general principle, control over the group process by the therapist should be kept at the lowest level compatible with maintaining a functional group.

The effects of control follow a curvilinear model. Some degree of control stabilizes a group and provides a structure around which the group can function effectively. As the level of control increases, a point is reached where the control becomes an inhibiting and stultifying influence. When control is too low, the group fails to maintain a focus and may become demoralized. Control is most constructive when it is directed at creating conditions for the enactment of therapeutic factors and the maintenance of a task focus. More structure is appropriate when the interactional capacity of the group members is limited. As mentioned in Chapter 7, there is some evidence that a modest degree of structure in the early sessions may foster higher levels of group cohesion.

Problems will arise for therapists who consider the main therapeutic impact to reside primarily in their own efforts. These therapists are liable to interfere with the therapeutic power available from the group system. Frequent use of interpretive statements to individual members will move the group into a leader-oriented style in which each member strives to find "the answer" from the leader. Instead, a major function of the therapist is to constantly promote therapeutic events between the members, a field of action that offers infinitely more variability. The therapist must have faith in the resources of understanding available within the group membership. By fostering member-member interaction, the therapist is enhancing the opportunity of members to help each other and to practice applying new psychological learning in a real social situation.

Stimulation of Emotional Arousal

Some therapists are personally very involved in the group process. They use high levels of personal self-disclosure and process control and tend to be aggressively intrusive into patients' emotional lives. They exhort the members to open up like the leader is doing. These efforts act as a stimulant to high emotional arousal in the group. This constellation of features describes "charismatic leaders," who by the force of their personality and demanding techniques will pull people into their influence. As will be discussed later in this chapter, such techniques may have beneficial results for some patients but carry a greater risk of negative effects. Some members in such groups report that they regretted saying too much, or that they were attacked by the leader or by others acting under the leader's suggestion.

On the other hand, leaders with quite low levels of personal involvement tend to have groups that are flat and uninteresting to the members. There is little danger of overtly negative effects, but the overall outcome is less favorable because members are not pushed to their maximum involvement in group work.

Professional Image

Therapists who present a positive professional image tend to have fewer dropouts and better overall results. The ingredients that have been studied most extensively include perceived expertness, as shown by a sense of competency and knowledge; attractiveness, as evidenced by a warm interactional

style; and trustworthiness, as shown by sensible comments and maintenance of confidentiality. Not surprisingly, patients want therapists who are
professional and appear to know what they are doing. These findings also
suggest that therapists might refrain from trying to become too fraternal with
their patients; a degree of professional distance is helpful, not harmful.

Therapist Self-Disclosure

Another important aspect of therapist style, related to professional image,
is that of self-disclosure. For practical purposes, it is most useful to look at
self-disclosure in terms of two categories of information: revelation of personal information or beliefs, and responses to group events.

Patients may want to know about their therapists' personal lives but
in fact do not really expect that they will find out. Considerable personal
self-disclosure will blur the distinction between the role of Designated
Leader and that of group member. The role of Designated Leader provides
a symbolic figure with whom important psychotherapeutic work can occur. The therapist who abdicates this position deprives the group of these
experiences. Therapists who find themselves straying into personal self-
disclosure should question their motivations. Such material will probably
not be therapeutic and may represent an attempt to reject the responsibilities of leadership or avoid group processes such as therapist challenge.

An exception to the expression of personal material is some reference
to general human experiences that may serve to align the therapist with
patient experiences. These experiences may include adjustment to the
death of a parent, a sense of accomplishment at graduation, and the pride
and pleasure one might take in children. Such statements are testimonials
more to the human condition than to specific therapist experiences.

The issue of therapist self-disclosure in regard to events happening
within the group is more complex. Therapists must first bear in mind that
any statement they make that implies a personal response or evaluation of
group events will have a strong impact on the members. Therapists should
evaluate and screen the level of their responses before committing them to
words. An appropriate guideline is always to delay and dampen the level
of responses, knowing that they will be magnified in importance by the
members. This guideline is not intended to violate the idea of therapist
spontaneity or genuineness, but rather is intended only to monitor and use
this dimension therapeutically.

The therapist may specifically use statements of approval to reinforce group norms or to mold interactional style as part of a general supportive and encouraging approach. Such statements of therapist approval are more appropriate in groups with more socially dysfunctional members. The therapist must be careful to attend to all group members; overtly "playing favorites" can be harmful. Therapists may inadvertently give the appearance of favoritism in a subtle fashion if they become influenced by group dynamics that may promote or criticize the role of a particular member. Of course, members may develop ideas about preferential treatment that can provide a focus for useful therapeutic work.

Operant Conditioning and Modeling

In Chapter 3, the use of operant conditioning techniques and the modeling of desired behaviors were discussed. These influencing processes operate whether or not the therapist is specifically aware of them and play a significant role in shaping the group atmosphere. It is useful to try to bring them into full awareness. Members are acutely attuned to the nuances of therapist behavior. Glances toward or away, nods, aha's, approving chuckles—all will serve as effective reinforcers. A kicking foot, a clenched fist, and a fleeting look of concern will all register. An impassive face that reveals no reaction to group events models an inhibited affective style. Beginning therapists should pay close attention to these behavioral issues so that their behaviors can then be brought under conscious control and used systematically for their effects. This is not to deny spontaneity or to promote a highly manipulative approach; but the therapist must be prepared to apply clinical judgment in filtering responses in the service of therapeutic goals.

The therapist can effectively encourage an interactive group process, promote self-questioning, and focus issues through the subtle use of brief reinforcing interventions. Consider one-liners such as "Joan would understand that" "The same as Henry?" "That sounds important" "Can you say that again?" "Uh-huh" "Go on" "That theme seems to keep cropping up" "More negative expectations" and so on. Such "quiet" interventions are almost subliminal but serve to maintain the group action and gently keep it on track.

Use of Homework

One general task for the therapist is to systematically promote application of therapeutic work. Outcome is improved when group learning is actively applied to outside circumstances. Evidence that patients have been thinking between sessions about issues raised in therapy is a good prognostic sign. The importance of continuing group work throughout the week should be stressed beginning in pretherapy preparation and regularly throughout therapy. Many patients find it helpful to keep a daily journal with their ongoing thoughts about issues raised in the sessions. Often, this then becomes a habitual process that helps them to keep a watchful eye on their psychological state.

Therapeutic homework not only maintains the continuity of therapy but carries an implicit message that the patient must shoulder a portion of the therapeutic responsibility. Patients' claiming that they have no recall of a preceding session should be taken as clear and specific evidence of resistance and addressed as such. The therapist should note the issues involved in the "forgotten" episode and then watch for their reappearance in the present session. The issues in question will almost always reappear, and with their reappearance the hidden material will gradually become evident. This undramatic approach to the mysterious amnesia is usually more productive than exhortations to remember.

The general theme of applying group experiences and learning to outside situations applies to all types of groups. However, another category of homework relates to specific behavioral tasks. Different types of therapy may use homework in varying ways. Those with a strong behavioral component may incorporate homework assignments that are designed to address specific behaviors. Counting or recording specific behaviors in diaries almost always results in a marked drop in the frequency of those behaviors. Those with primarily a psychodynamic orientation will assign specific homework tasks that focus on critical intrapsychic issues or their interpersonal or behavioral consequences. For example, a man dealing with a prolonged grief reaction to the death of his father contracted with the group to go to his father's grave and speak the words he never had the chance to say. He returned the next session to report a poignant and healing experience.

It is useful to recall for the group from time to time that the purpose of therapy is not just for the patient to change *within* the sessions, although evidence of such change is usually a good sign. The purpose is also, and primarily, for the patient to alter outside relationships and circumstances. It is a fantasy born of resistance for patients to anticipate that they will get better during therapy and then change their behavior afterward. The process of applied change must begin promptly and regularly.

The therapist should monitor how patients apply group experiences outside the group. Unfortunate situations can occur if the patient attempts to apply group behaviors inappropriately. In general, psychotherapy groups deal with issues involved in close relationships, not necessarily those that pertain to the working place or an impersonal public setting. Patients may misjudge the timing of their application attempts and try out behaviors suitable for close relationships with their employer or neighbors, with unfortunate results.

Intervention Skills

Conducting group psychotherapy entails the development of an expanded repertoire of intervention skills. Much of this repertoire can be built on experience in individual psychotherapy. The major additional task is to learn to address aspects of the group system and not just individual members. In this way, therapy is conducted through the group process, and an expanded array of helpful experiences is made available. The use of interventions directed at a member that would work well in the individual therapy format may interfere with the development of the group culture.

Attention to Process

The therapist must strive to understand the interactional process going on in the group. This involves a constant struggle to avoid being caught up solely in the content of the material. At times, the therapist will be very much an interactional member of the group, but she must be able to back out of the group and view it as an observer. The therapist should make this shift every few minutes during a session so that it becomes second nature to think on a double-track system. The therapist is, at one level, attending to the words and the content themes and, at another level and at the same time, looking at the process through which the material is being presented or handled. Working at the latter level involves addressing the question "Why are these persons talking to each other in this fashion right now?" Systematically looking around the group at each member on a regular basis may trigger useful ideas about the meaning of the interaction. The therapist should give consideration to what is going on in the here and now of the group exchanges.

The leader is well advised to think constantly about four levels. First, the leader might practice thinking of the possible meaning of what is going on in terms of the whole group (Is one person expressing or containing group issues). Second, the leader needs to ascertain whether members are speaking as part of a subgroup. Third, the leader can reconceptualize the action in interpersonal terms (What has gone on between two members?). Finally, the leader can consider whether an intrapsychic focus is likely to be most relevant. Remember that moving to this level without considering the other three levels often means that group and interpersonal cues may be missed. Once a theme or issue is in focus for the therapist, it is wise to wait a bit. Often, a member will catch the same issue and the leader can simply reinforce what that member has to say. This approach is based on using the group interaction as the vehicle for change more than on making direct therapist interventions.

The therapist should resist the temptation to offer quick interpretive explanations. The initial task is to describe what is happening. For this purpose the use of a systematic approach is very helpful. The focus is less on the content of the material being discussed and more on the process between the members. The process often throws new light on the meaning of the content. In some ways it is easier to do this in groups than in individual therapy, because the therapist can back out of the action inconspicuously and watch how members are dealing with each other. Reviewing videotapes of sessions is a useful method for developing this perceptual skill.

Silence often descends on a psychotherapy group and may have many meanings. Some patients report that silence is comforting because it allows them time to be with their thoughts and apply what has been happening in the group to their own circumstances. Others experience silences as enormously anxiety producing. The therapist needs to make a decision as to whether the silence is a "working" silence or an "avoiding" silence. Generally, prolonged silences early in a group are nonproductive. They lead either to more resistance or to a sense of futility. Some therapist intervention is appropriate, even if only nonspecific ("It looks like people are lost in thought. Would anyone like to share those thoughts with the group?") or having only an implied connection ("We fell silent just as Ann was talking about her sense of disappointment about not getting more direction in the group. Is that something that's on other people's minds as well?").

In the more advanced group, silences may carry more specific messages. Often the silence in this context has to do with a state of resistance regarding the nature of issues being addressed. This resistance may take the form of anxiety about pursuing such topics or may reflect a stubborn quality of not responding to the leader's pursuit of sensitive matters. As with all states of resistance, these instances of silence are a good sign that important matters are under consideration. Sometimes it is useful to simply reflect, "I guess it's not easy tackling these issues that go way back." Generally, aligning techniques are most effective, especially when directed at what the members are experiencing in the silence. Apocryphal stories are told of entire sessions being spent in silence. Such circumstances may raise interesting theoretical questions, but they are not likely to be of enormous help to the members.

Clarification Versus Interpretation

One basic way of thinking about therapist interventions is to categorize them as involving primarily clarification or interpretation. Both approaches may be used to address focal issues. Clarification seeks more information about the issue or situation. Interpretation draws attention to some aspect of the situation and offers either a direct or an implicit opinion as to its meaning or significance. Both clarification and interpretation introduce a component of structure and control into the process by their focusing action. However, they differ in the way they do this (87).

The basic intent of clarification is to promote an opportunity for a response that is determined by the patient. This encourages patient autonomy and also promotes an alignment with the patient's inner world that enhances empathic bonds. By enabling more information to be generated, clarification allows situations to be understood in more complex ways. In Chapter 9, the mechanisms of self-disclosure and interpersonal feedback were described. In a group situation, these interactional processes allow enormous scope for effective use of clarification questions. When properly applied, clarification leads to more effective conflict resolution. "I may not entirely agree, but at least I understand your situation better." The therapist does not need to feel compelled to come up with accurate interpretations that will produce immediate insight. By massaging the interaction with clarification questions, the therapist promotes the interpersonal learning cycle.

The goals of interpretation are similar in nature to those of clarification. An opinion is offered to promote a new awareness and thus "confronts" the patient's existing understanding of self or situation with an alternative possibility. The interpretive process should not be seen as an adversarial process with an implied contest of wills. If it becomes that, it will usually fail in its intent. It is better to think of this process in a technical fashion as a way of opening new channels for thought. This approach is different from clarification because the answer is implied in the interpretive message. Thus, the patient is presented with the need to compare two viewpoints. This may make it easier to accept or reject the suggestion, rather than to explore the issue.

Recent studies in individual therapy suggest that interpretive techniques overall do not promote the therapeutic task as effectively as clarification. Interpretations that are given when the patient is in a closed-off state result in more defended responses, indicating closure on the subject. However, interpretive techniques do result in further exploration when the patient is already in an open and accessible state. In other words, when the patient is already searching for alternative explanations, interpretations are more likely to be constructively received. This attention to openness is in keeping with a long psychotherapeutic tradition that emphasizes the importance of timing in regard to interventions. The idea of looking for patient openness—or, in the language of the generic model, when the patient's state of Self-Relatedness is open—is a useful clinical guideline for judging when to use confrontations. Paying close attention to the immediate state of Self-Relatedness may save the therapist from getting caught in nonproductive efforts to hammer home a point when the patient is quite impervious to penetration. A judicious delay might be in order until a shift to openness is perceived.

Once the therapist has embarked on a given course of action, it is important that she stick with it unless it was clearly an error to have done so. In particular, if the intervention has touched an important and emotional issue for a member, that member should not be left hanging with the reaction. The therapist owes it to the patient to follow through. Therapy is a deadly serious business and not a place to throw out stray comments without being fully prepared to live with the consequences. If, on the other hand, the therapist's intervention emerges as not productive, she might as well acknowledge that to the group so they do not spend valuable time trying to live up to the therapist's expectations of what is important.

Whole-Group Interventions

The qualities of the group system have been referred to many times throughout the preceding chapters. Each developmental stage has characteristic themes and related emotional tone. The affective climate of the group will surge into strong patterns, perhaps covering several aspects of the spectrum within a single session. Sometimes the therapist only becomes aware of these swings because he reacts to them personally. As a guideline, any time the therapist feels a strong reaction to the group, it is helpful for him to take a deep breath or two and cognitively back out to consider what is happening within the group system. Bion's three "basic assumption" states, which were described in Chapter 9, may be reviewed. Is that group member who is doing all the talking speaking just for herself, or is she speaking a group message without perhaps even realizing it? What is the dominant interpersonal theme in the air? Can the group, or at least some of its members, be placed somewhere in the Structural Analysis of Social Behavior (SASB) space? Is the group split into two subgroups having different positions on the theme?

Once the therapist has a handle on a group quality, whether emotional in nature or thematic in content, he is in a position to consider a group-level intervention. "If I'm reading the situation right, it seems to me that there's a lot of sadness in the air today." "It sounds like Janet's talk of seeing herself as unworthy of anyone's attention is echoed in a lot of the members." "I wondered if the sense of not getting enough from parents might be connected in here with this being our third-from-the-last session."

It is useful here to recall the idea of a group system. If the leader is on target with the focus, then it is likely that the intervention will apply to many group members and will serve to reinforce further exploration of the underlying issues. The leader can try an intervention and then listen carefully for the response of the group over the next two or three minutes. If the group explodes into an energetic continuation of the topic, the intervention is on target. If the group suddenly becomes silent and tense, the intervention is probably on target but perhaps the timing was off a bit. Or the leader may just have to persevere and keep the group focused on the issues underlying the intervention. If nothing seems to happen, the leader needs to wait and think.

As a general rule, it is probably best to consider a group-level intervention as the first choice. Such an intervention requires the therapist to keep a sharp eye on the whole group at all times or to identify a subgroup theme. Next in priority, an interpersonal intervention can be considered, something going on between two or more members, and finally an intrapsychic focus. Of course, a whole-group intervention may have as a goal the stimulation of internal thinking, so all levels need to be kept in mind. "The group feels like it's in a tug-of-war over whether to get closer or stay pretty much separate. I wonder if this is a parallel to the difficulty many of you have described about how hard it sometimes is to get in touch with what you are experiencing in your own reactions in the group." "The group has taken quite a swing into how bad things could be; sounds rather like how hard you can all be on yourselves as well without much reason."

Timing of Interventions

The question of timing is crucial to effective interventions. The most accurate and eloquent interpretation given at the wrong time will be wasted. The usual problem is making an intervention too early. Perhaps with some anxiety that something needs to be said, the therapist will move in too quickly with a lengthy statement that takes the pressure off the group for developing its own initiative. A good rule of thumb is that an interpretation should be made just before the members are about ready to put it into words anyway. If that is the case, then more often than not, a simple stimulus question will enable members to develop their own interpretative thought. An approach that encourages patients to reach their own conclusions provides an autonomy-developing style that can be transferred to outside situations. A good therapeutic outcome is one where patients can think back on therapy as a process by which they learned to understand their problems on their own with the encouragement of the therapist. This point is particularly relevant to group therapy, in which any given member has the advantage of receiving reflective or interpretative statements from anyone in the group. By holding back, the leader leaves the field open for helpful statements from other members and thus promotes the therapeutic factor of altruism.

Once an interpretation has been made, it is important to carefully monitor whether the result was further opening up and exploration or, on the other hand, a state of greater defensiveness and withdrawal. The result usually is evident within the next few minutes. This careful tracking of the state of Self-Relatedness will indicate to the therapist the accuracy of the timing judgment.

Application of SASB Concepts to Leadership Behavior

The SASB circumplex provides a convenient screen to test for the interactional nature of therapist interventions. Most therapist actions and responses are characterized by interpersonal styles on the right side of the circle (review the SASB circle on the flyleaf). For groups that are more advanced in their development or with higher-functioning patients, most interventions will be characterized by qualities in the upper-right quadrant. In early group sessions, at times of increased group stress, and with lower-functioning patients, more of the interventions will be drawn from the lower-right quadrant.

It is inevitable that every therapist will experience from time-to-time a surge of emotional response to group events. At times, this is clearly recognized, and one can purposefully respond with full awareness and firm clinical judgment. At other times, an overdetermined reaction is only recognized a few minutes after it has occurred or sometimes after the session is long over. It is important that the therapist learn from such experiences. Some patients are just plain exasperating, and if there are several in a group, the therapist may need to take a lot of deep breaths to keep his reactions under control. It can be helpful to review the patient's history and refresh one's understanding of the origins of the behavioral patterns being enacted in the group. Such a review will also make it easier to detect these patterns at an early point so that the personal response can be predicted and therefore mastered. Responses that are complementary to the dysfunctional behavior will only serve to reinforce those patterns. A solid cognitive understanding of the issues can be very helpful.

Some issues produce a reaction within the therapist because they press on areas to which the therapist is personally vulnerable (countertransference). For example, pleas for assistance may be hard to refuse even though they may reinforce excessive dependency. Critical remarks may trigger anger because they echo one's own parental patterns. The need to take control of a group situation may conflict with dimensions of passivity within the therapist. Apprehension about closeness may result in an overly distant therapeutic style. The first step in such situations is to recognize that they are taking place. The therapist has a responsibility to address issues that are interfering with sound clinical judgment. A knowledgeable clinical supervisor can be very helpful. Peer supervision seminars can also be effectively used. Experiential training workshops at conferences may offer an opportunity to work through some issues on neutral territory. Personal psychotherapy may also be an important option. The discussion that follows uses the SASB system to identify some common therapist problems.

Therapists may under unusual circumstances occasionally use controlling maneuvers in a highly specific manner. However, if used consistently, these maneuvers will reinforce patient compliance and passivity and work against developing member autonomy. Remember the principle of com-, plementarity: control will predictably elicit a submissive response. A therapist shift to a distancing, separating, or ignoring stance (represented by the top of the SASB circle) will threaten the quality of the Therapeutic Bond and may sap group cohesion. A shift of this kind is a sign that something is not going right and needs to be addressed at an early point.

A shift to an attacking or blaming stance (represented by the left side of the SASB circle) is almost always a sign that the therapist has lost the basic therapeutic attitude with the group or a member. This shift is often revealed through the use of poorly constructed interpretive interventions. The language may be subtly critical or demeaning, or the nonverbal vocal quality may unconsciously leak a quality of guilt-inducement or a sense of exasperation or anger.

Clarification and interpretation have interesting differences when placed within the SASB space. Clarification interventions are primarily characterized by freeing up, affirmation, and approach (represented by the upper-right quadrant of SASB circle). These interventions are positively motivated and designed to elicit a patient response that enhances autonomy. "Can you explore a bit more what you meant by that idea of fearing to get close?" [Feel free to open up]. Confronting interpretations that are presented as ideas or suggestions for consideration also lie in this area. "Have you ever considered that there may be a connection between your present fears and those bitter memories you were telling us about from the time of your parents' divorce?" [What do you think?]. Such interventions will contribute to further introspective thinking.

However, it is not unusual for interpretations to shift toward a more controlling posture (represented by the lower-right quadrant of the SASB circle). "You may not have thought of this, but it is clear to me that your recurrent patterns of leaving your partners on short notice represent a childlike avoidance of facing issues" [Please give some thought to what I know is wrong with you]. The comment may be technically quite accurate, but the process has a strong control element. Patients may conclude that they just do not know how to understand things without the therapist there to keep them on track.

Critical comments may also be inserted under the guise of interpretation that portray a judgmental and critical attitude that may trigger defensiveness. "It seems that you have again failed to appreciate how you become trapped in these self-destructive relationships" [stupid]. A nonverbal tone of irritation may contribute to this attitude. The valence has now shifted toward blame (represented by the lower-left quadrant), which will predictably elicit a resentful response, if not an angry counterattack.

Responses that lie on the negative side of the interactional spectrum may be interpreted by patients as attack or blame and should not be part of the therapeutic repertoire. Such responses seldom have a positive effect and serve only to further alienate or shut down group interaction. This does not mean that the therapist might not on occasion align with a group member's perception that some of that member's behaviors are unwarranted; however, care should be taken that such alignment is about specific behaviors, not about the person in general. The use of confrontational techniques must be seen as a technical decision, not a vehicle for personal attack. This is a boundary line that may easily be breached.

Thus, both clarification and interpretive interventions may have the same interactional process message. However, confrontational techniques are more liable to contain alternate or mixed process messages that may be less therapeutic in nature. There is some advantage, therefore, to considering carefully which method to use. If the therapist is in doubt, the active clarification approach has less potential for misuse. Of course, a middle ground exists in which clarification techniques are used to direct attention to a particular issue in a manner that is essentially interpretive. "You said earlier that you couldn't stand your father. Now you are feeling quite angry with Dan. Could you clarify for me how you see the two of them as being alike?" [Go ahead and make your own linking interpretation].

Therapists might also use the SASB system to contemplate the nature of their own reactions during a group. Often, the therapist's reaction is a reflection of a similar process going on in the group. Think of a situation in which you felt uncomfortable or uncertain about your response to a group event and try to locate this internal response state in one of the SASB quadrants. Using the composite SASB circle, determine what the key words trigger as you look at yourself and at the group and its members. Often, the therapist's internal reactions are an important source of information about the nature of the group at that moment. Sometimes the affective responses the therapist experiences come before a cognitive recognition of the issues, so it is important for the therapist to pay attention to them.

An attitude of benign professional curiosity represents a Rogerian position that is drawn from the upper-right quadrant in the SASB circle. "I am positively interested [Affirm] in what you have to say about yourself [Disclose]. Indeed, I find your situation interesting and a challenge to understand [Approach]. Can we work on it together? [Free Up]"

When the therapist experiences a strong urge to take care of the patient or the group—a strong need to provide something—she has shifted toward an interpersonal style marked by protection and control (represented by the lower-right quadrant in the SASB circle). When this occurs, it is probably a good indication that the therapist should pause and ask herself, Are these people as helpless or lacking in resources as I currently see them? Such reflection might allow the therapist to see a way of shifting up to a clarification response (represented by the upper-right quadrant of the SASB circle). A Protect position automatically carries with it the expectation of a Trust response from the patient or group, with the implication of not being able to do for oneself.

If the therapist finds himself moving into a critical-response mode to the group or to one of the members and has visions of laying down the law, straightening the group out, or discharging them forthwith, a flashing red light should metaphorically flash in front of the therapist's eyes. Interventions made from this position (represented by the lower-left quadrant in the SASB circle) are likely to be nonproductive and possibly damaging. They encourage a submitting response and pull both the therapist and the group into a more enmeshed relationship, with control issues underlying the process. This is a no-win situation that is likely to lead to Self-Blame, perhaps for everyone involved.

Sometimes the therapist will convey to the group or to a member a feeling of distance, lack of involvement, or boredom (represented by the upper-left portion of the SASB circle). Although not as dangerous as Blame, this position is not likely to be helpful and will sap group energy. It may result from a group situation in which the members are treating themselves the same way, that is, with Self-Neglect.

Therapist Neutrality

In the discussion earlier in this chapter, the supportive model was characterized as having a more interactive therapist stance as compared with the interpretive model, which is characterized by greater neutrality. However, in all therapy, the therapist must be alert to problems when a strong personal reaction to group events is experienced. The therapeutic task is to address the psychopathology underlying dysfunctional behavior. To find oneself reacting strongly to a patient indicates a loss of perspective and will have a significant impact on the therapeutic process. This loss of perspective is of relevance in all treatment groups but is of particular concern when the intention is for the patient's relationship with the therapist to be an important therapeutic focus.

The intent of therapist neutrality is to preserve the "as if" quality of the therapeutic situation. Control of personal responses helps to maintain a frame around this artificial situation. The task of the therapist is to accept the patient's material and assist the patient in the process of understanding it. This requires that the therapist be loyal to the therapeutic system, not aligned with or against the patient.

These comments do not imply that the therapist need be unresponsive—only a blank screen or a reflecting mirror. An empathic attitude remains important, as do warmth and concern. However, an overly reactive stance renders the therapist vulnerable to being misinterpreted and may foster attempts by the patients to negotiate special alliances. The goal might be described as detachment without insensibility.

It is easy to lose neutrality in groups. The group will exert a powerful suction on the therapist to join with the members' views regarding difficulties and ideal solutions. Several issues can be identified that might lead to a loss of therapist neutrality.

Denial of separateness.   The therapist's situation is in many ways a lonely one, and the therapist may try to break out of this self-imposed role. A group setting may intensify this type of reaction. Everyone else is relishing the fruits of universality, and the therapist must watch as an onlooker, forbidden to fully partake. This reaction may be particularly acute when termination is addressed.

Avoidance of specific transferences.   Therapists may find themselves reacting to particular expectations of the group. They may want to protest their lack of perfection when being idealized in the engagement stage. When therapists are the subject of group criticism in the differentiation stage, they may want to plead their essential goodness. They may want to be seen as providing the most important therapeutic ingredients in the interpersonal work stage. And in the termination stage, they may not want to be the depriving parent. Such reactions may represent personal areas of relative vulnerability for the therapist.

Therapist self-centeredness.   The therapist may experience some need to promote a particular view of life or to develop a group of personal followers. Acting on this need not only leads to undue control being exerted but also violates the technical task of understanding, not determining, the direction of change. Some therapists find it difficult to refrain from an excess of exhibitionistic behavior, going well beyond a small touch of the theatrical that may insert energy into the group. Such behavior may entertain a group, and indeed make converts, but also undermines the importance of the members themselves doing the hard work.

Personal reactions (countertransference). The question of therapist reactions to psychodynamic material is too broad for an extended discussion here. The literature on individual psychotherapy has much to offer in this regard. In groups, a powerful and rather primitive set of pressures, such as those described by Bion, can develop. These are rooted in basic human concerns for acceptance, recognition, protection, and self-esteem. Therapists may find themselves reacting to such material in an uncomfortably strong manner. Such reactions may be an important clue to understanding what has been going on. But the therapist's reaction may be too strong. Coming out of a group session, one may realize that the nature of an intervention was uncalled for or overdetermined. Intrusive thoughts about the group between sessions may indicate that an area of personal sensitivity or vulnerability has been approached. In such situations, some form of supervisory consultation is indicated. This consultation may be of a formal nature or simply a discussion with a knowledgeable colleague.

Because strong personal responses are common in groups, it is important that the group therapist have a sound background in individual psychotherapy and some exposure to experiential group training. At the very least, with such a background, the clinician will be alerted to problematic areas or issues. If these issues continue to interfere with sound clinical judgment, regular supervision, preferably with an observational component, should be considered. More formal personal training or a therapeutic opportunity may be of value.

Cotherapy

The use of cotherapists has been discussed in Chapter 6 in the context of group composition issues. The argument was made that the presence of two therapists increases the complexity of the group system, so that in time-limited groups in particular, keeping the field of action as clean as possible has advantages. Some examples were given of reasonable rationales for the use of cotherapists. However, cotherapy should not be chosen as a way of addressing therapist insecurity. Cotherapy demands greater skill and experience, not less.

Two cotherapists form a couple or a team; they are cotherapists together. The cotherapy relationship itself will develop over time and often does so in concert with group development. As the group enters the differentiation stage, cotherapists often find that they too have things to sort out. It is crucial, therefore, that cotherapists work with a sense of mutual respect and openness. This must be the case even if they are unequal in experience. Such a relationship atmosphere provides the base for mutual support and acknowledgment.

Much has been written about cotherapists' serving as interactional models for the group members. In fact, it is probably important that the basic tone of the relationship be harmonious and collaborative, more than it be a demonstration of the specifics of communication technique. Cotherapists must be able to communicate effectively. This is much easier to accomplish when they share a basically similar theoretical position about how they understand relationships and how their group is to be led. Time needs to be scheduled and jealously guarded for at least a brief talk before each session and particularly afterward for an informal debriefing together. There must be a commitment to address tensions between cotherapists at an early point. Tensions from within the group will inevitably be transmitted onto the cotherapy relationship itself, and constant reparative efforts will be needed. In general, such efforts are best handled outside the group. In some circumstances, for example, when cotherapy tensions are directly reflective of group tensions, it may be helpful to reflect how these tensions have been addressed by the cotherapists. But such a move would be done only with some prior discussion and as a planned therapeutic technique. When cotherapy is working well, it can become a stimulating opportunity for peer supervision and, for many therapists, a way of addressing threatened burnout or the loneliness of a private office practice.

It is not uncommon for power imbalance to emerge surreptitiously between cotherapists. This may take the form of competitiveness, with constant interruptions or corrections between cotherapists. Sometimes the imbalance takes the form of excessive passivity by one cotherapist or a mutual codependency that hampers effective proactive therapeutic interventions. Such trends need to be addressed firmly even though the confrontation may raise uncomfortable issues. These control tensions often arise during the differentiation stage. A well-functioning cotherapy team can be very effective in assisting the group to address and work through these issues. When one cotherapist is the focus of group pressure, the other is in a position to keep the group actively at the task of conflict resolution.

Cotherapists need to be constantly balancing their activity levels. This does not mean that they do the same things, but both should be seen as important contributing figures in the group interaction. It is not uncommon for cotherapists to play somewhat different roles in the group. Indeed, they may decide to work together for that very reason. This often arises on the basis of female and male cotherapy pairs. Often, cotherapy is chosen for that very purpose, for example, with adolescent or couples groups. Such a pairing presents the group with a parental image of authority that may prove effectively evocative of important early family images for the members. This provides much opportunity for transferential attachment patterns. It also provides the possibility of attempts by the members to split the leaders into positive and negative roles.

Patients often present with firm opinions about the gender of the therapist they desire. This belief may carry with it positive opportunity for constructive identification. But it may also serve to avoid addressing gender-specific relationship issues within the therapy situation. A mixed-gender cotherapy pair may be one way of addressing this. The same-gender therapist may be seen as providing support and serving as a safety factor that makes it possible to deal with important issues through the other-gender therapist (or vice versa).

It is strongly advisable for cotherapists to know each other and to have some choice in working together. This is clearly particularly relevant for groups in which interpersonal/psychodynamic approaches are to be used. Cotherapists are also encouraged to interview prospective group members together, even though this demands extra clinical time.

Cotherapy is often used for training purposes. Most commonly, this takes the form of an experienced clinician's working with a trainee. The group members need to know that this is the arrangement. The imbalance of experience means that the roles initially will be somewhat skewed. The possibility of inappropriate competition with the senior cotherapist or excessive deferral by the junior one must be guarded against. The frame of the teaching experience must include an opportunity for pre- and postgroup discussions. Most groups take pride in seeing the junior therapist demonstrate a steady increase in effective interventions. I always make sure that I am absent for a session or two after the group gets well established so that the junior cotherapist has a chance to assume full ownership rights.

Cotherapy can be effective and satisfying. However, there is no empirical evidence that it results in more effective therapy, though this may be in part because it has not been extensively studied. It certainly does introduce more complexities into the therapy task and doubles the financial cost. Because of the increased intensity, most inpatient units and partial hospitalization or day treatment programs routinely use cotherapy. The opportunity for regular and frequent staff discussions and debriefings makes this realistic. It is likely that outpatient groups will increasingly be expected to be solo led.

Concurrent Group and Individual Therapy

There are various ways by which a patient may be intentionally seen by more than one therapist. *Combined therapy* refers to the patient's being seen by the same therapist in individual and group treatment. *Conjoint therapy* denotes that the patient is being seen by different therapists simultaneously. And *concurrent therapy*, a more global term, refers to either of these cases (88).

The practice of patients being seen in both individual and group psychotherapy concomitantly with the same therapist is likely to be less common in third-party payment situations. If such *combined therapy* is undertaken, arrangements must be set up with clear boundary guidelines. The individual sessions are best used primarily to rework and deepen material stimulated in the group and not to replace the group as the principal source of new material. This arrangement may be helpful in preventing the premature termination of a difficult patient. The group setting then allows the exploration of the interpersonal implications of material identified in individual sessions. The individual interview provides the opportunity for a more detailed examination of transference/countertransference reactions. The group setting, with a more diffuse focus on the therapist, may offer routes to resolution. Evidence of secrecy between the formats should be pursued, as it frequently masks a pattern of avoiding relevant issues. It is prudent to establish the expectation that the prime responsibility for reporting individual material to the group lies with the patient, but that the therapist may on occasion help that process along if required. It is generally an error to add individual sessions in response to the emergence of resistance in an ongoing group.

Individual therapists may refer patients to another therapist for group as an addition to their individual therapy (i.e., *conjoint therapy*). The same principles of open communication apply as in combined therapy, but the risk of tension and splitting between the two settings is increased. This risk can, to some extent, be minimized by insistence that there be direct and regular communication between the two therapists. The presence of such an agreement is helpful whether or not such communication routinely takes place. In time-limited group psychotherapy, it is more common to insist that the group be the only active therapy. It is advantageous to keep the system as simple as possible to compensate for the limitation of time.

One common reason for concurrent therapy is to provide management of medication. A convenient approach is to schedule time for a regular individual visit before or after each group session. Each group member would be assigned one of these sessions. In the course of 2 months, all members could then be seen. This arrangement can be used when the therapist is also monitoring medication or when a psychiatrist is performing the medication function and another professional is running the group. In the latter circumstance, it is important that the treating professionals have a positive collegial relationship and mutual understanding of the value of each treatment component. Otherwise, the patient may get conflicting messages about the value of one or the other that can subtly undermine both.

Such a bimonthly individual session, if conducted by the group therapist, can also be used as an opportunity to reflect with the patient on group events and to review general goal directions. The spacing of the visits makes it less likely for there to be problems between the two formats.

Prevention of Negative Effects

No therapist wants to do harm. However, many patients terminate their group experience before they have had a chance to benefit from it. Others report, even years later, that they experienced their therapy as personally damaging. This experience is usually related to a Focal Incident involving self-esteem issues that led to a lasting effect of demoralization or unresolved anger.

Premature termination from therapy groups is quite common, with a substantial percentage of patients leaving the group before termination. (This happens to about the same extent in individual therapy.) The majority of patients who drop out do so within the first six sessions. This suggests that selection, composition, preparation, and entry factors are responsible. Unplanned termination later in a group's life usually involves either a specific upsetting incident or resistance to addressing specific problem areas. An additional unfortunate effect for those who terminate early is that they may be discouraged from seeking further professional help in the future.

Errors of judgment or dangerous situations that predispose to negative effects can be identified, as discussed in the following subsections. Remember the ancient nostrum *primum non nocere*—above all do no harm (89).

Selection and Composition

Some casualties are directly the result of errors in clinical judgment made before the group begins. These errors involve questions of assessment and group composition described in Section II. Patients with a marked paranoid style may be put in a position where a negative experience is inevitable. The stimulation of the group environment usually exacerbates such qualities, which in turn produces a negative reaction from other members. Thus, both the group and the individual suffer. Similarly, patients who use extremely brittle denial may be unable to use group interaction constructively and antagonize the group. Major schizoid traits may be interpreted by the other members as resistance or implied criticism, and the patient may find himself in a scapegoated position that exacerbates preexisting doubts about social competency. A serious misalignment of expectations about therapy will create problems and may on occasion result in the individual's eliciting a rejecting response from group members that has a harmful effect.

Early Group Events

Not belonging.   In the early sessions, the group must develop cohesion. Central to this process is a sense of belongingness. An active experience of being outside of the group culture and not belonging has the potential for a powerful negative effect. The therapist has a specific responsibility to monitor for this sort of development. The issue must be addressed promptly.

Excessive self-disclosure.   The revelation of highly charged factual material, such as incestuous experiences or violent crimes, and potentially highly charged information, such as one's sexual orientation, can be harmful if occurring before the development of a strong supportive atmosphere. The group may find it overwhelming and, to preserve an emerging sense of cohesion, may isolate or attack the individual.

Early conflict. As with the revelation of highly charged factual material, the early eruption of significant conflict before the group has become consolidated is likely to be poorly tolerated and lead to early dropping out. Groups with early conflict have difficulty developing a sense of cohesion. A possible exception to this is adolescent groups, in which early confrontation of the leader is common.

Attack or Rejection

The experience of being attacked or rejected is the single most important predictor of negative effects. Patients may report years later the damaging effects on self-esteem of an attack or criticism they received in a group. The confrontational process of the differentiation stage becomes dangerous when there is a perception that it is driven by the intent to harm, disgrace, or reject the recipient. The therapist must be on guard for such qualities, which may lead to an active scapegoating situation. This group phenomenon can be particularly damaging because the individual is left alone to face the entire group. An intense and unresolved process of scapegoating entails serious risk for both a negative effect and premature termination. Although most likely to occur at an earlier point in the group's life, scapegoating may emerge at any time in response to group stresses.

Unresolved Affective Issues

Many Critical Incidents in a group are characterized by heightened levels of affect. Because such intensity may be threatening to the group members, a powerfully felt statement may be met with silence. Being left "up in the air" with no response can be a devastating experience. It may be interpreted as a rejection of the individual or a condemnation of the subject matter. In states of high emotion, there is more susceptibility to distorted interpretations, so the therapist may need to intervene to bring the group back to the issue so that the affective dimension can be diffused. Otherwise, the involved individual may resolve never again to risk so much.

An added danger is that a person may leave a session having misinterpreted the meaning of the group's response, convinced of his or her own stupidity or worthlessness, and perhaps with thoughts of self-destructive behavior. Toward the end of any highly charged session, it is helpful to have a brief go-around to assess how the members are reacting and to promote closure. It may be appropriate for the therapist to ask an individual member to stay after the session so that an assessment can be made of clinical safety.

Leadership Style

A related danger stems from an aggressively confrontational style such as that often associated with charismatic qualities that demand followership. The danger of this style lies in the possibility of leading some members into levels of self-disclosure or risk taking that they are not able to tolerate. They may leave a session only to recognize that they have gone far beyond the bounds they consider appropriate, regret this in a shameful or fearful manner, and never return. Over time, the memory of the event increasingly takes on the qualities of an attack in which they were the helpless victims. As a result, they may experience an enduring sense of having been violated and of vulnerability, which could lead to an unwillingness to trust in other therapeutic situations. A similar situation may result when a therapist unwisely encourages excessive self-disclosure.

Sexual Relationships Between Members

The emergence of overt sexual behavior between group members is always a serious matter. This is not because of issues of morality, though that may be a consideration. An ongoing intimate relationship between two group members largely precludes their effective use of the group. They will have secrets to be kept from the group and will have difficulty maintaining a "therapeutic attitude" regarding their own relationship. A therapy group is not real life; it is a simulation. When that distinction is lost, the learning potential drops. It is incumbent on the therapist to resolve the situation. The circumstances may be discussed in the group with a particular interest in the extent to which this "acting out" is driven by group dynamics. A meeting with the involved members outside of group is also useful to reach a decision about who should terminate from this particular therapy group.

Some such episodes involve irresponsible actions by members who take advantage of the naïveté or distress of others. Unfortunately, those who are victimized often have had similar experiences before entering the group and view their present victimization as further demonstration of their own vulnerability and inability to master their environment. Thus, the experiences may exacerbate an already tarnished sense of self-esteem.

Termination

The stress of termination, if not handled appropriately, may result in a panicky sense of abandonment or dissatisfaction that may interfere with a constructive internalization of the group experience. Sometimes under the stress of termination, compensatory and destructive decisions may be made, such as impulsively deciding to become involved in other relationships or to act on an increase in suicidal thoughts. All of this underlines the need to deal persistently with termination issues. The therapist's reluctance to deal with separation may contribute to these problems.

SECTION IV

Group Models for Clinical Service Systems

CHAPTER 12

Planning for Clinical Group Programs

*G*roup psychotherapy is particularly well suited to larger service systems. A setting in which a number of clinicians can refer patients to groups provides access to a larger flow of patients. This makes it possible to develop groups for special purposes without having to wait until enough potential members can be accumulated. Most clinicians are now connected with a larger system in some manner. This shift in service delivery organization has made the development of group treatment programs more practical. Such an approach requires careful planning, and this chapter reviews the sorts of decisions that need to be considered.

Developing a Group Program

A service system cannot simply establish a group program without careful planning. The first crucial step is to secure unambiguous support for the idea from senior administrative sources. It must be clear that it is administrative policy to promote groups. Such a commitment is most evident with the appointment of a group program coordinator. Finding an experienced clinician to undertake this role as a major time responsibility will go a long way toward achieving program success. This role is a highly political one because it involves negotiations with all aspects of the system. A collaborative and facilitating approach is essential. Programs will fail or succeed on this appointment.

The next step is to assess the resources available within the clinical staff complement. This assessment needs to be done carefully. It is not adequate to make casual inquiries about who has done groups before. It would be better to begin with a small core of more experienced clinicians and expand later than to attempt to include all clinicians out of democratic motives. The core group of staff can then be a resource for program planning purposes.

Some staff preparation and training would be useful. Such training is most pressing if the available skill level is relatively undeveloped. Pressing inexperienced clinicians into group work without preparation is a recipe for problems, if not disaster. At the least, the program will get a bad reputation; at the worst, group casualties may begin to appear. If most of the group clinicians are well trained, the in-house program may focus more on specific interests and skills. A common training experience will also promote a collaborative atmosphere.

Some forum for clinical supervision should be available. In a larger program, this may entail a formal clinical supervisor's meeting regularly with the clinicians either individually or, perhaps even better, as a group. The role of the supervisor should be clearly seen as separate from the responsibilities of an administrative supervisor. Regular staff meetings at which group issues are discussed can be very helpful. Group psychotherapy has the ability to pull therapists into group process entanglements, so access to an arena in which issues can be nondefensively reviewed is important.

At the system level, it is useful to take a longer-term perspective on the planning process. Developing groups on the spur of the moment to respond to an immediate perceived need will in the end prove frustrating. It is more stabilizing to think of the group program in terms of an annual planning approach. Although one need not be totally inflexible in this regard, this approach encourages the development of a group system that responds to the ongoing needs of the clinical population. The system should try to avoid offering particular types of groups only sporadically. Certainly, for the most commonly used groups, it is better to estimate the number required in a year and to plan accordingly. This approach creates a sense of continuity over time that is reassuring to referral sources and to the group psychotherapists alike. Forward planning can accommodate to time constraints for clinicians and adjust to planned absences or rotations as well as to seasonal changes in patient load.

Another system decision to be made pertains to the use of cotherapists. Use of cotherapists will make a considerable difference in the professional resources required. The review of this issue in Chapter 6 suggests that cotherapists be used only when there is a clear rationale in terms of the patient population being served. Two poorly trained cotherapists are no better, and probably worse, than one well-trained therapist.

Yet another aspect of developing group programs concerns how they are marketed within the service system. Here, the networking expertise of the program coordinator is crucial. Possible referral sources must be kept informed of the status of the groups. One good way to inform referral sources is with a regular bulletin that lists the titles of all groups, their current status, and when new admissions can be accepted. In a large system, a weekly bulletin might be considered. Smaller systems may get by with a bulletin at longer intervals. It should be possible to present this information for several months in advance. The descriptive information at the beginning of each group model in Chapter 13 provides an idea of how to develop group descriptions. It is also helpful to have experienced staff responding to referrals and making appropriate triage decisions regarding what group would be most suitable for a given patient. This is not a job for the junior member of the team. Well-trained staff can, based on a relatively brief interview, make more accurate decisions about the most appropriate program.

The formal nature of such program functions will depend on the size of the program and the number of referrals to be processed. There are advantages for marketing to both referring clinicians and patients in developing theme-oriented groups that have clear objectives. Obviously, the coordinator needs to be responsible for responding to requests, concerns, or ideas from those in the larger system. A checklist for assessing the readiness of a system to initiate a group psychotherapy program is presented in Table 12–1 (90). Both the time required for a coordinator and the frequency of a group status sheet are underestimated.

Assessment of System Needs

Is it possible to predict the overall service needs of a given system? Predictions are always tricky, but one can come up with some educated guesses. First, service statistics for the preceding year should be reviewed and the following issues, among others, considered:

- How many patients were seen in what format for how long?
- What is the distribution in terms of age, gender, marital status, and socioeconomic level?
- Is a diagnostic breakdown possible?
- What is the need for acute treatment to avoid inpatient care?

Table 12–1.   Group Program Readiness Checklist

1. Administration has given a public mandate for the development of a group psychotherapy program.

2. A group program coordinator has been hired and has been given protected time for administrative functions.

3. A regular group status sheet is produced and circulated to referral sources.

4. Groups have been developed for the most common conditions seen in the clinical setting.

5. Treatment models have been selected on evidence-based criteria.

6. Each group has a clear written description of the goals and the referral criteria.

7. All patients referred for group go through a screening and orientation session.

8. Pre post testing is routinely done and satisfaction ratings obtained.

9. Arrangements are in place for the training and in-service development of group therapists, including regular scheduled clinical supervision (supervisor or peer).

10. Adequate space and clinician time resources are available.

11. Group therapists are allowed adequate time for the extended charting/contact activities required.

12. The benefits/fee structure provides an option for a trade-off of three group sessions for every individual session and an enhanced reimbursement for group therapists.

Source.   Adapted from Crosby G, Sabin JE: "Developing and Marketing Time-Limited Therapy Groups." *Psychiatric Services* 46:7–8, 1996. Used with permission.

■ What is the balance between patients needing relatively brief acute interventions and those needing longer-term care?

■ What are the conditions of coverage provided by the system?

Such information may not be available in an accurate or comprehensive form if the system is new, but reasonable assumptions can usually be made. Note that these questions focus on the needs of the target population, not the interests or skills of the clinicians.

Based on this information and on consideration of the psychotherapy dose-response relationship graphically presented in Figure 1–1, a general sense of the service load can be made. Of this total, what percentage can be managed in groups? Here is where the commitment to the use of groups comes into force. Some systems provide the vast majority of their psychotherapy using a group format. Others may take the position of supporting group approaches but in fact use these formats for only a small percentage of the caseload.

Hypothetical use of staff time in a "typical" general mental health service system is presented in Table 12–2. The breakdown into crisis management, time-limited, and longer-term time categories is taken directly from the time dimensions discussed in Chapter 1. The staff load is first calculated based on use of individual therapy only and is then recalculated with a major part of the load handled in group format. Twenty percent of patients in the crisis management category are treated in brief 8-session groups like that described in the Crisis Intervention Group model (see Chapter 13). Sixty-five percent of the patients in the time-limited group and 80% of the patients in the longer-term group are treated in a group format. This distribution would represent a major commitment to the use of groups. Nonetheless, Table 12–2 gives some indication of the size of service efficiency that could be achieved, representing substantial changes in resource utilization.

Several dimensions are common to all of the group models that are presented in Chapter 13 (Table 12–3). Although generally recognized, these dimensions are perhaps not always applied in a systematic manner and may be found in different combinations. When planning a group, therapists would find it worthwhile to review these dimensions (which form a continuum between the two poles) to be quite clear about what they have in mind. Does the plan match the needs of the patient population and the clinical resources available? Can these dimensions be used to design a group for a particular set of patients whom the therapist has encountered? Is a special group needed, or can the issues be effectively handled in a skillfully led general group?

A Model Group Program

In a busy clinical setting, one should not speak of starting groups, but of designing a group program. In Chapter 6, the advantages of closed versus open groups and the usefulness of some degree of homogeneity were described. A group program permits these questions to be addressed in a systematic manner. The following sequential criteria might be used as guidelines in thinking about what a given system might require:

Table 12–2.   Hypothetical utilization of staff time comparing individual versus group modalities for 100 patients

Treatment (by time category)	Number of sessions	Number of patients	Staff time: individual therapy (hours)	Percentage of total staff time	Staff time: individual and group therapy (hours)		Percentage of total staff time
Crisis intervention	8	50	400	20	32	(10 patients in 1 group, 2 therapists)	3
					320	(40 patients individual)	30
Time-limited	25	35	875	43	150	(24 patients in 3 groups, 1 therapist)	15
					275	(11 patients individual)	27
Longer-term	50	15	750	37	100	(12 patients in 1 group, 1 therapist)	10
					150	(3 patients individual)	15
Total		100	2025	100	1027		100

1. Consider a brief crisis management group as a good place for many patients to start. Indeed, for many of these patients, this kind of group will be the only treatment required. A rapid access group with continuously changing membership and a limit of six or eight sessions for any one member could be used. Such a group requires a highly structured approach and attention to immediate coping strategies. A crisis management group can serve as a useful holding environment in a larger service system that combines the functions of active treatment, extended assessment, and triage. It may be useful as a mechanism for obviating hospitalization.

2. Try patients who require more intensive psychotherapy in time-limited groups (12–25 sessions) as a way 1) to evaluate capacity to use the group format effectively, 2) to assess motivation, and 3) to determine whether there is need for longer-term treatment. A substantial majority of patients will find this type of group sufficient.

3. Use a closed format for time-limited groups, with the possible exception of offering some groups, especially those with a more structured format, the opportunity for signing up for a second course.

4. Strive for general-purpose groups to the extent possible. This type of group provides the most efficiency in managing a broad spectrum of referral problems. For example, a system might want to have constant accessibility to general time-limited interpersonal groups that can serve a broad segment of the nonpsychotic population. Certainly, groups for depression, eating disorders, and anxiety disorders (including panic disorder) are likely to be in high demand. Parenting and marital therapy

Table 12–3. Dimensions for conceptualizing group models

1. Members with high interactional capacity vs. members with low interactional capacity
2. Homogeneous composition vs. heterogeneous composition
3. Focus on limiting time vs. time-unlimited perspective
4. Emphasis on supportive techniques vs. emphasis on interpretive techniques
5. Focus on managing the group process vs. focus on understanding the group process
6. Focus on specific symptoms vs. focus on the person of the patient
7. Focus on the present vs. focus on the past
8. Focus on behavior and cognitions vs. focus on affect and interpersonal meaning

are also likely to be frequently requested. The general interactional capacity of the members may be used to develop two streams: one with a high degree of structure for those with lesser capacity, and the other with a focus on psychological understanding and learning from group interaction for those with higher capacity. Both would be time-limited and would incorporate active supportive psychotherapy techniques.

5. Consider what specialized, quite homogeneous time-limited groups are required. Some groups may address a psychoeducational need, such as for an eating disorder, or a specific skill, such as assertiveness or anger management. Groups may be developed for populations at risk such as those with postpartum conditions, those who have experienced acute loss of a spouse or a child, or those adapting to a major medical illness. Intensive time-limited groups are typically composed of patients with greater dysfunction and higher symptom distress levels. At the very least, the approaches used in such groups might be drawn from a technical spectrum including cognitive-behavioral treatment, interpersonal psychotherapy, and psychodynamic treatment.

6. Carefully assess patients' needs for longer-term group treatment. The decision to place a patient into a longer-term group is perhaps the most critical decision of all, in part because the utilization of clinical resources increases significantly with this kind of group treatment. This would be the point at which some sort of formal review/second opinion process might be introduced. The psychotherapy dose-response relationship in Figure 1–1 (see Chapter 1) suggests that from the point of view of a functional program, long-term therapy can be considered to begin somewhere around 6 months. It is predictable that about 15% of patients entering a mental health program might require such services. Longer-term groups might work best with a slow-open admission policy, or perhaps segmented time periods during which new members are admitted.

7. Clarify the intent of the longer-term group. If the purpose is to provide intensive psychotherapy, composition decisions need to be carefully made. (For example, patients with personality disorder who have serious dysfunction and are high service utilizers may need 1 to 2 years of treatment.) If the purpose is to provide maintenance and support, perhaps forever, as with the schizophrenic population, the composition decision is made based more on level of psychosocial functioning than on diagnosis.

8. Keep careful statistics over time that will provide guidance as to the best balance among these options.

The criteria outlined above regarding the time components of psycho-therapy can be built into organizational structures. For example, by a limit being placed on the number of individual crisis-oriented sessions, a specialized service component can be designed for this purpose with a mandate to keep a very clear, specific focus and have the goal of reestablishing stability, not effecting major psychological change. A portion of this work could be done in a group format. Then, a specific decision could be made to shift the patient into a more intensive, specialized but time-limited program, a format to which groups are well suited. Clear criteria would be required for patients to move into longer-term treatment. Many patients who require such treatment could be managed in a group format.

For the referral process after assessment to work effectively, there must be specific criteria regarding the goals of each service. A clear general group description is a good starting point. However, more specific inclusion/exclusion criteria may be required. Above all, it is important that a "dumping syndrome" (i.e., placing patients inappropriately into groups for service system convenience) not be allowed to develop. Here, the role of a group coordinator can be crucial. *Every* instance of mismatch between intake assessment and treatment selection should be noted and reviewed. Such instances of mismatch are generally a result of inadequate criteria or lack of a suitable program, not just poor judgment. Over time, such occurrences should gradually decrease as greater clarity is achieved.

The first task in developing a group format is to write out a brief formal description that could be used for general programmatic purposes. This description should, in lay terms, explain the group to a potential referring source. This process begins with selecting a name that truly reflects the central purpose of the group. The description of each model in Chapter 13 begins with such a summary. These descriptions were developed based on the guidelines listed in Table 12–4.

Education and Preparation of Patients

Resistance about increasing the use of groups will come from two sources: patients and staff. Patients are likely to be skeptical about a referral for group therapy. Their principal exposure to groups might well have been through media presentations where humor or sensationalism was the dominant force. The first mention made of the possibility of group treatment is a critical point, and a positive and constructive attitude must be demonstrated.

Table 12–4.   Guidelines for group descriptions

1. Title that reflects in lay terms the nature of the group (no jargon)
2. Target population (e.g., age, situation, disorder)
3. Special inclusion or exclusion criteria
4. Goals/skills that the group will address
5. Some indication of the format of the sessions, especially any special features
6. Frequency of meetings and duration of the group, and whether open or closed
7. Starting date
8. Referral route

Any comment suggesting even slightly that groups are being recommended because of cost pressures will predictably elicit a sense of outrage.

A consistent process of education should be built into the system. This process might involve including articles about the use of groups in publications for members of the healthcare plan. Handouts can be available to give to patients once the idea of group treatment has been raised. The Patient Information Handout in Appendix 9 is an example. Clinical staff should be alerted to the importance of taking proactive measures to inform patients about groups. Patient concerns are predictable and universal and should be sought out. It is helpful to have a working knowledge of the outcome literature, such as that discussed in Chapter 1. Patients should know that group psychotherapy is as effective as individual psychotherapy. The clinician can identify specific advantages of a group approach for the patient. For example, that it is helpful to talk about one's problems with others who will understand them. That tackling problems together provides more ideas and feedback. That problems in the interpersonal area are particularly well addressed in groups, where there is a chance to learn from actual interactions.

Resistance from staff is often more subtle. For example, the director of a busy student health service professed great interest in increasing the use of groups. At the end of 6 months, three suitable candidates from such a fertile source had been found! Usually, a dearth of referrals is related more to professional than patient concerns. Again, a systematic effort to educate, as well as availability of clear referral criteria, is indicated. Use of outcome or performance figures may also be helpful. Cultivating good collegial relationships is, of course, essential.

Group Records

Good record keeping is a necessary part of clinical practice. The recording of group therapy events is a more complex task than the recording of individual sessions. The Group Report Form (see Appendix 10) discussed later in this chapter should be completed immediately after the session while the experience and the sense of involvement are still alive. A delay of even an hour produces a drop in the accuracy and immediacy of the records. Trying to write up a group session the next day or a week later is not only unsatisfactory in terms of recording events accurately but also less satisfying in terms of reviewing the important aspects of the session. Time should be set aside to write up the session. Fifteen minutes is a bare minimum, and for a new therapist 30 minutes is more realistic. The time needed for writing up the session should not be squashed in while keeping the next patient waiting. It should be considered as part of the time allotment for the group and carefully preserved as such.

Just as time is needed at the end of a group session, so a few minutes should be taken before each session to review notes from the previous group session. (The Group Report Form, discussed below, is designed with that function in mind.) The purpose of spending a few minutes recalling the previous session is to place oneself back into the group atmosphere. Patients may spend hours mulling over what had happened in the preceding session and come in ready to continue where they left off. Therapists, on the other hand, have seen a week of patients in between. Many of these patients are likely to be working on issues with generally similar themes that require related therapeutic strategies. Everyone has had the experience of catching oneself halfway through an intervention with the sickening realization that, while the intent may have been correct, the facts belonged to another patient. Taking a few minutes before a group session to reorient oneself to "the lay of the land" at the end of the previous session is very helpful.

Service Program Requirements

Service programs differ in their requirements regarding record keeping. Some require a full note for each member after each group. Others specify only that there be a brief entry along with the record of attendance. The latter is preferable in time-limited groups, in which the patient is enrolled for the entire sequence of sessions, as well as in longer-term groups. Crisis intervention groups need more complete session entries in each chart because the attendance situation is much more variable. Of course, any unusual situation should always be recorded in the individual chart.

Group Report Forms

The one-page Group Report Form (see Appendix 10) is a practical method for reporting both the group-as-a-whole and its individual members. The form has intentionally been kept to one page to force the therapist to abstract themes. This results in more efficient and effective group records than does a lengthy anecdotal summary that may occupy several pages but is lacking in focus.

The names of members and therapist(s) are placed in the circle of boxes in accordance with the seating arrangement during the group. Lines can be drawn between the boxes in the chart to indicate the most prominent interaction patterns among members, including the therapist. This simple directional pattern is quite revealing of group process patterns. Within each box, the main issues related to the individual are summarized, whether these are raised by the patient or by the therapist. By being allowed only limited space, the clinician must summarize important themes and not get into too much detail.

The remainder of the page is used for group-level comments. The categories listed are for the purpose of stimulating ideas and are not necessarily to be exhaustively reported for each session.

Major themes.   The therapist should stand back from the group and consider the few principal thematic topics that were discussed during the session. Understandably, this will eliminate a lot of detail and allow one to focus only on the main issues around which the session was organized. In most sessions, three or four areas will be covered. It is useful to provide brief examples and to try to identify triggering events that result in a shift of theme.

Focal Incidents.   The therapist should list and briefly describe the few episodes that stand out as being of particular importance. Such episodes are usually heralded by the emergence of strong affect. The therapist should go around the group and think of events that seemed relevant to each member. Focal Incidents often involve self-disclosure, insightful breakthroughs, an important exchange between two members, or a unified group reaction such as an attack on one member or the leader. These episodes can be briefly identified as an "aide-mémoire" for later use.

Therapist issues. Major events involving the therapist should be identified and recorded. Material recorded can include evidence for transferential and countertransferential reactions. A brief comment might be made of the main features of therapist intervention style. If there are cotherapists, they should review the quality of their collaboration and comment on issues to keep in mind for the next session.

Supervision comments. The therapist should record supervision comments, including ideas from the postgroup discussion or formal supervision session. These comments might involve the meaning of some group events or thoughts on technique or therapeutic strategy.

For next session. After having thought through the session in order to write it up, and after having discussed it with observers or a supervisor, the therapist should make a list of issues to consider before entering the next session. Consideration might be given to, for example, structural issues such as attendance or tardiness; content areas for follow-up; issues that predictably may come up or should be brought up; aspects of technique to consider; strategies concerning any given patient, such as the need for more support or more confrontation; aspects of the group climate or norms to be addressed; or procedural announcements. Sometimes the listed areas represent hot issues generated immediately after the session that should not be lost. The list should not be too long; probably including five or six items is enough.

Most clinical services require an entry on each member's individual chart for each session. This entails considerable paperwork following each session. One convenient format is the Group Member Summary Form shown in Appendix 10. This format facilitates brief entries for a single patient and has the advantage of providing a quick review of preceding sessions with a minimum of paper. It is also a handy reference when completing Discharge Summaries. This form would replace the function of the boxes in the top half of the Group Report Form. The structure of this form could be easily simulated by computer entries.

Another group report form, also shown in Appendix 10, has the same multisession layout as the Group Member Summary Form. The Group Session Summary Form would be primarily for the use of the therapists, using the same categories as listed above. Of course, the Group Member

Report Form itself could also be used to record only group-level events for a given session. It has the advantage of replicating the visual space of the group and encouraging use of arrows and boundary lines to represent group structures.

Small Programs and Private Offices

Small service programs or clinicians in a private office may feel some pressure to admit patients continuously. However, most patients can be maintained on a waiting list for several weeks if they have a concrete starting date assigned. For example, a clinician might contract to provide two general-purpose groups based on the Interpersonal Problems Group model (as described in Chapter 13). If these were to be scheduled in 16 session staggered blocks, a new group could begin every 8 weeks. Such a system would be able to handle an average weekly intake load of about one patient per week. Those patients requiring more therapy after a time-limited group could move into a single longer-term group with a slow-open admission policy of filling empty slots as they arise. With this three-group mini-program, a substantial flow of patients could be handled over the course of a year.

A number of clinicians might collaborate on a group program. Referrals are routed through a common assessment procedure, at which point they would then be spread among the members of the group. This approach would allow for the development of more specialized groups.

Each practice situation has its own characteristics, but the principles described in this chapter should help to clarify the most effective and efficient organizational route. Clinicians might do well to promote the idea that their ability to do both individual and group psychotherapy gives them a "value added" advantage.

Professional Ethics and
the Group Psychotherapist

Group psychotherapists are bound to the professional ethical standards of their primary discipline. Two sets of issues present themselves to today's clinician: 1) How are the well-established ethical guidelines for individual clinical work adopted to the group environment? and 2) What are the ethical implications that arise when working in a managed care environment?

Ethics and Group Psychotherapy

The following ethical concerns apply to all psychotherapy and all psychotherapists, but take on added features in the group context (91):

1. Patients have the right to receive information about the nature of the group treatment and the possible risks. The information sheet discussed in the pretherapy preparation section of Chapter 6 (see Appendix 9) contains a general introduction to the nature of the group therapy environment. This material should be augmented with a discussion of the theoretical orientation of the specific group to which the patient is being referred. The introductory description of each group model in Chapter 13 provides some of this information, but the description should be amplified in discussion with the patient. This discussion can be combined with some comments about the relationship between the patient's presenting complaints and the type of treatment chosen. It is also useful to review alternative approaches that are in common use and to explain why the treatment in question has been chosen. The therapist must be clear that he has a responsibility to intervene to prevent anyone from having a negative experience and that the patient has a right to terminate the group at any time, though the patient is requested to discuss such thoughts with the group before actually terminating.

2. The patient should be maintained in therapy only as long as clinically indicated. Although this guideline is applicable to all types of therapy, it must be coninually kept in mind in group therapy, where issues specific to the group context can make judgments about termination more complex. There may be strong attachment bonds to the group that make leaving difficult and make talking about leaving just as difficult. The therapist may be reluctant to bring the topic up lest another member or two seize on the idea and consider leaving as well, even if they are less ready to do so. In closed groups, the original contract will have spelled out when the group is to end, but individual circumstances may make it relevant to question that time limit for a given member. For example, an error in assessment may have occurred and the approach being used may prove not suitable for the patient. Presenting this situation to the individual and to the group may be difficult, as discussed in Chapter 9.

3. Discrimination on the basis of race, color, sex, sexual orientation, age, religion, national origin, or physical handicap is addressed in most professional ethical guidelines and is strictly prohibited. This guideline

must be reconciled with the development of groups for specific target populations. Groups are frequently composed according to these very criteria. Reconciling these two aspects is perhaps less of a problem in a private office but can become a sensitive issue in a larger service system where there are finite resources.

4. The therapist is covered by the usual guidelines regarding confidentiality, but these do not apply in the same way to the group members. The expectation of confidentiality should be spelled out in writing and repeated verbally both to the individual and to the group in the course of the first session so that it is clearly understood and the reasons appreciated. Any hint that this guideline has been broken should be discussed directly and immediately in the group and with the offending member. This area becomes less clear in inpatient units, where patients are expected to attend group but often are provided with limited opportunity for orientation. The therapist may need to intervene in inpatient or crisis intervention groups to caution a member about excessive personal disclosures, especially those of a factual nature about the member's life outside.

5. Sensitive situations can arise regarding information the therapist receives from or about an individual member in the group. For example, the pregroup Model Confirmation Letter (see Appendix 11) mentions that phone calls between sessions may be shared with the group at the therapist's discretion—that they form part of the larger frame of the therapeutic situation. The therapist must use some caution in how to apply this guideline. A first step would be to check with the patient at the time of the call about how the information is to be shared with the group. The patient should be encouraged to bring the matter before the group himself. If the patient does not do so, the therapist may make an oblique reference later in the next session to something that might be discussed, and if the hint is not taken, the therapist might then identify the event and encourage the member to elaborate on it.

   Another sensitive situation arises if the therapist obtains information about extragroup socializing. If there is a clear negative response from the member to the idea of sharing the contact with the group, then there needs to be a serious discussion with the member concerning the original condition. It should be clearly spelled out how a repeat of the extragroup contact will be handled, and a clinical note should be made summarizing the discussion. Repeated problems of this nature might be grounds for discontinuing a member.

This discussion is based on contacts that have significant treatment implications in relationship to the type of group being conducted. The more the focus of the group is on learning from the interactional group process itself, the more care must be taken. Remember that actions may speak louder than words and that all extragroup contacts need to be carefully considered by the therapist even if no immediate action is contemplated.

6. The clinician must be aware when the needs of the patient are beyond her clinical competence to effectively manage. Consultation must be sought at such times and appropriate referrals made. Group psychotherapy embraces a wide range of diagnoses and techniques, and few clinicians will be skilled in every one. Hiding behind a general competence in running groups may mask areas of deficiency in specific areas. The interpersonal support or stress of sitting in a group may create a situation in which a member begins to reveal important information that was not discussed at assessment and that alters the implications of the original treatment plan. In such situations, if the subject cannot be pursued adequately in the group, it is best to take the patient aside after the session and review the matter in more depth.

7. Sexual intimacy is prohibited between professional and patient. Popular fantasies to the contrary, it is much less likely to happen in the context of group therapy than in individual treatment. However, the therapist has a responsibility to pursue the implications of sexual behavior between group members if it occurs. The therapist's role is not to condemn or support it, but to understand the situation and be sure that one or other of the participants is not being taken advantage of or acting out issues arising from the group. Handling of such situations is discussed in Chapter 9.

Ethics and the Managed Care Environment

The clinician working in the managed care environment is participating in a complex ethical arena. Clinicians see their primary responsibility as being to their own patients, and this historical tradition of the healer is fundamental to a trusting and collaborative therapeutic alliance. However, the other side of this situation also needs to be considered. Historically, many people have not had access to adequate health care and may receive access to a much broader range of services because the managed care organization has a responsibility to provide the care to the population it serves. Indeed, it may have the resources to do so better and in a more timely and equitable manner than an individual practitioner could hope to do. These two forces may at times seem in competition, and balancing them can be difficult.

A few general principles about how a managed care system operates might be helpful. Ideally, these principles can be incorporated into accreditation guidelines. They will not prevent disagreements but may help a collaborative resolution process evolve. Issues related to the following situations are being challenged through the legal process, and one can anticipate the emergence of more universal guidelines over time.

1. The role of the clinician as a patient advocate should not be altered by the system of health care in which the clinician practices. This does not mean that the patient necessarily should have access to every possible treatment option, but that clinicians not be prohibited from presenting their assessment of the treatment options most indicated.
2. Healthcare system allocation guidelines that restrict choices beyond normal cost-benefit judgments should be established at a policy-making level. The clinician can then be clear about the nature of rationing guidelines and can explain these to the patient.
3. The input of clinicians should be incorporated into the process of developing service guidelines. The sign of a more mature organizational structure is when clinical viewpoints are sought and considered. There can then be a minimum of middlemen between patient and clinician.
4. A formal timely and accessible appeals mechanism should be in place for situations in which the clinician believes a serious clinical error is possible.
5. The focus should be on cost-effective delivery of health care, not on arbitrary withholding of care. In terms of group psychotherapy, a reasonable guideline is to provide a trade-off (a "flex," in today's parlance) of three group sessions for every one allowable individual session.
6. Patients should be fully informed about benefit limitations.

It might be helpful to recall that Hammurabi, king of Babylon (d. 1750 B.C.), introduced laws that limited doctors' fees and punished those who injured their patients.

Training of the Group Psychotherapist

The finding of few differential effects between various kinds of therapy has led some to assume, erroneously, that anyone can provide group psychotherapy if he has common sense and a benign attitude. The first error is to assume that experience with groups of relatively healthy group members, such as a training group, prepares the clinician for work with patients with higher levels of psychopathology. As healthcare systems become more selective about who receives more intensive care, the level of severity in patients seen for treatment is increasing. Consequently, properly trained clinicians are increasingly essential to provide adequate levels of care. Untrained therapists are likely to have more dropouts, experience more management problems, and obtain lower satisfaction results. This realization is leading larger healthcare systems to invest more in training and continuing education programs.

The second error is to assume that if clinicians have had reasonable training in individual psychotherapy, they can make the transition to group work without much preparation. Acting on this assumption frequently results in a leadership style that attempts to do individual therapy in a group setting. This approach will sap group cohesion and lead to an increased rate of dropping out. The therapist may have difficulty containing an increasing level of group tension. This may lead the therapist to become either frustrated at not being able to do what she wants to do because of the group context or excessively anxious to the point where she cannot do anything with much conviction. The result will be dissatisfied patients and disillusioned therapists.

Comprehensive training of a group psychotherapist involves various components. All of these components may not be found in one setting, and sometimes the clinician-to-be must search for the range of experiences. Formal group training is available in some professional programs and in some communities, but many clinicians find themselves in the work force with limited preparation. As the use of groups expands in larger systems, there is pressure for more formal certification procedures such as that provided by the National Registry of Certified Group Psychotherapists (91).

Clinical Supervision

The most important, and the most available, component of clinician training centers on systematic supervision. Such supervision may begin with an opportunity for the supervisor to observe a group and meet with the leader after each session. This procedure is best set up for a definite number of consecutive sessions, preferably at least a dozen. Only over this length of time can the observer begin to get the feel of how a group evolves. Perhaps the most important aspect of this experience is to try to understand what is happening for the whole group, not just the individuals. The therapist can, it is hoped, provide some sense of what it was like in the actual group room. Many programs have observers rate aspects of the group interaction, such as who talks to whom, or track themes or critical incidents. It is an advantage to have a supervisor also watching with the trainees.

Various formats can be considered for the trainee's first group. There are some advantages to pairing a trainee with an experienced group clinician. An important one is that the trainee can be reassured that there is no pressure to be particularly active early in the group. The most important task of the trainee is to become comfortable with the group atmosphere and try to think of what is going on in the whole group and between members, not the individual problems of each member. Such a focus begins to make the trainees aware of the rich interactional possibilities in the group field. They can be encouraged to regularly scan the entire group to gauge the reaction of each member and try to establish a group theme. They will learn to sit with the group interaction as it develops and resist the urge to do something that might derail the natural development of the group. The trainees are encouraged to try out some clarification or linking interventions by modeling on the senior therapist. They will have time to develop their own style with more experience. As the group moves on, the trainee can become increasingly involved in the leadership task. It is important with this model to allow at least 30 minutes, if not an hour, after the session for a full debriefing on the experience.

Other programs will have trainees run a group as cotherapists. Although this can be effective, it runs the risk of problems arising between the two therapists. Both will be anxious about being in a group and about being observed by the supervisor, a field rich with competitive or avoidant possibilities. Certainly, with this model, on-site live supervision is strongly indicated, or at least the use of videotaping so that the supervisor can see what is actually transpiring.

A regular supervision seminar where group issues and problems from several groups can be discussed from a more theoretical point of view is very helpful. It also provides a structured group experience in its own right, with the problems being experienced in the treatment groups often being reproduced in the seminar context. It is strongly recommended that each trainee have experience leading several groups, preferably of different types so that a broad frame of reference can be established (92). For at least one of these, the trainee should conduct the group as a solo therapist.

Experiential Training

An opportunity to be a member of a group is an invaluable component of the training experience for the beginning group psychotherapist. Ideally, this experience would be in a format that could extend over time for at least 4 or 5 months. This format allows the trainee an opportunity to become engaged in a group, experience a deepening of the group involvement, and then go through the termination stage. Such an experience is a rich opportunity to learn both about groups and, often, about self. Although the group is expressly described as a learning group and not a therapy group, the participant generally finds it quite evocative of personal issues that engender an introspective process. In training programs it is generally best if the group leader is an experienced clinician who has only tangential connections with the program so that participants do not feel that they are in a situation where they are being evaluated for their competence. There should be very clear and specifically outlined guidelines about the leader's reporting to the training director only in regard to attendance.

National and local meetings of group psychotherapy associations generally offer experiential group opportunities of a more time-limited nature. Experiential training provides an opportunity for the individual trainee to determine if group work is of interest. Some people take to groups automatically, others have to work at it, and still others find it aversive. It is best to determine where one fits, and experiential training is a good place to start.

Didactic Education

Formal course work is available in many larger centers. The American Group Psychotherapy Association (AGPA) has recently developed a formal curriculum for a 12-hour introductory course that has a broad selection of key readings. (This curriculum is available from the AGPA at the address provided in note 90.) Many continuing education programs also offer basic and advanced courses. The more established group training programs require around 90 hours of course work.

This book covers most of the topic areas in established training programs. A solid grounding in the theory of small-group functioning equips the therapist to develop group approaches for different patient populations using a variety of theoretical models while remaining true to the effective use of the small-group environment.

Didactic programs provide an opportunity to conceptualize the issues. Supervision and experiential training address the development of skills and techniques. The National Registry of Certified Group Psychotherapists requires an introductory course and 75 hours of supervision, as well as 300 hours of experience. Continued reading and experience are required to adapt the generic group to a full range of theoretical models.

CHAPTER 13

Models of Group Psychotherapy

*T*his chapter describes several practical models for conducting therapy groups. All of these models apply the principles of the generic model of psychotherapy described in Chapter 2. However, they address different parts of that model in different ways. For example, the Interpersonal Problems Group model places great emphasis on developing the Therapeutic Contract through an extensive assessment procedure with detailed feedback, whereas the Crisis Intervention Group model provides only a single introductory sheet before the patient joins the group. In the Panic Disorder Group, therapist interventions stay focused on behavior and cognitive goals, whereas in the Antidepression Interpersonal Group there is a major focus on interpersonal patterns, including those manifested in the group itself. In other words, varied therapeutic techniques have been developed for selected patient populations, but all should be tested against the generic model in their application and molded to meet its expectations.

The material from Chapters 3 through 11 is applied selectively depending on the goals of each group and the capacity of the members. This approach should be thought of as getting the best "asset allocation mix" for a particular set of group members. All groups contain the same potential ingredients, but these ingredients are used in different combinations. The presence of common therapeutic features is the main reason that there has been so much difficulty in the psychotherapy research literature in establishing differential effectiveness between various approaches (93). The situation is even more striking in group psychotherapy, because all group formats will be saturated with the impact of common therapeutic factors that operate quite independently of efforts to provide a specific theoretical treatment. That is the main reason why there has been an attempt in this book to separate group dynamics from psychodynamics.

A seemingly endless variety of group models have been proposed. The models presented here have been chosen to exemplify a reasonable range of different types of group structure. The various models may be modified for specific patient populations. No day treatment model is included because these programs usually offer a complex mixture of different group techniques. The development of a therapeutic milieu in day programs or inpatient units is an important topic that goes beyond the scope of this book (94).

No specific model for patients with major early sexual or physical abuse is provided, although issues related to early abuse are addressed in the context of Adult Children of Alcoholics in the Substance Abuse Group model (95). Severe abuse histories are commonly found in patients presenting for psychotherapy, and the subject needs to be carefully assessed in every patient. Clinically, the issues raised by such early traumatic experiences produce profound difficulties in adult attachment and self-esteem. These are themes that flow through all intensive psychotherapy. Specialized programs may be of help for some patients in the earlier phase of treatment to facilitate recognition of the past, break through denial, and establish a therapeutic alliance. Many patients are able to achieve this in general psychotherapy groups as well. It is certainly common for abuse issues to emerge in some form during the course of treatment in almost any therapy group. It is important that all group psychotherapists be prepared to address such material or know when a referral elsewhere is indicated. The later phase of treatment for these patients merges into the mainstream of serious psychotherapy.

Nor is there a model that addresses the treatment of patients presenting with issues of psychological adaptation to major medical illness. Recent work has supported the impact of stress on the immune system and the value of psychological support in influencing the progression of malignancy. Other work has shown the value of psychotherapy in reducing risk in coronary heart disease. These studies have revitalized the interest in the psychosomatic/somatopsychic interface and have led to an increase in the use of groups in medical settings (96). In terms of group management, these groups rely heavily on the supportive therapeutic factors, accompanied by varying degrees of psychoeducation, lifestyle enhancement, and self-management techniques.

The idea of utilizing different group models for specific target populations will be new to some clinicians. Most clinicians use a mix of theories and techniques that they have acquired over time through training or continuing education workshops, or through day-to-day experience. Interventions are drawn from this repertoire on the basis of clinical hunches. There is quite solid evidence that psychotherapy, including psychodynamic psychotherapy, achieves better results when it is guided by a clear set of strategies. Every clinician operates with an internal protocol of what he or she plans to do. Protocols in the form of practice guidelines or manuals make these expectations more explicit.

The models described in this chapter can be seen as a type of practice guideline but fall short of constituting a treatment manual. They are formats to serve as general designs, not rules to be slavishly followed. The use of such models also emphasizes that different patient populations respond best to specific types of interventions. It is now expected that the practitioner will have more than one approach to offer and can shift comfortably into various techniques as required. Alternatively, a good network with other clinicians who have specialized skills might suffice. This versatility requires augmented training for all of us but at the same time opens up greater opportunities. We can expect the clinical research literature to begin to provide more detailed confirmation of the value of specific approaches for specific conditions over the next few years.

As noted above, the list of models presented in this chapter is not exhaustive, and the practitioner will see within them various components that might be linked for a given special clinical population. Such efforts to tailor the group ingredients for a selected population are encouraged. There are advantages to committing such guidelines to writing as a personal reference outline before beginning the group.

The first three models—Interpersonal Problems Group, Antidepression Interpersonal Group, and Panic Disorder Group—are at the higher end of therapeutic intensity. All three can be said to be insight-oriented, although the nature of the insight varies. In all three, the patient is asked to make connections between internal events and interpersonal behavior at psychodynamic, interpersonal, or cognitive levels. These models use extensive assessment procedures to develop a focus for therapeutic work, and the therapists are active in maintaining that focus. All expect active therapeutic activities between sessions and immediate application of group learning to current outside situations. They therefore have admission criteria that stress motivation and reasonable interpersonal capacity. All three formats have an established track record for effectiveness and together encompass a major part of the intensive time-limited group psychotherapy spectrum.

The next two models—Crisis Intervention Group for outpatients and Inpatient Ward Groups—have a brief crisis orientation. The goals of these groups are much more restricted: reestablishment of basic self-control, mastery of a current situation, and resumption of functional social roles. These groups may also serve a screening and preparation function, on the basis of which members may be referred for additional treatment.

The next two models are designed for longer-term care. The first of these, the Personality Problems Group, is an intensive treatment program designed for patients with severely dysfunctional personality disorders that combines cognitive-behavioral approaches with a self-psychology orientation. The other, the Community Support Clinic, is a maintenance program for severely mentally ill patients designed to keep them functional within the community and prevent decompensation.

Finally, programs for special populations—Eating Disorders Information Group, as an example of a psychoeducational approach, and Substance Abuse Group—are described. These models are intended as examples of how groups might be designed for the needs of a particular type of patient. The chapter closes with some comments about the function of self-help groups and their interface with other group models.

The group formats discussed in this chapter cover many possibilities and can be used for creative thinking about the therapist's particular clinical setting. The small-group format is a flexible vehicle for delivering a wide variety of treatments to just as wide a variety of patients. The list of models presented below will, it is hoped, encourage the development of more examples.

Interpersonal Problems Group

Formal Description

The Interpersonal Problems Group is designed for adults over the age of 18 who have experienced recurrent significant problems in their close relationships. The group provides a format for intensive discussions of current and past relationship patterns and how these have affected self-esteem. The connections with earlier experiences, particularly those in the family of origin, are explored. Special attention is paid to the nature of relationship patterns established within the group itself. The group meets weekly for 90 minutes for 20 sessions. Patients must be available for the entire sequence of sessions. No new patients are admitted after the third session.

This group model is designed as an intensive general psychotherapy group to address problems that lie primarily in the interpersonal and self-image range. The principal theoretical orientation is interpersonal/psychodynamic. This group operates much as do traditional longer-term psychotherapy groups, but with modifications related to the time limit. It incorporates many features from the individual brief dynamic psychotherapy literature. Attention is paid early in the group to the development of group cohesion to provide a supportive dimension as discussed in Chapter 3. A strong interpretive component is expected, primarily through the focusing activities of the therapist, as described in Chapter 11. The length of the group may vary from 12 to 26 sessions, with the longer end of this range providing more time in the interpersonal work stage.

It is anticipated that most of the patients would have significant elevation on anxiety and depression symptom scales but would not be in the severely incapacitated range. Most of the six personality dimensions should be in the higher range and the rest in the middle range, as discussed in Chapter 5. In particular, at least a middle range would be expected on Psychological Mindedness and Quality of Relationships. Heavy loading in a Conduct Disorder direction is a relative contraindication to participation in this type of group. General life adjustment in the last 2 years should not be severely impaired: ratings on the Global Assessment of Functioning Scale (Axis V in DSM-IV) and the Global Assessment of Relational Functioning Scale should not be lower than the midpoint.

Most patients with issues of person loss through death or separation can be effectively treated in this group model. This model is also suitable for many patients who have suffered physical or sexual abuse. The main issue would be the degree to which the trauma is available for recall and discussion. Of course, the more general features of psychosocial adaptation might rule some patients out. Patients who are having difficulty recompensating following a major stress are good candidates for this type of group. Often, the stress will have been of a nature that pressed specifically on vulnerable psychological areas.

Examples

A 36-year-old professional woman experienced major depression and low self-esteem for 2 years following a divorce. She was on an extended leave from her job and doubted that she would be able to return. Major issues concerning the need to have someone to depend on emerged during the assessment interview.

A 42-year-old man presented with symptoms of depression and hopelessness with active suicidal ideation but no specific plans. He described a succession of unsatisfactory relationships with women, the latest of which had ended 6 months before, when he and his wife divorced. This divorce occurred after a 2-year marriage in which the central issue was his inability to allow himself to tolerate the increasing expectations of intimacy from his wife.

A 23-year-old university student presented with symptoms of anxiety and depression that were interfering with her ability to study, as a result of which her previously high grades were falling. Her assessment interview centered on her realization that she had conducted her life with the primary goal of meeting the expectations of her professional parents, and she was beginning to wonder who she was as a person. She was preoccupied with ruminative thoughts about what she would do after graduation.

A 33-year-old man presented with surging waves of anger that he was afraid were going to get out of control, though this had not actually happened. In the assessment, he linked these anger surges to stresses caused by his experiences with his current employer that replicated experiences with his intolerant and critical father. He was in danger of losing his job over these matters, and his generally negative interpersonal style had contributed to two divorces.

A 55-year-old administrative assistant described severe levels of anxiety and despair. She initially attributed these symptoms to work stress that centered on a demanding but unsupportive boss. Further questioning revealed that her mother had recently relocated from a distant city and was now living a few blocks from her. Her mother's relocation to such a close proximity had reactivated earlier issues that the patient had "solved" by getting as far away from her parents as could be achieved on the North American continent. The increased proximity triggered fears of intrusive enmeshment with her mother, and the woman began having long-dormant nightmares concerning sexual abuse from her now deceased father, for which she blamed her mother because she had not intervened.

Although there are likely to be stress issues in the recent history of most patients presenting for treatment, it is best if these are not of a major, ongoing nature during the time this group will be meeting. For example, dealing with the acute phase of a pending separation or involvement in the daily care of a dying parent would make optimal use of the group difficult.

Groups with a higher supportive dimension would be indicated. In addition, the patient's understandable immersion with current difficulties may occupy a lot of group time to the detriment of the work of other members.

Personality issues are also likely to be present given the focus on interpersonal relationships. Patients with marked Cluster A features will find this type of group difficult. One would want to test carefully for motivation and capacity to participate. Patients with high levels of problems related to Cluster B features are appropriate candidates but may be difficult to contain in this format if they have a recent history of impulsive self-harm and frequent use of emergency facilities. Patients with Cluster C features are quite appropriate candidates if the overall level of decompensation is not too severe. Thus, this approach will be suitable for many patients with personality disorder depending on their capacity for interpersonal work.

The Interpersonal Problems Group is able to accommodate a wide range of adaptational problems. The general nature of the group makes it a useful component in a service system because the admission criteria are quite broad and it is an efficient vehicle for providing intensive psychotherapy. The group could be designed for a variety of target populations based on gender or age categories, such as abused women or university students, or based on adult developmental stages.

Therapeutic work is centered on the experiences in the group process. Therefore, all efforts to keep the frame of therapy very clear are helpful. It is wise to insist that no other talking therapies be undertaken during the period of the group. Brief medication management visits would be acceptable, but it is best if the group leader not be responsible for these, as discussed in Chapter 11.

Management Strategies

Assessment.   The full protocol outlined in Chapters 4 and 5 is used. This protocol should include a careful review of significant relationships during the assessment interviews. Particular attention is paid to the assessment of personality and interpersonal patterns, and the use of appropriate questionnaires is encouraged. A feedback session is used to sensitize the patient to recurrent patterns and to stimulate an introspective attitude. These patterns may become the basis for a list of Focus Areas, as discussed in Chapter 5. It is most satisfactory to schedule this feedback session to take place 1 or 2 weeks before the start of the group so that the material is fresh. The pretherapy handout material is discussed in some detail to develop a clear picture of how to get the most out of the group experience. Because the implications of time are going to be in sharp focus for this group, it is useful to be very precise regarding time boundaries. A sample Pregroup Confirmation Letter is provided in Appendix 11. These pregroup activities are designed to ensure rapid immersion into the therapeutic task and help to establish a clear Therapeutic Contract as described in the generic model.

The early sessions.   The first-session protocol described in Chapter 7 is fully implemented. The goal is to have all members outline in some detail the personal and relationship issues that are of primary concern to them. Such an approach addresses the expectation in time-limited psychotherapy that there be a clear goal focus. If target goals or Focus Areas have been described in a formal report, this can be distributed at the end of the first session, with the request that members review it for accuracy. Some time can then be spent in the second session briefly going over these comments. In that way, the focus is reinforced. It can be helpful in the second or third session to have each member repeat his or her target goals as a reminder to the other group members about what to be alert to. If there is a new member joining the group in the second or third session, this second go-around can be nicely integrated by having the existing members by way of introduction summarize what they had said earlier. This introduction paves the way for the new member to do the same and helps keep the member from experiencing a feeling of being behind in the group process.

For the Interpersonal Problems Group, the target goals are couched in terms of relationship patterns, specific problematic or "toxic" persons from the past or present, specific traumatic events, and specific attitudes toward self. There is a general emphasis on integrating family-of-origin experiences with current problems. Because of the affect-laden nature of these target goals, the therapist must walk a fine line between maintaining the intensity and containing the level of affect. This is best done by a continuous use of process debriefing interventions throughout the life of the group but most actively in the early sessions. In this way, a collaborative approach to Therapeutic Operations is promoted.

The therapist focuses during the engagement stage on the rapid development of a cohesive group atmosphere by reinforcing the supportive therapeutic factors and emphasizing issues across the external group boundary. This approach enhances the development of a positive and strong Therapeutic Bond. The elaboration of individual issues is utilized more for working toward these group goals than for immediate insight.

The level of therapist activity is usually rather low in this stage and primarily of a reinforcing and facilitating nature.

Group conflict.   The focus on group interaction established at the start will push the group into the differentiation stage within a few sessions. The therapist may model a more confrontational stance and encourage statements of personal opinion and intermember challenges. As in the engagement stage, individual issues are handled primarily in terms of their contribution to the stage task. If this shift in group atmosphere has not occurred by the sixth session, a full review is in order to identify the reasons for the delay. The purpose of reinforcing, and to some extent accelerating, this stage is to allow the maximum amount of time in the interpersonal work stage. Therapist activity level may be somewhat higher so as to be sure that the more confrontational atmosphere is regularly debriefed. Critical attitudes about the therapy or the therapist should be fully explored.

Interpersonal work.   The focus then shifts to a greater emphasis on introspective work concerning the connections to the Focus Areas established at the beginning of the group. In the Interpersonal Problems Group model, these themes are constantly related to intragroup events; the group works extensively with the here-and-now interpersonal action within the room. Therapist activities may increase as the stage progresses to ensure that target issues are kept in focus, though such activity is used only to the extent required. This focusing activity is built primarily around events in the group that parallel patterns from past or current relationships. There should be a general expectation that issues raised in the group will be applied at an early point to external situations. Such an expectation is a transparently open effort to ensure that In-Session Impact experiences are integrated into Post-Session Outcome changes.

Termination.   At the midpoint of the group, the therapist makes a clear statement that the group is half over and reminds the members of the date of the final session. A formal review of goals is conducted at this time. This review is designed to reinforce the focus, to identify goals that have not yet been addressed, and to allow the development of new goals. At each session thereafter, some reference is made to the session number, the number of sessions remaining, or the date of the last session.

This process sets the stage for dealing with termination issues, and termination themes may be dealt with as such from that point onward. The last four sessions must be viewed primarily through the lens of termination. Active exploration of the impending end provides an opportunity for dealing with deep issues of personal responsibility that go to the heart of self-image and relationship balance.

The final session is structured with a go-around of individual final words to ensure that the full impact of termination is experienced. An individual follow-up session is scheduled in 4 months to review progress and to act as an encouragement for ongoing psychological work. If formal questionnaires were used during assessment, the symptom questionnaires are repeated at the second or third session from the end, and the full set of questionnaires are repeated prior to the follow-up meeting.

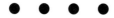

This protocol helps to package the group experience tightly. It ensures that maximum use is made of the limited time available. The principles are those of standard interpersonal/psychodynamic therapy. These are amplified by a detailed assessment process that focuses on interpersonal phenomena and the full use of the therapeutic factors inherent in an interactional group. The format applies the principles of the generic model in a systematic manner. Ambitious goals for major psychological change are promoted.

Antidepression Interpersonal Group

Formal Description

The Antidepression Interpersonal Group is designed for patients who have experienced repeated episodes of major depression and may have a history of significant dysthymia as well. This group model is not suitable for patients with a bipolar diagnosis or severe psychotic depression, nor for those experiencing acute major suicide risk. The group begins with a full exploration of the depressive syndrome and its impact on members' lives. This includes attending to daily lifestyle patterns that will help to combat isolation. The focus then shifts to the connections between depression and interpersonal relationships. These connections are seen as a complication of depression, and no assumptions are made regarding cause or effect. An intensive but semistructured approach to the current nature of important relationships is used. Group interaction is emphasized. The focus remains on current and future problems, and extended discussion of topics related to past experiences is not encouraged. Medications are not managed within the group. The group meets weekly for 90 minutes for 16 sessions. No new patients are admitted after the third session.

The format of the Antidepression Interpersonal Group model has been adapted from the interpersonal psychotherapy (IPT) model of dyadic therapy developed by Klerman and Weissman for the treatment of depression. This approach has been used in numerous research studies and was one of the formats considered in the National Institute of Mental Health (NIMH) Treatment of Depression Collaborative Research Program. This format has consistently produced positive results with few side effects and is associated with a low dropout rate. In comparative studies, it appears to have about the same effect as cognitive-behavior therapy of depression, with a suggestion that it might have better longer-term effects. Even in serious major depression with marked endogenous symptoms, IPT has produced results very similar to those with antidepressant medication. The Antidepression Interpersonal Group model adapts the basic IPT strategies for application in a group format. A protocol for applying IPT in individual therapy has been comprehensively laid out elsewhere by Klerman, Weissman, and colleagues (97). The clinician should have training and experience in applying this model to individual therapy before applying it to a group context.

The prevalence of major depression in the general population is estimated to be between 3% and 5%. This disorder is a major contributor to overall health costs (98).

The Antidepression Interpersonal Group approach would be suitable for any depressed patient, including the particularly difficult dual-diagnosis patient population suffering from depression/dysthymia where major characterological issues are anticipated. These issues tend to center on obsessional features, often combined with avoidant, dependent, or passive-aggressive qualities. Dysthymia results in lengthy suffering, with inhibition of personal potential and disturbed relationships. It is estimated that 80% of patients with dysthymia will eventually have a major depressive episode. The group format described here is particularly indicated when there are significant interpersonal problems that are associated with the depressive symptoms or that serve as triggers for major depressive episodes. The goal is to use the general effects of the group environment to address these broader features as well as the depressive symptoms themselves.

Patients with depression or dysthymia usually present with an extensive history of trials on various antidepressant medications. It is helpful to have a good working relationship with a psychiatrist who is particularly interested in the pharmacological management of mood disorders. Otherwise, considerable group time might be spent in speculating about what combination of medicines each member has tried. With a clear boundary between group focus and medication focus, such conversation can be kept to a minimum at the beginning and then firmly transferred outside of the group.

Example

A 47-year-old man was referred with a 3-year history of severe depressive symptoms accompanied by suicidal ideation but no specific attempts. His work performance was impaired, and at the time of the referral he was on an extended medical leave of absence. The onset of the depression coincided with separation from his wife and eventual divorce after a 12-year marriage in which she was described as extremely controlling and unaffectionate. The patient acquiesced to her settlement demands and realized in retrospect that he had made a serious error, leading to loss of most of his assets. Subsequent to the separation, major work stresses also developed, with the threat of bankruptcy. During the assessment process, the patient described the recurrent nature of his passive patterns with both business colleagues and earlier intimate partners. He was able to apply this awareness to a new relationship and to his business situation. As he found himself able to become more assertive, his depression lifted and his self-esteem improved.

A 36-year-old woman was referred with an 8-year history of dysthymia and three episodes of major depression, the most recent having begun 6 months before the referral. A variety of antidepressant regimens had been tried, with only partial effectiveness. The initial onset of depressive symptoms occurred shortly after the premature death of her mother in a boating accident. As the oldest child, she had felt responsible for looking after the family and acknowledged that she had never allowed herself to really grieve the loss. The most recent depression appeared to have been triggered by the death of an aunt to whom she had always felt particularly close.

Conceptually, IPT strategies can be located midway between interpersonal-psychodynamic psychotherapy and cognitive-behavior therapy. The focus on basic patterns in relationships and on a category system for understanding them is very close to the cognitive-behavioral idea of schemas that determine the psychological meaning of relationship events. The use of four categories of associated stress (grief and loss, interpersonal disputes, role transitions, and loneliness and social isolation) permits a clear focus to be maintained. The therapists will be working primarily on the supportive side of the supportive-exploratory continuum as outlined in Chapter 11. Therapist interventions include active focusing and confrontation of issues, with efforts to clarify patterns of interaction, but with less use of interpretive interventions. Current stresses and current relationship issues are emphasized. Reinforcement of coping strategies and mobilization of current resources are used along with active elicitation of the relevant emotional reactions.

The basic format of the Antidepression Interpersonal Group model could be applied to a somewhat broader patient population with a combination of general anxiety and depressive symptoms. The symptom focus would expand, but the basic strategies would be the same. From this perspective, IPT could be seen as a more structured version of the Interpersonal Problems Group model with a more consistent use of supportive techniques for a rather similar, though more dysfunctional, patient population. It might be seen as a way of combining the historic focus on general interpersonal phenomena in the interpersonal/psychodynamic tradition with the increasing emphasis on symptom-based treatments that is now expected in many service settings.

Management Strategies

Assessment. In the assessment interview, the clinician must probe into the circumstances surrounding the onset of the major depressive episode(s). The process begins with a careful search for possible triggering events, which are usually found in the interpersonal realm. Depressions occurring around the time of relationship breakdown are particularly common. Often, situations involving the management of anger are implicated, along with echoes of difficulties with assertion. Such critical incidents may activate dormant dysfunctional thoughts that then escalate in intensity. Getting a very precise time line is helpful in assessing whether the interpersonal component is a likely cause or an effect of the depressive state. If severe depressions emerge quickly with no evidence of triggering issues, a strong biological component is likely and the use of medications is indicated, including prophylactic use. However, even for these patients, the strategies included in this group may be helpful. Depressive symptoms and interpersonal functioning are seen as constituting an interactive cycle in which one will influence the other no matter which comes first. In the assessment, the clinician should try to identify coping strategies used by the patient and the positive assets they bring to the therapeutic task. Also, the clinician should inquire about seasonality, because seasonal affective disorder has a specific treatment approach (i.e., light therapy).

The focus of the group will be on current situations, not on exploration of the past. However, the detailed pretherapy workup focusing on past relationships that is used in the Interpersonal Problems Group model is still indicated (see Chapters 4 and 5). This survey will lay the groundwork for addressing current interpersonal issues. Questionnaire measures of relationships may be helpful.

The early sessions.   The first task of the group is to review in detail the nature of the depressive syndrome that each member is experiencing. This review allows one to give the symptoms the specific name of a depressive disorder and to normalize the symptoms as part of that syndrome. The common features, epidemiological data, and treatment prognosis can be reviewed. Careful review of the depressive syndrome is especially important because so many of the neurovegatative symptoms interfere with daily functioning (see Table 4–3). Suicidal ideation is included in this discussion as a common component of major depression. Many members will be on medication, and the principles of pharmacotherapy and drug side effects may be discussed. Detailed individual prescription information is best left to an outside prescribing physician.

The use of a daily journal is encouraged to help maintain a focus on application to the patient's current situation. The discussion of the impact of depressive symptoms will lead naturally to a review of their impact on daily lifestyle. A review of overall lifestyle may be useful (see Appendix 13) and can be incorporated into goals tracked through journal entries. Some therapists may choose to use the journal as a review mechanism at the beginning of each session and at the end of each session have patients enter goals for themselves to work on in the coming week. Therapists may vary in the degree to which they focus on specific written material rather than simply maintain a consistent focus on goals relevant to the depression.

Clarification of interpersonal patterns.   After the early tasks are addressed, the group moves on to an in-depth review of the relationship patterns that emerged during the assessment process. One format for structuring this review is to have each member write an autobiographical statement that focuses on interpersonal information.

The work sheets provided in Appendixes 6 and 7 are also useful in structuring the understanding of relationship issues. Current relationships, including recently ended ones, are emphasized. In some situations, there may be included a significant other from the past about whom the patient is having intrusive thoughts; that is, the person is very much a living presence, even if not actually with the patient now. This might take the form of a delayed grief reaction. Rating relationships on the three dimensions of the Structural Analysis of Social Behavior (SASB) system provides an organized format for thinking about the nature of the interpersonal issues. It will become evident during this task that key relationships are the focus for negative cognitions that distort or exaggerate the situation. These patterns may be usefully labeled and discussed, a process that would bring an applied cognitive component to the task.

The goal of this exercise is not to promote a detailed reliving of the past, but rather to address several key operational issues. First, recurrent patterns in relationships over the lifeline should be identified. Second, this information should be applied to the context of previous depressive episodes to determine if a consistent pattern can be found. Third, this historical information should be grounded in current relationships, especially those most connected with the onset or maintenance of the present depressed state. Fourth, the primary problem area should be defined in terms of the four categories described in the interpersonal model (see discussion on the Interpersonal Problems Group earlier in this chapter). Here, this group model diverges from the Interpersonal Problems Group model in that for the remaining duration of the group the focus remains primarily on the present and future state of current relationships, and less on a direct reworking of old material.

The process of reviewing the details of each member's relationship history will take several group sessions. This is not time wasted. Members will learn more about themselves as they listen to others' stories. An interactive process is to be encouraged in this task. The outcome of this segment of the group is a clear agreement from each member in terms of what interpersonal contexts are to be the principal focus and what problem categories are involved. It is usual to have more than one category seen as quite relevant; sometimes all four are in play. It is useful as a reference point to rank the categories and the main issues involved with each in the daily journal.

Management of the differentiation stage.   With the passage of time in the group and the focus on relationship experiences, the group environment will start to be viewed in a more critical evaluative manner. The difficult nature of the task of addressing major depression will also become apparent. This is an important transition for the group.

The tasks of this stage revolve around a more confrontational and assertive stance between members that is likely to press directly on vulnerable personal characteristics of many of the members. The process can be mediated through three techniques. First, the leader provides verbalized support for the importance of "coming to grips" with issues and emphasizes the role of feedback in this process. Such support serves to normalize the group's experience and to reinforce that the group is on track. Second, the leader draws parallels between the group process and the issues of difficulty in assertiveness and sensitivity to disagreement or anger that many members mentioned as an aspect of the interpersonal features of their depression. The group is pictured as a place where such ideas and behaviors can be tried out. The confronting nature of this stage of group development is used to reinforce the importance of addressing negative cognitions in the psychopathology. Finally, the leader explores the self-critical nature of the response to acknowledging negative thoughts and to being more assertive. A clear overlap with cognitive-behavioral perspectives will be obvious. These interventions help to deepen the work of the group and lay the foundation for more intensive exploration of relationship issues. The meaning of leader challenge is not extensively explored, but instead is accepted and managed.

Application of the four problem categories.   The semistructured approach used to this point helps to move the discussion directly into the nature of important relationships. It bypasses a lot of anecdotal information and focuses on interpersonal meaning. The role of misperceptions and beliefs about relationships is emphasized. The goal is to increase role mastery by an active exploration of alternative ways of understanding the situation.

Each of the four problem area categories has its own set of strategies based on the IPT protocol. These provide an overview of ways to approach mastery of each problem area. The basic therapeutic strategies for each category are listed. As the group moves into a more interpersonal work style, it is important that each member keep his or her own category priorities in mind and the issues involved in them. For most members, more than one category will be relevant, so much cross-learning can occur. Regular use of a daily journal will also help members to adapt the group experiences to personal goals.

A number of sessions may be spent on working through a particular problem area, making full use of the group as a supporting and reflecting vehicle. A problem-solving approach is adopted, moving from identification of how the problem area applies to each member, to what their expectations and perceptions are of the problem, to consideration of possible alternative ways to handle the problem area, and then to attempts at new behavior. The first two categories, grief/loss and interpersonal disputes, are particularly common and deal directly with relationship issues. Role transition issues often complicate the relationship situation or may in themselves be the principal challenge. Patients with longer-standing problems with social isolation and major difficulties with sustaining meaningful relationships will have more difficulty in addressing these deficits. However, if they can become involved as group members, they may experience a degree of acceptance and closeness that is quite motivating for them. In some ways, a group setting is likely to be more helpful than individual therapy in this regard.

Interactional work between the members continues to be important. The presence of the modest structure supplied by the written material does not mean that the process is heavily leader controlled. The therapist's principal activity is maintaining a focus on relevant issues and encouraging group exploration of these issues. The presence of many common themes makes it easy to use whole-group interventions that label these themes and promote further exploration of them. As the group progresses, it may shift into more existential themes concerning the values and meaning given to one's life. The focus on current adjustment should regularly include a review of general lifestyle issues that were raised in the beginning sessions: "How to develop a nondepressing lifestyle." Prolonged preoccupation with the past should be seen as resistance to current application. The expectation still holds that the ideas presented in the group will result in application to real situations outside of therapy.

Termination. Termination in the Antidepression Interpersonal Group is handled much as described in the Interpersonal Problems Group model. Patients with depression or dysthymia are often quite sensitive to attachment loss issues, so dealing with termination openly is a further way to achieve a targeted approach to important issues. The relapse prevention strategies described in Chapter 10 are also used.

All three mainstream approaches to the psychotherapeutic treatment of resistant depressed states (cognitive-behavior therapy, IPT, and brief psychodynamic therapy) have been reported to have significant recurrence rates. There is therefore a growing interest in longer-term maintenance efforts. The Antidepression Interpersonal Group format could provide an efficient mechanism for delivering maintenance treatment, for example, with a monthly "Maintaining Your Interpersonal Health" session. Such a program might be designed as a review session to which graduates from several groups could be referred.

The Antidepression Interpersonal Group is an integrative model that combines features of supportive group therapy with an established treatment for depression and dysthymia. The format could be readily adapted to other difficult patient populations, because the principles of IPT are increasingly being applied to diverse conditions. The content focus can vary, and the timing of the sequential progression through the protocol may be judged clinically according to group cohesion and the capacity of the members. The model makes full use of the interactional properties of the small group without moving into interpretive techniques. The emphasis on supportive features and on a modest degree of group structure makes it less likely that the group will get into management problems that might have harmful effects.

Panic Disorder Group

Formal Description

The Panic Disorder Group is designed for adults over the age of 18 who have a history of panic symptoms of at least 6 months' duration associated with marked impairment of general psychosocial functioning. The group emphasizes the use of self-management relaxation techniques and cognitive strategies to combat negative thought styles, as well as exposure to feared situations. Attention is also directed to issues of general lifestyle. Group interaction is emphasized. The group focuses on current and future problems; discussion of topics related to past experiences and problems is not encouraged. The group meets weekly for 90 minutes for 16 sessions. No new patients are admitted after the third session.

This group model is used as an example of a cognitive-behavior therapy (CBT) group approach. It can be modified to address the needs of other targeted patient populations as discussed at the end of this section. Full use is made of the supportive features of the group discussed in Chapter 7. However, the intensive application of cognitive-behavioral strategies requires a significant degree of patient initiation in applying the material between sessions. Thus, the format must be considered to be among the more demanding of the group models from the patient's perspective. Depending on one's viewpoint, the cognitive-behavioral elements of this group model may be seen as more or less stressful than interpersonal/psychodynamic therapy, but both in different ways use challenging interventions as a major component.

The group is of substantial duration (i.e., 16 sessions) because selection criteria emphasize serious dysfunction. Programs of this length, particularly when they try to capitalize on group interaction to reinforce the material, inevitably will move into a further stage of group development. It is important, therefore, that the therapist be prepared to manage this effectively. Management will center on maintaining a clear distinction between group dynamics and psychodynamics. Because of the requirement to review individual status at each session, it is best to keep the size of the group at a maximum of eight members.

The Panic Disorder Group is an example of a group composed on the basis of a specific diagnostic category (99). Panic disorder is one of the most common of the anxiety disorders and is associated with considerable general effects on physical and emotional health.

Management Strategies

Assessment. The Panic Disorder Group is designed for people who experience panic attacks, not simply high levels of chronic anxiety, and are seriously dysfunctional because of them. Panic attacks are associated with certain symptoms (Table 13–1), a number of which are related to the hyperventilation that commonly accompanies an attack. The attack is characterized by the sudden onset of severe, almost paroxysmal, symptoms that often lead the individual to think that he is going crazy or is going to die. The severe phase of the attack usually does not last more than a few minutes, though this may seem like an eternity to the person experiencing the attack. The diagnosis of panic disorder requires the presence of panic attacks that occur "out of the blue" without specific situational triggers. Most patients

Table 13–1.   Symptoms of panic attack

A discrete period of intense fear or discomfort, in which four (or more) of the following symptoms developed abruptly and reached a peak within 10 minutes:

1. Palpitations, pounding heart, or accelerated heart rate
2. Sweating
3. Trembling or shaking
4. Sensations of shortness or breath or smothering
5. Feeling of choking
6. Chest pain or discomfort
7. Nausea or abdominal distress
8. Feeling dizzy, unsteady, lightheaded, or faint
9. Derealization (feelings of unreality) or depersonalization (being detached from oneself)
10. Fear of losing control or going crazy
11. Fear of dying
12. Parasthesias (numbness or tingling sensations)
13. Chills or hot flushes

Note: A panic attack is not a diagnostic disorder in itself, but panic disorder cannot be diagnosed in the absence of panic attacks.

Source.   Adapted from American Psychiatric Association: *Diagnostic and Statistical Manual of Mental Disorders,* 4th Edition. Washington, DC, American Psychiatric Association, 1994, p. 395. Copyright 1994, American Psychiatric Association. Used with permission.

will, in addition, have attacks precipitated by specific situations or relationship stresses, particularly separations. The diagnosis also requires the presence of persistent cognitive symptoms of fear of further attacks and a significant change in behavior because of this fear. Major depression, substance abuse, and suicidal thoughts are often associated with panic disorder.

The most common association of panic attack is with agoraphobia (i.e., anxiety about being in places or situations from which escape is difficult or where help is not available, such as crowds, or an enclosed space such as a car or elevator). This condition results in avoidant behavior and, at its most severe, to a homebound state. Determining the details of the first attack may be instructive.

This careful approach to diagnosis is helpful when designing groups for specific populations. For example, in the case of panic disorder, consideration must be given to medications (tricyclic antidepressants or anxiolytics) that are helpful in reducing the incidence of specific attacks. Medications are particularly useful at the beginning of treatment, but high relapse rates are found when they are discontinued. A common treatment regimen is to begin with medications to get the severest symptoms under control and then to institute CBT while tapering the medications. CBT is directed at the fears that perpetuate the avoiding behavior and involves self-mastery techniques as well.

The first session. The protocol used in the first session is that described in Chapter 7, but the content deals primarily with the symptoms of panic and their effects on restricting activities. Disclosure of this information may be associated with anxiety about how the others will respond and with negative or critical views of self. This reaction is the usual material of early groups and is handled in the same way. Because anxiety reactions are likely to be triggered by the stress of the first session, the use of a *microlab pairing technique* could be considered. Members are asked to move into pairs and are given the task of introducing themselves and their main problems to each other. Each member of the pair then introduces the other to the group. This technique provides a supportive method of getting directly into important areas and addresses the common avoidance characteristics of panic disorder patients. A psychoeducational review of the features of panic disorder and of the principles of treatment can be integrated into the first one or two sessions. This review might focus especially on the "learned alarm" reaction (i.e., the escalation of anxiety as a response to early anxiety symptoms). A discussion of medications and side effects is also useful.

Daily journal. The first session includes a serious discussion about the importance of homework for enabling one to make use of the cognitive strategies to be covered. A daily journal is used. Keeping a journal helps the patient identify recurrent patterns associated with symptoms as well as track response to treatment. It is also a good method to reinforce the importance of homework application of the material being covered in the sessions. In all cognitive approaches, the skills being taught must be translated into actual behavioral application outside the session. Journal sheets can be developed that focus on panic symptoms and the usual phenomena associated with them, as well as providing space for general comments. Journals must be reviewed in group sessions to demonstrate the importance attached to them by the therapist. Such review is best done at the beginning of each session. Even without a journal, a weekly systematic check-in is useful to monitor application of group learning.

Self-management techniques.   The early sessions are a good opportunity to introduce strategies for managing anxious states. Such strategies include training in progressive muscle relaxation and diaphragmatic breathing exercises. Therapists with experience in guided imagery or meditation techniques may include these techniques. After a couple of sessions, it can be helpful to introduce a controlled stimulation of anxiety by purposeful overbreathing, spinning, or exercise (interoceptive exposure). The relaxation techniques can then be used to control the symptoms.

These self-management techniques also help to dampen background anxiety levels that may trigger panic attacks. They provide an early experience in gaining some degree of self-mastery. It is helpful to include relaxation exercises in a few sessions, perhaps at the end of the session as a way of preparing to leave. Refresher courses can be interspersed throughout the group's life. Patients are encouraged to practice these skills on a daily basis.

Lifestyle patterns.   The onset of both depression and anxiety disorders is influenced by general background stress levels as well as specific triggering events. Levels of stress can rise subtly, with the individual not being aware of change over time. Often, relatively simple steps to reduce stress and introduce a more balanced lifestyle can be helpful in providing enough relief to permit the use of more specific therapeutic efforts. The Life Style Inventory (see Appendix 13) is an example of a handout that can be used to structure such a discussion.

Negative automatic thoughts.   The cognitive consequences of the panic states are explored in parallel with the self-management techniques. The initial focus is on the catastrophic consequences of panic attacks and on the fears about what others will think if they see the patient's anxiety. The patient needs to know that these negative automatic thoughts are learned patterns and that they actively influence how the anxiety experience is understood. It is important that members practice identifying when these thoughts are occurring, how to interrupt them, and how to create personal coping statements that can replace or counteract the negative ones. Beliefs should be reframed as predictions and assumptions, not absolute facts. The role of negative thoughts in triggering anxiety, in augmenting the degree of anxiety, and in maintaining protective behaviors should be identified.

These strategies can be rehearsed in the group and, indeed, applied specifically to group situations where anxiety is stimulated. Often, having members work in pairs on such exercises is helpful.

It is rare to find patients whose negative thoughts apply only to the panic situation. Usually, by the time treatment is sought, these thoughts have been generalized to many aspects of life. This information will be of use later for structured exposure to feared situations. Once the core panic-related cognitions have been reviewed, the cognitive triad and the 10 common cognitive distortions that were discussed in Chapter 5 can be introduced.

Management of group development. The presence of structure in the early sessions promotes rapid cohesion within the group. The open group process and the use of pairing exercises increase a sense of intimacy. These features often will lead the group system to the point of needing to deal with differentiation-stage phenomena earlier than in more process-oriented groups. This paradoxical situation is one for which many CBT therapists are unprepared.

The best orientation when group tension rises is to apply group dynamics theory. The process of differentiation is based on differences and the need to be seen as an individual. Such features can be actively explored with the members. "It sounds like you don't see it quite the same way as Mary." "It's good to hear such a solid set of opinions." "The group is feeling more vigorous these days. That will be good for our work." "There have been a number of questions about how the group is being run. Does it seem like I'm pushing too hard? not giving enough direction? avoiding some important issues?" By calmly addressing the tensions in a matter-of-fact manner, the leader provides the members with a valuable opportunity to speak their piece, just what many patients with anxiety disorders need to do. This process material is not interpreted at the level of individual psychodynamics, nor are connections established with past experiences in the family of origin. This group is not based on an interpersonal group model.

Self-directed exposure. A key component of treatment, particularly for phobic avoidant behavior, is exposure to the feared situations. This technique is introduced after the members have achieved skills in relaxation and cognitive interventions. Patients are asked to make a list of all the circumstances they can think of in which fear of a panic attack interferes with participation. The situations on the list are then ranked into a hierarchy of importance according to the distress experienced. Patients then design a program for themselves of systematically addressing each situation beginning at the bottom of the list (i.e., with the least-distressing situation). This task may be carried out in pairs, both within the session for planning purposes and, perhaps, in outside application. A daily journal is helpful in keeping track of efforts to expose oneself to the feared situations.

Addressing interpersonal applications.   As the group moves into the interpersonal work stage, patients will feel more need to express personal thoughts. This is a good opportunity to shift to the behavioral consequences of the negative cognitions. The therapist should elicit a clearer description of just how limited the scope of life has become for the members. Often, there is a pattern of reinforcement of dysfunction by well-meaning family members. Such matters are particularly salient for patients with major agoraphobic symptoms who have developed a pattern of avoiding situations they fear might trigger a panic attack.

This area can be addressed by shifting the cognitive focus to the maladaptive expectations the patients have of others and of themselves. Introducing the theme of achieving increased autonomy, with an emphasis on taking small steps toward doing more on their own, is often helpful for patients. The therapist can promote an active use of group discussion with feedback and ideas. Often, examples of interpersonal difficulties are evident within the group itself and can be examined as they arise. There are multiple opportunities for modeling, coaching, role playing, and monitoring within a group. The more members can be of help to each other, the better. The therapist will need to use tactful interventions to keep the focus on behavioral and cognitive change. The program may include designated sessions that family members are encouraged to attend. Such sessions might include a psychoeducational component about panic disorder, as well as reference to the importance of distinguishing between helpful and harmful reinforcing behaviors.

Termination.   Because the Panic Disorder Group format is designed to last for several months, members have the opportunity to become quite connected. Therefore, the termination process must not be neglected. Some CBT therapists recommend a gradual tapering of sessions, though this is not so easy to do with the group format. In addition, the "fading," or "thinning of the reinforcement schedule," approach avoids the valuable task of addressing the impact of termination. There is the fear that doing so will produce a recurrence of symptoms, which indeed it will often do. But better to deal with this directly in the group than let it happen afterward.

Perhaps a middle ground is best. There is general agreement that termination is certainly a time to introduce relapse prevention strategies, as noted in Chapter 10. With the CBT approach, there may be some advantages to scheduling group follow-up sessions at gradually increasing intervals for reinforcement purposes. These sessions should be formally scheduled, and a definite termination date should be set so the sessions can be used also to work through the meaning of taking over treatment for oneself.

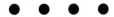

The general features of the Panic Disorder Group protocol can be summarized as follows. Group management uses structured discussion of presenting complaints, weekly review of progress between sessions, management of group development, and direct discussion of termination stresses. Specific techniques include use of a daily journal, psychoeducation, self-management exercises, control of negative thoughts, direct exposure to feared situations, and examination of interpersonal consequences in terms of reinforcement patterns.

Adaptation of Strategies to Other Targeted Populations

The strategies of the Panic Disorder Group model, summarized directly above, can be adapted to other targeted populations. There are a number of useful treatment manuals that patients can obtain and use as workbooks for a variety of symptom areas. In many cases, there is a therapist manual as well (100).

Major depression.   Cognitive-behavioral groups for major depression would place special emphasis on negative cognitions (101), but the other strategies also can contribute. (See section on Antidepression Interpersonal Group model earlier in this chapter for a discussion of the assessment and management of major depression.)

Obsessive-compulsive disorder.   It is now believed that obsessive-compulsive disorder (OCD) has historically been underdiagnosed and that the lifetime prevalence approaches 3%. OCD requires greater attention to behavioral challenge through exposure to feared situations and prevention of the usual responses. Somewhat less emphasis would be placed on cognitive aspects. Behavioral approaches are more likely to be helpful when the patient has rituals in addition to obsessive thoughts. Note that severe OCD is often accompanied by major depression. The choice of medication would shift to a serotonin reuptake inhibitor such as clomipramine or fluoxetine. Medication is best tapered and discontinued well before the group ends. Long-term maintenance of improvement appears to be significantly better with behavioral strategies than with psychopharmacological ones (102).

Simple phobias. A approach similar to that used for OCD can be used for simple phobias, for which the primary focus would be on relaxation training accompanied by exposure in vivo to the feared situation (103). Briefer groups of up to eight sessions are generally adequate, and the groups purposefully stay in the engagement stage throughout.

● ● ● ●

Panic, agoraphobia, major depression, OCD, and simple phobias all respond to cognitive-behavioral interventions using a time-limited approach. With the exception of major depression, they do not respond as well to general interpersonal/psychodynamic techniques, particularly in the shorter term. For patients with major problems in the interpersonal sphere, graduation to an interpersonal group might be indicated after achievement of some degree of mastery over the habituated cognitive and behavioral symptoms.

Consideration might also be given to a formal integration of cognitive-behavioral and interpersonal strategies. For example, a group could begin with an emphasis on self-management strategies and lifestyle and cognitive approaches and then introduce interpersonal techniques at a later point. Or the more structured and less structured components could be separated into segments within each session. This type of integration is also discussed in the context of the Personality Problems Group model.

Crisis Intervention Group

Formal Description

The Crisis Intervention Group is designed for the management of patients in acute crisis situations. It can accommodate patients with a wide range of nonpsychotic problems but would not be appropriate for patients with acute psychosis or hypomania. The group provides an opportunity to talk about current stresses. It utilizes a supportive approach that emphasizes practical techniques that foster immediate mastery. The Crisis Intervention Group is not an insight-oriented psychotherapy group. The group meets weekly for 90 minutes. Each patient referred may attend up to eight sessions over a 3-month period. Patients are encouraged to come regularly for the first three or four sessions and may then space their attendance. A regular turnover of group membership will occur.

An alternative title for this group might be the Rapid Access Group. This model was designed with the experience at a large urban hospital in mind. The model is suitable for a relatively unselected patient population presenting through emergency rooms or the intake service of outpatient clinics. Patients are also referred from a short-stay inpatient unit that works in close collaboration with the Emergency Room. Patients from other inpatient units sometimes come to the group during the week before their discharge. The Crisis Intervention Group can thus be used to avoid or shorten inpatient admissions (104).

The theoretical approach is strongly supportive in nature, with few opportunities for more exploratory work. Referral patterns indicate a heavy representation of major personality pathology of all kinds among the relatively unselected patient population described above. In suburban settings, one might expect to have a different balance, with more acute stress reactions and fewer characterological difficulties. In such situations, the goals of a Crisis Intervention Group may be more ambitious, closer to those of a time-limited group.

Crisis Intervention Groups always utilize cotherapists, preferably of both genders. It is helpful if one of the cotherapists is quite familiar with community resources, perhaps having a background in social work or community nursing. The nature of referral problems is quite diverse, as is the coping capacity of the patients. At times, one leader may need to actively look after an upset patient or divert an inappropriate referral elsewhere. Unusual management situations often arise in the group, and having two heads thinking about how to manage them can be essential. Co-leadership also provides a basic level of safety when dealing with referrals who might have received a less than comprehensive assessment.

The Crisis Intervention Group program is not for therapists who want to create the perfect group. On the other hand, it allows one to work with a wonderfully wide range of humanity, with all its foibles and eccentricities. It seems best, as learned from experience, that the cotherapists adopt a respectful but not too heavy-handed approach to group management. While not abandoning professional responsibility, the therapists need to be able to sit back and enjoy the interplay of the patients, each with a unique and interesting character. This stance helps the therapists to maintain a therapeutic attitude.

Example

A 47-year-old woman was referred from a medical ward 1 week before discharge. She was creating chaos among the nursing staff because of her demanding behavior and imperviousness to any suggestions for self-care. She arrived in a wheelchair, with massively edematous legs, and, even before the group had formally begun, proceeded to dominate the group conversation with a tirade of abuse about the system. It took some vigorous interventions to temper this torrent. She listened closely to the other members and became calmer. The next session she began talking about her fears of losing her children and how they all seemed to be turning against her. Her fantasy was that she might stuff them all back into her womb so that they would be little again. The therapists resisted an interpretive response. Over the next two sessions, the patient returned home and reported having a warm conversation with one daughter for the first time in several years. By her sixth session she reported that her children could not believe the change in her and that one of her sons was contemplating seeking treatment himself if it could be so effective. She was encouraged to join a neighborhood support group and did so before leaving the Crisis Intervention program.

The constantly changing group membership means that the Crisis Intervention Group will function in many ways like an inpatient group. Each session must stand to some extent on its own, though a degree of continuity is achieved through the focus on goals. The group will exist forever at an engagement stage–style of interaction. Evidence of a negative tone toward the leaders should be responded to at an early point and defused by a practical discussion of the issues. The group will have neither the capacity nor the structural stability to work through differentiation-stage issues, and it is harmful to encourage such work. The therapists need to directly acknowledge that insightful work will not happen except as an occasional by-product.

Management Strategies

Rapid access. All patients are seen for an initial evaluation within the department before referral to the Crisis Intervention Group. This evaluation is usually done by a clinician not attached to the group itself. Screening criteria are purposefully kept to a minimum. The patient should not be acutely psychotic or organically impaired. There should not be current major drug or alcohol abuse. Patients at extreme risk for suicide or violence cannot be contained in such a group. Otherwise, the group is open to most patients.

Patients are given an information sheet by the referring clinician that describes the group in terms of its primary goal of enhancing social coping (see Appendix 12). Providing such information can be seen as a modest attempt toward pretherapy preparation. Often, patients arrive with incomplete clinical information, so the first task may be to conduct an informal mental status assessment and clarification of basic referral issues. Finding out why the patient has come, in the patient's own words, can be quite illuminating and may not bear much resemblance to the ideas of the referral source.

Structured sessions. The sessions follow a consistent internal structure. This means that the Therapeutic Operations are driven by a higher level of therapist activity than in most groups.

1. Names are exchanged and the leader briefly reviews the purpose of the group and the attendance guidelines to reinforce the basic outline of the Therapeutic Contract. The new members are informed that they will have a chance to talk about their situations after the returning group members have reported. It is suggested that this will give them an opportunity to see the sorts of problems that are brought to the group.
2. A go-around for all returning members takes place. Each is asked to report on her week, with a particular focus on the goals established at the previous session she attended. About 5 minutes per patient is the norm, with allowance for unusual circumstances. In this portion of the group, the focus is clearly on one member at a time, with opportunity provided for questions or brief comments from others.
3. After all returning members have spoken, the new members are asked to talk about what brings them to the group and what they would most like to get out of the experience. This task is made much easier because they have already heard a range of problems discussed. It is unusual

for there to be much hesitation; indeed, new members are usually eager to finally get their chance to say something.

4. The remaining time is used to continue the group discussion, with active guidance from the leaders and always with practical coping strategies in mind. The amount of time will vary with the number of members and the amount of detail in the first go-around.

5. In the last 20 minutes of the group there is another go-around. Each member is asked to set some specific practical goals for the coming week. This is a greater task for new members. Goals are recorded by the leader in the session.

6. It is not unusual to have some administrative or clinical details concerning individuals to deal with after the session ends. At least one of the leaders must block off time for this purpose.

Maintaining a supportive atmosphere.   The supportive therapeutic factors are in full view. Members are encouraged to ask questions of each other, and exchanges of helpful suggestions occur frequently. Universalization is actively reinforced. The improvement in older group members is noted by new members. Affect is accepted but not probed.

A positive attitude is maintained. Major group process transgressions commonly occur. Some members will launch into controlling monologues, whereas others will demonstrate gross misunderstanding of the situations being discussed. There will be blatant denial of problems or displacement onto various agencies, authorities, or relatives. Such incidents are tolerated and worked with, not challenged. The goal is to maintain a positive Therapeutic Bond between the members and the leaders, along with a modest level of group cohesion. The group is used as a source of reinforcement to try new ways of coping.

Leader activity.   The leaders are benignly in control of the group process. Overly active members will be thanked for their contributions, and the conversation will then be shifted to another member. A firm focus on current adaptation is maintained. If a member indicates the desire to delve into past events or family-of-origin material, he will be redirected to what needs to be addressed in the present session. If affect begins to mount, the leaders will move into a more cognitive exploration of the issues. It is important that the therapist activity be built on an empathic attitude and gracious language. The control being calmly enacted is in the service of productive work, not a critical response to bad behavior.

Goal setting. Each session begins and ends with a discussion of goals. The focus is on quite concrete strategies that will encourage greater mastery. Patients have to be continually urged to keep their goals realistic and manageable and not to try to deal with everything at once.

Attention is paid first to basic daily routine: developing better sleep hygiene, getting out of bed in the morning, eating regular meals, and getting some modest exercise by taking walks. Utilization of available social contact opportunities is encouraged. This may involve, for example, contacting family, calling friends on the telephone, getting out of the house to go to the store, or going to a neighborhood recreation center. Proper use of medication may be reviewed.

When these basics are in place, goals may shift. Small relationship tasks may be undertaken—for example, to reestablish contact with a family member after an argument, to make a long-delayed appointment with a service agency, or to set limits with friends about making so many demands. Often, trying out ideas or rehearsing what to say in the session can be helpful.

Brilliant interventions are few and far between. An emphasis on positive strengths, support of the desire for change, and empowerment of the individual to talk openly about what might be most helpful often provide adequate opportunity for the patient to become more settled. Seeing other patients tackling the setting of goals is often quite helpful for defensive patients, allowing them to become more collaborative in their approach to treatment. Obtaining some order and mastery over daily routine will lead to a more positive attitude and better self-esteem.

Patient disposition. For a number of patients, a few sessions in such a group can get them back on track. They may stretch out their sessions to fill the entire 3-month period to give themselves time to follow through on their plans.

It is to be expected that some patients will come only for a small number of sessions and move on. They are contacted after the first missed session to check on their status and dropped from the roster after missing three sessions without contact. Such patients often say that they enjoyed the group and that things improved.

Another important function for the Crisis Intervention Group is to screen patients for ongoing therapy. The group provides an opportunity to test motivation and interactional capacity. It can be useful in determining what sort of program is indicated. In a number of instances it has provided a positive experience that convinced the patient to join a longer-term group.

This group model provides a useful buffer for referral sources who need an immediate response. For some patients, it is adequate treatment; for others, it allows an opportunity to assess suitability for additional treatment. The group environment is used for its general positive properties, not for exploratory or interpersonal work. A recent informal review of a year's experience indicated that about 20% of referrals either did not arrive or came for only one session. Almost all the others attended at least four sessions, and many attended six to eight sessions. These figures follow almost exactly the pattern of the utilization curve shown in Figure 1–1 (see Chapter 1). In the judgment of the therapists, about two-thirds of those attending more than one session appeared to have benefited from the experience.

Critical Incident Stress Debriefing

A different sort of group format is used for *critical incident stress debriefing* (105), an approach applied in disaster situations. The format is quite structured and deals specifically with preventing the development of posttraumatic stress disorder. The facts of the disaster situation are reviewed, participants are encouraged to begin verbalizing their reactions to the experience, the normal features of acute stress reactions are described, and a sense of community is fostered. These techniques are not those of a usual psychotherapy group. In critical incident stress debriefing, the intent is to contain and begin to channel the normal reactions to disaster, not to get into psychotherapeutic change. Often, emergency personnel and other community leaders have been trained in these procedures. The clinician should be careful not to get in the way, but to be prepared to accept referrals for those victims having more difficulty or to serve as a consultant.

Inpatient Ward Groups

Formal Description

Inpatient Ward Groups meet three times per week, on Monday, Wednesday, and Friday afternoons at 1:00 P.M. Unless there are specific reasons, it is expected that all patients will attend. Two groups are held simultaneously. One of the groups is designed to deal with personal issues that are related to hospitalization or that will complicate managing after discharge. The other group focuses on learning more about the illness that led to hospitalization and the skills needed in managing outside of the hospital. Both groups emphasize understanding how to gain some control over the situation that led to admission and how best to manage after discharge. (See alternative scheduling options below.)

Inpatient groups face many unique difficulties. Patient turnover is rapid, the level of pathology is high, motivation may be low, and the mix of problems is continually fluctuating. Investigations and treatments are in progress simultaneously, and often this produces scheduling problems. Psychotropic medications or ECT may interfere with cognitive functioning. Many different professionals are involved in the patients' care. As the average length of stay on inpatient units continues to drop, the level of pathology increases. In the face of all of this, groups remain an important feature of the inpatient milieu. Patients regularly report that they have received considerable help from the ward group experience (106). One study reported that the therapeutic factor felt to be most helpful was altruism.

Various strategies have been devised to make the most of this difficult situation. It should be clearly recognized that the group component of inpatient care is only one part of treatment; other treatments will deal with other aspects of the patient's overall treatment. The goals for inpatient groups need to be limited to realistic levels. They also have to be tailored to the nature of the unit. Most inpatient units are now designed for relatively short stays, with admissions longer than a few weeks being the exception. The model presented here has that type of setting in mind.

Long-stay units tend to focus on specific diagnostic categories that present major levels of dysfunction. For example, a core of severely ill schizophrenic patients require treatment directed at self-care and basic social skills. Units for patients with severe eating disorders, particularly anorexia nervosa, feature renourishment programs along with cognitive and educational groups and a family therapy component. These types of programs are designed to prepare the patient for ongoing outpatient therapy. The occasional inpatient unit specializes in treating patients with borderline personality disorder (BPD). Apart from such unique treatment programs, a better general guideline would be to keep patients with severe personality disorder as far away from a hospital bed as possible. Child and adolescent units have quite special needs, as do longer programs in correctional settings. Many of these longer-term programs are designed with formats similar to those of day treatment programs. The general group psychotherapy principles outlined in this book would be appropriate, with the added requirement of integrating the groups into the other aspects of the milieu setting. Often, a mix of structured and process-oriented groups is found.

Management Strategies

Selection and preparation of patients.   Patients should be selected to attend group only if they can to some extent stay seated and attend to the process. Most patients experiencing acute psychotic states or major depression can do so. Selection of mute, incoherent, or extremely labile patients is inappropriate. Acute mania is a contraindication until the patient begins to settle. It may be best to exclude patients with severe impulse-control problems until their volatility has decreased. Moderately demented patients may derive some benefit from the socializing stimulus, especially on wards with many other elderly patients.

One of the therapists should spend a few minutes with a patient before they begin the group to provide a brief orientation. Such orientation might consist of a description of when the group meets and what the main goals are. Basic ground rules concerning attendance, participation, and confidentiality are reviewed. A short handout might be considered.

Maintaining realistic expectations.   Inpatient Ward Groups are best conceptualized as remaining forever in the engagement stage. They are continually rebeginning and working to consolidate into some sense of groupness. Therapeutic factors from the supportive cluster—acceptance, hope, universality, and altruism—should be mobilized. A positive orientation should be encouraged, and the group should be purposefully discouraged from getting into the leader challenges of the differentiation stage. There is seldom enough time or group stability to hope to get through such material satisfactorily. The emphasis is on coping with current problems, not curing symptoms. Therapists will find useful ideas from the crisis intervention literature referred to earlier in the discussion of the Crisis Intervention Group model. The tasks include a controlled mobilization of affect with cognitive support; encouragement to clarify current issues and circumstances, particularly those surrounding the need for admission; and then promotion of a problem-solving review of alternative strategies. A broad scope of topics dealing with current reality, ranging from understanding the symptoms of schizophrenia to increasing self-awareness of the effects of the stress of a broken relationship, can be addressed. Often, goal setting initially might involve only the next 24-hour period and then be extended as the patient's clinical condition begins to settle. Discharge planning should be kept in mind from day one.

Two streams. It is most common to divide patients into groups based on a two-level system of interactional capacity. One group contains patients experiencing psychotic symptoms, including the effects of organic impairment. The other is composed of those patients who are able to talk more actively about themselves and interpersonal matters. There will always be some patients in a middle range of capacity who can be placed in either type of group, in part to balance attendance of the two groups.

Alternative scheduling options. Some programs with daily ward groups restrict entry to Mondays and perhaps Tuesdays only, thus achieving some degree of membership stability for at least a week. Because the patients are actually interacting throughout the day, such arrangements may allow the development of more advanced group work. Daily groups are able to maintain more continuity and are particularly useful on short-stay crisis units. Twice-a-week groups will clearly need to focus on one session at a time. Ward groups for patients with significant cognitive dysfunction are best limited to 45 minutes, and for patients in groups with an interpersonal focus, from 60 to 90 minutes.

Reflections of the ward milieu. Ward groups do not exist in a vacuum, but instead actively reflect ward issues. On short-stay wards, such issues usually involve specific ward crises. The groups provide a good opportunity for patients to debrief on incidents. They may also be a good place to pick up reverberations of general ward management problems. For this reason it is important that there be an open, positive understanding among the group leaders and the rest of the ward staff. Such an understanding is often achieved by having a ward nurse function as a rotating cotherapist along with a permanent experienced group leader. The policy on the organization of the groups needs to be clearly sanctioned and supported by the administration. The policy should include a firm statement against removing patients from groups in progress. On the other hand, groups should be scheduled when interruptions are less likely. One unit ran their groups from 10:00 to 11:00 A.M., right in the middle of ward rounds, and the therapists wondered why people kept being removed.

Using a single session.   Because of the rapidly changing membership in Inpatient Ward Groups, it is realistic to focus on what can be achieved within the time of a single group session. This perspective encourages a pragmatic focus on immediate coping issues. Continuity between sessions is an added bonus. A single-session focus also ensures that the leaders attend to basic group tasks of orientation for new members and preparation for the departure of leaving members without feeling guilty that more in-depth work is not accomplished.

Leadership issues.   Inpatient groups must be structured and focused through an active and positive therapist style, which reinforces the supportive therapeutic factors. The focus of the group is more on information than on affect. This cognitive focus can combine elements of psychoeducation, problem solving, and cognitive-behavioral techniques. A go-around format ensures that all patients have a chance to participate. The goal at all times is to reinforce mastery of affect, impulses, thoughts, and daily routine. The leaders should be alert to escalating affect and should move quickly to dampen this process. On occasion, a member might be requested to leave the group for a while until things settle.

Patients are encouraged to think about their treatment from a therapeutic standpoint. The here and now of the group is extended to the here and now of the patient's immediate life circumstances. Specific attention is paid to the events leading to admission. What clues can be used to identify problems early? How can the patients seek help before the need for hospitalization arises? How do they cope with current symptoms, and what is the role of stress in precipitating these? The therapists help the patients to try to identify negative cognitive styles that result in a deepening spiral of hopelessness and to challenge the validity of these automatic thoughts. What are the effects and side effects of the medication they are taking? Reference to discharge planning, including ideas about how to stay out of the hospital, is made immediately. Details of past history and dynamic interpretations are out of place. Sanction and support are given for patients talking among themselves between sessions, something they will be doing anyway. Members are continually being discharged, and managing without the relative security of the ward and facing outside stresses will be a constant theme. This focus will sensitize patients to treatment and self-management issues and, it is hoped, will increase their motivation to comply with outpatient arrangements.

Ward meetings.   Many units have regularly scheduled community meetings of all patients and most staff members. The large number of participants means that the meeting cannot function as a therapy group. A more suitable structure is that of a town-hall meeting with a chairperson and an agenda. The presence of this structure paradoxically results in greater freedom to participate because there is not the expectation that attention will be focused on every phrase. Topics can include planning of ward activities, management of the problems of living together through establishing daily goals, specific ward incidents, and information about procedures, meetings, and so on. Such meetings can be quite helpful in maintaining a sense of ward tradition and in mediating problems before they become too highly charged. Some specialized units may be able to develop a large-group format, with which more ambitious aims of a therapeutic community can be addressed.

Continuity with postdischarge groups.   A fully developed service system will have an array of groups available for patients being discharged. It may be advantageous for inpatients to attend a session of their future outpatient group while still in hospital, thus establishing a reassuring connection. Good communication between inpatient and outpatient therapists assists this process.

Personality Problems Group

Formal Description

The Personality Problems Group is designed for adults who have experienced long-standing problems in their close relationships, particularly problems of enmeshment and instability. These patterns will usually be connected with patients' low self-esteem and, often, a sense of confusion about their own identity. Periods of decompensation will have occurred with some regularity, often necessitating hospital admission because of suicidal thoughts or self-harm behaviors. The personality problems will have interfered with vocational adaptation as well. Shorter-term intensive treatments should have been tried with limited success. The group meets weekly for 3 hours. The first segment consists of a 1-hour block in which the focus will be on lifestyle, self-management, and behavioral and cognitive-behavioral techniques. Following a 30-

minute break, the second segment begins and consists of a 90-minute general group in which the emphasis is on learning from the group interaction itself. This segment emphasizes a focus on self, as well as interpersonal skills. (The two segments could be scheduled on different days of the week to provide more regular contact opportunities.) The group meets from September to June (approximately 35 sessions), and there is an option to continue during a second year. No patients are admitted after the first three sessions. No other regular formal psychotherapy is allowed. Medication management should be handled by psychiatrists other than those involved in the group.

This group addresses the needs of a patient population with severe and disabling personality problems (107). The format of the group combines two active ingredients: 1) self-mastery techniques and 2) exploration of how interpersonal relationships are managed, including how the individual experiences self in that context. The short-term goal of the group is to provide a containing environment to reduce utilization of other, more intensive resources. The longer-term goal is to develop higher-level coping skills to forestall recurrent catastrophic relationship situations and repeated bouts of self-destructive behavior. Such events often involve increased use of other medical resources.

The frame of the therapeutic process is an even more central concern than in most psychotherapy. No other active talking treatment is allowed, and medications should be managed by someone other than the group leaders. Cotherapy is utilized, and there is a strong preference for a male-female pair. The same therapists conduct both segments to maintain consistency. This group model requires experienced therapists. It would be better to provide low-frequency supportive maintenance contact than to attempt such a group without adequately prepared leaders.

Management Strategies

Assessment.   The patient population suitable for this extensive program will include a heavy loading on Cluster B characteristics. In terms of the six personality dimensions discussed earlier in this book (see Chapter 4), the group will have a high level of Emotional Reactivity. Most will be in the lower level on Quality of Relationships. They may be at either extreme on Extraversion/Introversion and will tend to fluctuate rapidly along the

Agreeableness axis, from exploitable passivity to angry distancing. Some may have many features of a Conduct Disorder, particularly because of high levels of self-preoccupation. The use of projective identification will be common. A strong loading on Conduct Disorder, particularly if accompanied by strong evidence of distrust and vindictiveness, should be a warning of caution, even when the group has been designed for treatment of severe problems.

The early phase.   It is expected that the group will take time to develop, and this process should not be accelerated. The accomplishment of a cohesive group is in itself a major triumph. One can anticipate that the members will be extremely sensitive to control issues, so the therapists are best to take a relatively low profile and not encourage the expectation that all results will come from their activity. The attitude should be that the most useful ideas will come from the members, because they are the ones who know most about what they experience.

The therapists will need to debrief routinely after sessions, with a focus on managing their responses to the projective provocations offered by the members. These provocations may include severe criticism and highly polarized views of the two therapists into good or bad parental images. The therapists are required to contain these affects as well as their own responses to them. At times of stress, the group may move into a consolidated emotional state like those described by Bion (see Chapter 9), and the therapists will experience the full force of this group affect. Debriefing should also include an exploration of the context in which the events occurred. This cognitive work will help the therapists regain a position of therapeutic balance. The nonreactive management of early anger is a most important task. Premature terminations are most likely to occur during this early phase. The therapists should think of this as a time when the patients are testing their capacity to stick with difficult issues without getting defensive.

The structured segments.   The question of control will be a particularly sensitive issue in the more structured first segment of each session. It might be helpful to conduct this first hour around a table to decrease interpersonal tension. It is best to structure this segment around personal vignettes that can be discussed from the standpoint of cognitive distortions. It is helpful to encourage members to bring in written descriptions, which can then be used as the material for discussion. This helps to bind affect and encourages a self-observing stance. Keeping a regular journal is expected of the members for their own use in thinking about things. Common themes will center on catastrophizing, rigid dichotomous thinking, untested assumptions about the reactions of others, and a constant theme of being the victim combined with callous disregard of others. Distorted belief systems about oneself and others will emerge. The first segment can also be used to discuss written autobiographies. As the group progresses, more specific attention to management of anger will be important.

The usual formal attention to thinking errors with a classroom atmosphere is not likely to be successful with this patient population. Massive noncompliance will occur as defenses are activated against authority. However, the basic strategies of cognitive work are helpful once they can be effectively introduced. They provide a mechanism that patients can use to delay responses and put relationships into perspective. Group interaction is to be encouraged, and the therapists need to avoid taking an evaluative position about the material being presented, even when it is quite dysfunctional in nature. The goal is to identify what has happened and what strategies can be devised to address such problematic situations.

Self-management techniques such as relaxation, meditation, and anger management may have the paradoxical result of tipping the patients into deeper anxiety or confusion. These techniques are better introduced later in the sequence after some preliminary cognitive control mechanisms have been adopted.

The process segments.   The process segments are managed as with any other group but slowly and carefully. If a table was used in the first segment, it is removed. Supportive therapeutic factors will appear, as usual, but more gradually and often in disguised ways. The therapists can cautiously reinforce these largely by identifying them, not by expressing an opinion about their merits. Interaction among the members should be strongly supported. External boundary testing will occur and can be a useful focus for discussion, not from the position of power but from curiosity. Such boundary testing is likely to involve lateness, missed sessions, subgrouping, seeking other treatment, emergency room visits, or phone calls. All such material should be brought into the group for discussion.

The misinterpretation of and overreaction to interpersonal events will respond only gradually to therapeutic efforts. Therapists need to understand this so that their inevitable impatience can be kept in perspective. These patients are experts at detecting negative vibrations and often react to such reactions in the therapists before the therapists themselves are aware of what they are experiencing.

It will be noted that the term *borderline* has not as yet been mentioned in the description of this group model. Despite its widespread use, the concept is sufficiently vague as to be of limited clinical meaning and is often used as a pejorative short-hand for the difficult patient who annoys therapists. Research studies clearly indicate that BPD is a multidimensional diagnostic category and is multidimensional in etiology. What does seem clear is that these patients experience strong and swinging emotional reactions in relationship situations that color and distort their interpretation of the motivations of others. For this reason, a central therapeutic factor is the therapist's ability to understand and tolerate the contradictory affective components of the patient's views of self and others.

The technique of reflective validation seems particularly useful for these patients, who suffer from severe defects in how they see themselves. The technique involves a restatement of what the patient is saying or experiencing about herself. For example, "I appreciate that it is hard to find yourself both longing for your father's approval and, at the same time, having a lot of angry feelings towards him" or "This sense of confusion you experience when that happens sounds like it makes you fear things will fall apart. Maybe you can just sit with it for a while here in the group and talk some more later" or "Your reaction to your boyfriend's departure is certainly understandable given the number of losses you experienced in your own family as a kid." Such interventions help the patient to clarify internal states and attach names to them. The therapist's restatements have a containing and calming function especially when the expected negative reactions from others do not occur. At least their experience of self can be understood by someone else. This is an experiential echo of the cognitive approach to the same phenomena in the structured segments.

The topic of suicide will be regularly introduced in the group by the members. It is important that the therapists feel comfortable with an open discussion of the topic. The key to this is an encouragement of a rational group process, not an escalation of alarm over the need to do something. An exploration of the context in which the thoughts arose may be helpful. The members need to know that the therapists are not going to be reliably available to answer calls 24 hours a day but that usual emergency resources are available. The therapists should be clear that they do not want such events to happen but that control ultimately lies with the patient. As with emotional responses in general, this sort of open discussion is usually quite calming.

It is to be expected that group interaction will become chaotic at times. The combination of high emotional reactivity and projective identification can lead to angry and, at times, vicious attacks between members, usually those having similar qualities that they project onto each other. The therapist must be prepared to assume control in such situations. The involved members are asked to be quiet, sit in their chairs, and take some deep breaths. The rest of the group is encouraged to continue without feeding into the controversy. The upset members may join the general discussion later. There may be small eruptions of the conflict later in the session that also need to be quickly modulated.

Example

A man in his late 40s had come to America at the age of 20. He still identified himself as an immigrant and lived in fear that if he had trouble with the law he would be immediately deported. He described a number of relationships with women who he felt, early in the relationship, were "the most beautiful, wonderful, loving people in the world"; but if they raised any expectations of him, he would immediately switch and terminate the relationships—"tell the bitches to get out of my life." In the group this dynamic was re-created with a younger woman with passive-aggressive and histrionic characteristics. In one session they both ended up standing and shouting obscenities at each other. Repeated and firmer requests were required to get them to sit down. Over time they maintained a truce and did not speak to each other, eventually tolerating some interaction. The man began making awkward but well-intentioned attempts at empathic comments to an extremely passive woman. Several months later another yelling match broke out but was quickly contained. The next session the man began speaking about his recognition of situations in which he would completely overreact with fear that he was in mortal danger and had to protect himself. This signaled a major shift in his level of openness and self-acceptance.

The advanced group.   As the group gradually adapts a more controlled interactional style, it begins to assume the features of a usual therapy group. The therapists find that they can be more active and reflective without triggering an immediate response. They will constantly strive to keep the focus on what the members are experiencing in the room. This here-and-now focus is designed to help the members identify, explore, and understand the nature of the interpersonal distortions that the members experience with each other. The usual progression is to move from expression of angry or distancing themes to toleration of increasing closeness.

The therapists can monitor this process by noting the frequency of periods of openness or vulnerability shown by the members. It is best not to mention these states early on, as the attention may shut them down. Oblique techniques might be used—for example, "It sounds like you are connecting with some important aspects of yourself like Henry did last session."

The process will fluctuate from a burst of intense activity to periods of resistance. Remember that the presence of resistance is a positive sign that core issues are being activated. An important function for the therapist is to act as a group memory—for example, to track for the group how similar issues are being resolved at increasingly functional levels as the group progresses, or to connect parallel themes between previous reports of outside relationships and what is happening now in the group. Even in the advanced group, interpretations are best used with caution and, if used, always presented in a tentative manner. A constant interest in how members are experiencing internal states helps to reinforce an increasingly differentiated sense of self and the complexity of that structure. It is also helpful to specifically identify for patients the nature of the changes going on within themselves.

Absences and termination. The selection criteria guarantee that severe attachment pathology will be highly prevalent among the group members. It is inevitable that there will be major reactions to missing members or absent leaders or to breaks because of holidays. These concerns may not be verbalized but rather may be acted out with absences, displaced anger, or decompensation crises. Such acting out should be anticipated, and if the subject is not brought up by the members, it needs to be introduced by the therapists. The purpose of this is twofold: first, to get an airing of the affective loading about the meaning of absences and, second, to think through coping strategies for the situation. For example, during a long weekend, how can each member organize her time to carry her through the period when the group would usually meet on a Monday?

The group will have to face periods of absences, often involving a number of members. The rationales are legion: "I had a cold"; "The bus was late, so I didn't want to interrupt the session"; "My mother called just as I was leaving"; "I forgot." A flurry of such situations suggests that the group is encountering some type of stress, often because of the challenge of shifting into a new developmental stage or beginning to address a new set of deeper issues. It is generally wise to consider such a flurry of absences a group phenomenon that is best addressed by the group itself. Rather than assume the role of schoolmaster, the therapist might show great interest in the fact that the number present is fluctuating and wonder what might be going on. The goal is to gently move the group into a serious discussion of what it means to have a lack of continuity. Examples might be used, such as that of a member who dealt with some personally very important issues in one session and what it was like in the next session to have several members who had not participated in it. A firm statement from the members that they want everyone present every session is an enactment of social negotiation and a strike against preoccupation with the self.

The idea of termination will activate similar but more powerful responses. If the group is closed, at least for a season, then the prospect of termination will automatically arise and can be processed in the group for several months before it actually occurs. If the group is slow-open, not the recommended format, then individual members will raise the topic. There are clear advantages to being able to address this loaded topic as a routine matter built into the time frame so that it can become an unavoidable group issue.

The Personality Problems Group model uses a multimodal approach. The structured segment of each session provides practice in ways to manage personal reactions and thought styles. The use of a structured segment also provides a safer approach to fostering self-revelation without triggering a destabilizing affective response. In the process segment, similar material is addressed from an experiential perspective beginning with a focus on self states and self definition. The traditional group psychotherapist might see the combination of cognitive and self-focusing components as a breach of therapist role expectations that will confuse the members. Such confusion does not appear to result. The interactional stance of the therapists toward the individual is similar in both, while the degree of group process structure varies. The two segments tend to complement each other by providing an opportunity for different types of experiential learning.

The course of severe personality pathology is chronic, with the pathology tending to burn out in level of intensity over time. It is to be expected that future stressful situations will rekindle problematic behavior. In other words, relapse is predictable. A similar situation is encountered in the Antidepression Interpersonal Group model. Consideration could be given to an ongoing maintenance program for the Personality Problems Group. For example, a monthly session might be scheduled that would be structured as a go-around discussion of how events and relationships have been managed and what is coming up in the next month that could be better managed with some preplanning. Reinforcement of cognitive-behavioral techniques could be incorporated. This format can be cost-effective if admissions, emergency visits, and office visits are contained. Because of the sensitivity of this group of patients to alterations of the frame of therapy, it would be wise for such programmatic decisions to be made in advance, not added at a later date.

Community Support Clinic

Formal Description

The Community Support Clinic model is designed for patients with an ongoing major mental illness, primarily schizophrenia or severe bipolar illness, that interferes significantly with basic community adaptation. The group is supportive in nature and focuses on activities of daily living and basic socializing skills. Management of medications is handled in the sessions, and a psychoeducational component concerning use of medications and their side effects is included. The clinic is held weekly for 2 hours. Frequency of attendance will vary according to clinical status and will be addressed as part of the group discussion. Patients may come weekly or at longer intervals as indicated.

The provision of adequate programs for patients with major psychiatric illness is a challenge to the mental health care delivery system. Too often it has been relegated to secondary status as not being worthy of the attention of experienced professionals. The mentally ill make up a substantial portion of the inner-city homeless population. This group model is not referred to as a "medication group" because the task for the program goes well beyond simple medication review. Long-term follow-up is effectively, probably preferentially, provided through group programs.

Patients with chronic mental illness have many issues in common. The use of long-term medication is necessary but produces many problems, and patients need support in adapting to and managing the inevitable side effects. Most of these patients have significant problems in daily living in terms of both residential placements and employment. Many lead desperately lonely lives, and it may be useful to encourage, rather than discourage, extragroup socializing. In this way, closer attention can be paid to the realities of daily life and how they may be addressed.

The organization of these groups must take into account that attendance is expected to be both perpetual and episodic and that a psychiatrist is required to handle prescriptions. The goal is supportive in the sense of helping the patient to master and cope with current problems; this does not mean that issues are ignored or handled with simple reassurance. This approach should involve problem solving, with active use of homework tasks between sessions. There are many ways to organize long-term care programs. The essential features are planning for long-term attendance and ready accessibility to treatment resources in situations of impending decompensation. The model described below has been successfully operating for over two decades with minimal need for hospitalization.

Management Strategies

Clinic organization.   This community support program is called a "clinic," not a "group." A particular block of time is available each week, for example, an afternoon from 2:00 to 4:00, to which are assigned a substantial number of patients. A total of 30 or more can be accommodated on the roster of a given group, with the anticipation of a weekly attendance of about 12. There is probably an advantage to having separate groups for patients with schizophrenia and mood disorders. These patient populations can be combined, but the adaptation issues, as well as the medications, are somewhat different.

The clinic is staffed by two outpatient staff members who are well connected with community resources. The patients may attend the clinic at varying frequencies but always attend the afternoon clinic to which they are assigned. Those recently discharged or experiencing decompensation may come weekly, whereas others who have been stabilized on long-term medication may come monthly or even quarterly. The clinic serves as a home base for all of these patients. Over time, there is enough intermingling that they get to know most members of their clinic. Coffee and maybe cookies are provided, and serious talk about how things are going is expected.

This program model provides the structure for "transference to an institution." The clinic continues forever, even though the staff members, as well as many of the patients, may change. It remains as a supportive resource to be used as required. At the same time, it provides coverage for large numbers of patients with efficient use of staff time (108).

Management of medication. Medication review and prescription renewal require the presence of a psychiatrist. This process can be handled in various ways.

1. One of the leaders is a psychiatrist, or the psychiatrist is in attendance for a portion of the group. The session begins with a go-around for members to "check in" regarding how things have gone since their last attendance. It is carefully noted just how long it has been since their last visit. This process of checking in provides an opportunity both to assess overall functioning and to detect a deterioration in mental status. Routine prescriptions may be completed in the group, or, if there are indications for concern, a patient can be seen privately. When patients are being maintained on depot medication, they can leave the group to receive their injection in an adjacent medication office and then return. The psychiatrist should be able to manage a good number of patients within the first hour of the group, certainly as many as or more than could be seen individually and with a longer opportunity to see how patients manage themselves in the social context of the group.
2. Patients can leave the group session for an individual medication assessment with the psychiatrist and then return.
3. Individual medication interviews can be scheduled before and/or after the group.

The important feature is that all aspects of care, including monitoring and administration of medications, are carried out during the same time slot

Management of the group process. The Community Support Clinic provides a rich mixture of group therapeutic factors, primarily those drawn from the supportive cluster. Interaction should be encouraged and often centers on telling stories of current experiences. Over time, these groups can deal with quite powerful personal issues, which often involve coming to grips with diminished functioning and quasi-dependent status. The intent is to provide an opportunity to talk about and discuss how to manage the difficult experience of having a major psychotic illness. Interpretive techniques are not appropriate. For these types of groups, it is best to select staff who have supportive and nurturing qualities, prefer active solutions over psychological metaphors, and know how to benignly but firmly set limits.

Content focus. Topics will largely arise from the initial go-around. There will be an ongoing focus on the need for medication and the management of side effects. Successful maintenance in the community is dependent on regular use of medications, so this topic must always be addressed when presented to enhance compliance. Other major topics will involve how to access community resources or deal with bureaucracy; personal safety; social isolation and relationship issues; and, sometimes, patients' thoughts about themselves and the meaning of their lives. A review of local news or community events is also welcome. Family, friends, or even managers of patient residences can also be welcomed at these clinics, where they may learn useful methods of maximizing adaptation. The "expressed emotion" literature indicates the importance of maintaining a positive emotional tone in interactions with the patient and the deleterious effects of a negative emotional environment (109). With this in mind, some programs encourage family members or other caregivers to attend.

This simple clinic structure puts the group experience at the heart of the program. It provides a method for supporting and monitoring a sizable clinical load in a flexible manner with predictable time management. Above all, it provides a known resource for patients whose lives otherwise often have little predictability.

Eating Disorders Information Group

Formal Description

The Eating Disorders Information Group is designed to provide accurate information about anorexia nervosa and bulimia nervosa, with the overall goal of fostering attitudinal and behavioral change. The format is a mini-lecture followed by an opportunity for discussion and questions. The material will be of help to the patients in understanding more about eating disorders and in learning straightforward ways of helping to control eating behavior. This is not an active treatment group, and no individual counseling is provided. The group meets weekly for 90 minutes for eight sessions. Handouts and recommended readings are made available.

Treatment for anorexia nervosa and bulimia nervosa must be multifaceted and integrative. Components from various theoretical orientations are used and are tailored to the individual needs of the patient. For the seriously ill patient, normalization of eating, restoration and stabilization of weight, and maintenance of the patient's physical health take precedence. Psychological approaches, including at various times individual, group, family, and marital psychotherapy, address the issues that precipitate the development of the eating disorder and that serve to perpetuate it. A number of specialized group treatment formats for eating disorder patients are available. These include psychoeducational groups, cognitive-behavioral groups, support groups, intensive interpersonal groups, groups in multimodal day programs, inpatient groups, and continuing care groups.

The suitability and sequencing of the different therapies will vary among patients. A useful treatment philosophy is to begin treatment with the least intrusive method and advance to more intensive measures as the patient's response indicates (110). For those patients presenting with early symptoms of bulimia nervosa, involvement in a psychoeducational group may suffice. The approach is a relatively simple and low-intensity treatment measure. Follow-up studies have found clinically significant changes in dysfunctional attitudes and eating behavior. Psychoeducation also forms an integral component of all treatment programs for eating disorders.

Management Strategies

Group composition. Anyone interested in learning more about eating disorders would be welcome in a psychoeducational group. If such groups are held as part of a general public service, a wide assortment of motivations will bring people to the sessions. Some will come because eating disorders are widely reported in the media and on the mind of most young women. Others will attend because they are concerned about other family members or friends and want to know what they can do to help. Many will have early symptoms of an eating disorder and either have personal concerns or are responding to concerns expressed by friends or family. A smaller number will be having significant difficulty with an eating disorder. When the group begins, the leader will generally not know what the membership balance is. In psychoeducational groups that are conducted as part of an eating disorders program, the situation will be more predictable.

Structure of the sessions. Sessions are primarily didactic and directed according to a predetermined agenda of topics. Personal self-disclosure from the participants is neither expected nor solicited. The group leaders focus their activity on imparting information and promoting discussion and eliciting questions and opinions about the specific topics presented. Questions are welcomed in the service of learning more about the syndromes. The leaders must continuously guard against slipping into a therapeutic mode. For many participants, there will be a pattern of secrecy about eating behaviors. So even though little interaction takes place between members, the nature of the material and of the questions asked brings with it a strong sense of universality and acceptance that such forbidden topics can be explored.

Content areas.   Attention is directed at providing descriptive information about eating disorders and dispelling myths and misconceptions. An effort is made to identify and correct distorted cognitions associated with eating, self-esteem, and interpersonal difficulties. The goal is to promote a normalized relationship with food and eating. Written informational material and recommended readings are helpful. Topics that are commonly included in a psychoeducational program are listed in Table 13–2.

The Eating Disorders Information Group model is an example of a psychoeducational group. The basic format can be used to develop groups with other topic areas, such as depression, the range of anxiety disorders,

Table 13–2.   Psychoeducational program for patients with eating disorders

1. Basic features of anorexia nervosa and bulimia nervosa
2. Multidetermined causes of eating disorders
3. Body controls regarding weight (set point theory)
4. Physical complications
5. Eating disorders and depression and anxiety
6. Effects of starvation
7. Importance of normal eating patterns
8. Ineffectiveness of dieting, bingeing and purging
9. Coping strategies for urges to binge
10. Body image, self-esteem, and close relationships
11. Social pressures for thinness
12. Food myths, good nutrition, and well-balanced meal plans

Source.   Adapted from Davis R, Dearing S, Faulkner J, et al.: "The Road to Recovery: A Manual for Participants in the Psychoeducational Group for Bulimia Nervosa," in *Group Psychotherapy for Eating Disorders.* Edited by Harper-Giuffre H, MacKenzie KR. Washington, DC, American Psychiatric Press, 1992, pp. 281–310. Copyright 1989, Ron Davis et al. Used with permission.

substance abuse, and other medical illness. Of course, all groups, and particularly cognitive-behavioral and social skills groups, have a component of psychoeducation. In psychodynamic groups, the psychoeducational component may be disguised in the form of clarifying interpretations. It is also important to keep the generic model in mind. Even in quite structured psychoeducational groups, the development of a positive alliance between the leader and the participants and a sense of group cohesion result in greater benefits.

Substance Abuse Group

Formal Description

The Substance Abuse Group is designed for patients with a history of major substance abuse who have successfully completed detoxification and stabilization programs. Sobriety must have been maintained for a minimum of 6 months, though 12 months might be preferable depending on the extent of previous substance abuse. This is an active psychotherapy group that deals with topics related to the nature of personal relationships and self-concept. It is expected that members will be abstinent from all alcohol or other substance use. The group meets weekly for 90 minutes over a 9-month period running from September to May. No new members are admitted after the third session. The group ends in May, but the members may individually consider a second year in the program for the following September.

The treatment of alcohol and other substance abuse in America moved into the mainstream of therapy in 1970 as a result of Congressional legislation and has assumed increasing importance with the wide prevalence of illicit drug use. Every community now has a variety of programs, often subdivided by drug of choice, that fall under the self-help label. Formal inpatient treatment programs for detoxification and the initiation of treatment are common. Most of these programs rely heavily on the 12-step model that originated with Alcoholics Anonymous (AA). Many use group leaders that themselves have a history of substance abuse but who have long maintained sobriety or abstinence. Group-based treatments form by far the largest component and are the preferred format. The group model described here is suitable for the later phase of recovery after the addictive behavior and the acute effects of withdrawal are under established control.

Several basic principles underlie all approaches to the treatment of substance abuse (111). First, abuse is not simply a symptom of other illnesses; it is the primary condition. Symptoms such as depression and anxiety should be seen as the result, not the cause, of abuse. For the great majority of persons who abuse substances, total abstinence must be the goal. Effective psychotherapy can seldom take place in the context of continuing use. Particularly in the earlier phase of treatment, a specialized program devoted solely to substance abuse is indicated and may be necessary to effectively break through denial.

An intensive treatment program is indicated for the first few weeks. This program is commonly based on residential care but may occur through a day treatment facility. Most patients attending will be under some sort of formal or informal duress. Denial of the extent of the abuse problem and the fantasy of returning to controlled use will be common. During this stage, psychological subtleties take a backseat to the necessity of acknowledging the problem and maintaining abstinence. Often, several weeks are required following withdrawal before there is stabilization of both physiological and psychological functioning. A direct and confrontational approach is necessary and is best provided by an active group culture. Firm attention to boundary violations is important, as is the expectation of involvement in self-help meetings. It is best that the group environment be restricted to these basics, so exploration of personal issues is not encouraged. The confrontive group can also be enormously supportive in managing anxiety and promoting motivation for change.

Following an intensive program, a period of reintegration occurs, lasting for several months. Intensive use of self-help meetings, as well as supportive therapeutic groups, is indicated during this period. The focus on sobriety and on managing the sequelae of the substance-abusing period in the members' lives is maintained. The group work during this reintegration period usually centers on relationships with family and friends and on work circumstances. Themes of guilt, shame, depression, and anger can be anticipated. The group approach is primarily supportive in nature.

Once sobriety and general social adaptation have been stabilized, some members will want to move into more traditional psychotherapy territory. It is important that this not be introduced too early in the recovery process. To do so would give the implicit message that sobriety might not be the most important task—that sorting out personal issues will solve the problem. A minimum of 6 months is necessary, and a full year is desirable, before formal psychotherapy should be considered.

Group psychotherapy is not the same as a self-help 12-step program. It is important for the therapist and the members to understand the differences so that the two formats can be complementary and not in competition. It is helpful if the therapist understands the language and basic principles of the self-help approach and clearly articulates the difference in expectations. In group therapy, for example, regular attendance is required, and the focus is on experiential learning from the group process, not acquiring information or specific skills. Interaction between members is expected, not a succession of individual monologues. The question of extragroup contacts will be looked at closely and discouraged. The approach will deal more with individual and specific issues than with the commonality of having the same addictive history. For this task, it is helpful for the therapist to have experience in both addictions and group psychotherapy. Patients need to be assured that there is no incompatibility with attending AA programs simultaneously with formal group psychotherapy.

The actual group management will share many features with the Interpersonal Problems Group model described earlier in this chapter. The therapist is active in developing a cohesive group atmosphere by modeling responsiveness and interest. One of the major advantages of a group approach is the capacity to function as a containing environment. Maladaptive patterns can be expected to emerge at an early point and must be addressed directly and early in a supportive manner. Often, the 12-step philosophy will be used as a defense against dealing with group process. The therapist may need to be active in promoting attention to painful self-states. Because there is a danger that such self-states will precipitate further substance abuse, constant debriefing on the experience within the session is important. The possibility of greater intimacy in the group will elicit distancing reactions to defend against dependency, and there is likely to be high sensitivity to hostility. These process events are, of course, the common material of all psychotherapy. In these groups, however, the members are frequently highly experienced at masking their difficulties and managing relationships to their immediate advantage. The connections between substance abuse and relationship stresses are constantly kept in focus and often involve parallel issues in the partner. There must be constant attending to the theme that abstinence is essential and that the individual is responsible for the first drink, after which loss of control is predictable.

The model described above typically entails 30 to 40 sessions, with the possibility of a second course. Generally, major substance abuse has deep roots and the patterns are well entrenched in the fabric of social and personal relationships. Consideration could also be given to having this later phase of treatment take place in a general psychotherapy group.

Adult Children of Alcoholics Group

Formal Description

The Adult Children of Alcoholics (ACOA) Group is designed for patients who have a family history involving parents who had a severe problem with alcohol or substance abuse. The patient will have a history of significant problems in the area of personal relationships and self-esteem. The group focuses on how patterns derived from childhood continue to have a damaging effect on present relationships. The group meets weekly for 90 minutes for 16 to 24 sessions, with the exact number of sessions established in advance for any given group. Patients must be available for the entire sequence of sessions. No new patients are admitted after the third session.

This model is very similar to the Interpersonal Problems Group except that the membership is homogeneous for substance-abusing patients. The ACOA concept of the "adult-child" incorporates some of the basic concepts of psychodynamic theory with a language structure reminiscent of transactional analysis. The application of these ideas generally follows a 12-step model, as in the ACOA special-interest groups aligned with Al-Anon. The incorporation of ACOA concepts provides an immediate connection for the members that is helpful in addressing the stigma and secrecy that often accompany such childhood experiences. The externalization of blame addresses the guilt and shame and allows a more forgiving attitude toward self. The homogeneous composition combined with the release of long-standing painful emotions ensures a rapid development of cohesion. For many participants, involvement in this engagement-stage experience of universality and acceptance is adequate for initiating a process of mastery. The 12-step structure helps to anchor and contain the experience.

The potential liability of the ACOA approach concerns the ACOA "label" itself and attendant rationales that may serve to stereotype the issues, much as the family of origin may have placed the child in a proscribed role. This labeling has the potential to perpetuate a sense of self in negative and deviant terms. There may also be a message, either direct or indirect, that these problems must be addressed only within the ACOA framework and to do otherwise would be letting the movement down. This situation is parallel to that discussed above regarding the importance of maintaining an open boundary between AA and other 12-step–based self-help approaches and group psychotherapy.

Management Strategies

Assessment. A full history must be obtained regarding the role of alcohol and other substances in the patient's life. Very often these patients themselves have difficulty with substance abuse or have partners who do. Sometimes the facts around these issues may indicate that substance abuse per se is not the problem, though poor relationships and self-image are a major concern. Self-diagnosis must always be confirmed by seeking factual information from the patient and other caregivers and third parties.

Attachment pathology. The common themes in ACOA psychotherapy groups revolve around the nature of close relationships, with a particular weighting on issues of trust and control. This is the universal material of psychotherapy. When the depth of dysfunction is more severe, there will be overlap with the features of BPD.

Intimate relationship patterns frequently center on an enacted dichotomy. The patient assumes the role of compulsive caretaker whose self-worth depends on maintaining control by attending to and placating the other. The partner exhibits out-of-control behavior that calls for control yet continuously harms the patient. To maintain the balance of the system, the patient must hide all symptoms, yet experiences self-critical and shameful thoughts that things are not going better. Shame is an affective state that is particularly well addressed in group psychotherapy, where the internal world can be opened up to response from others (112).

The therapist. Psychotherapists in general must be alert to excessively strong urges to take care of others. This potential is increased in ACOA groups, in which the common defense is one of helplessness and needing to help. It may be hard for the therapist to withstand the suction from the group to come to group members' rescue. The blurring between the self-help traditions and group psychotherapy becomes particularly apparent in this situation. That danger is possibly also a good reason for considering mixed groups in which patients with family histories of substance abuse are combined with other members who have some of the same patterns but with different antecedents. This might help the ACOA members to avoid dogma and speak about their own experiences.

The role of self-help movements in the treatment of substance abuse raises many interesting and sometimes controversial issues. The best guideline for the group therapist is to carefully think through the differences and the similarities and to share these with the patients. A collaborative approach will allow comfortable referral for intensive psychotherapy from self-help ACOA programs and use by the therapist of self-help groups as an adjunctive modality.

Self-Help Groups

Participation in self-help groups has increased rapidly over the last three decades. It is estimated that 9 to 12 million people belong to self-help groups in the United States, more than attend formal mental health services. The nature of self-help programs has shifted over time, with fewer personal growth groups and more targeted groups, but the overall numbers continue to increase. Such programs exist in a loosely defined, relatively unbounded area. They are largely self-governing and self-supporting, offering full accessibility and no charge. It has been suggested that these programs are a response to the decreasing role of social institutions, such as the church, that historically have provided social support within the community.

Studies of a variety of support groups clearly indicate that these groups provide a rich mixture of the supportive therapeutic factors and create a highly cohesive group environment that encourages, or in some cases demands, powerful self-disclosure statements (113). These groups provide abundant opportunity for modeling on others and for learning by hearing of the experiences of others—all ingredients that are likely to provide support and promote change. Some self-help groups also have quite powerful rules that are reinforced by being authenticated by other members or controlled by punishment, such as with the threat of being excluded.

Although there are many features common to all self-help groups, different self-help groups use quite different mechanisms that go well beyond simple social support. Most self-help groups are designed for a particular symptom or condition and use mechanisms that are appropriate to that target. AA, for instance, addresses the alcoholic's sense of personal power by insisting on the acceptance of being subject to a higher power. Recovery Incorporated invokes tight rules of order to gain cognitive control to help contain a tendency to overreact to interpersonal issues. Even groups that deal with bereavement do so in quite different ways, depending on the nature of the loss. In many ways, self-help groups operate on principles that are almost the opposite of those in formal psychotherapy groups. They rely on a global core ideology, not complex psychological theories. They do not use the group interactions except in joining together to address external behaviors or situations. They reduce the role status of leaders, who usually suffer from the same affliction as do all of the members.

The wisest approach for the clinician is to respect and support self-help efforts. By maintaining a collaborative relationship, the clinician can refer patients who would benefit from self-help, and be available to the self-help movement when members present problems beyond the group's capacity to manage. It is useful to advise patients that they may need to try several self-help groups before they decide on the one that seems right for them. It is probably not advisable for clinicians to become involved in training self-help group leaders. Each self-help system has its own mechanisms and strategies that have been refined over time for that particular population and should be respected. The request for input may reflect a desire on the part of self-help facilitators to become therapists, which, if acted on, would undercut their value as self-help leaders.

Appendixes

Appendix 1

Global Assessment of Functioning (GAF) Scale

Overall	Symptoms and psychological functioning	Social and occupational functioning
100	100 **No symptoms**	100 **Superior functioning in a wide range of activities**
90	90 **Absent or minimal symptoms** (e.g., mild anxiety before an exam)	90 **Good functioning in all areas,** occupationally and socially effective
80	80 If symptoms are present, they are transient and expectable reactions to psychosocial stressors (e.g., difficulty concentrating after family argument)	80 No more than a slight impairment in social and occupational functioning or school functioning (e.g., infrequent interpersonal conflict, temporarily falling behind in schoolwork)
70	70 **Some mild symptoms** (e.g., depressed mood and mild insomnia)	70 **Some difficulty in social or occupational functioning,** but generally functioning pretty well; has some meaningful interpersonal relationships
60	60 **Moderate symptoms** (e.g., flat affect and circumstantial speech, occasional panic attacks)	60 **Moderate difficulty in social, occupational, or school functioning** (e.g., few friends, conflicts with peers or co-workers)
50	50 **Serious symptoms** (e.g., suicidal ideation, severe obsessional rituals, frequent shoplifting)	50 **Serious impairment in social, occupational, or school functioning** (e.g., no friends, unable to keep a job)
40	40 **Some impairment in reality testing or communication** (e.g., speech is at times illogical, obscure, or irrelevant)	40 **Major impairment in several areas, such as work or school, family relations** (e.g., avoids friends, neglects family, is unable to work; child frequently beats up younger children, is defiant at home, is failing at school)

(continued)

Global Assessment of Functioning (GAF) Scale
(continued)

Overall	Symptoms and psychological functioning	Social and occupational functioning
30 20	30 Behavior is considerably influenced by delusions or hallucinations or serious impairment in communication or judgment (e.g., sometimes incoherent, acts grossly inappropriately, suicidal preoccupation)	30 Inability to function in almost all areas (e.g., stays in bed all day; no job, home, or friends)
	20 Some danger of hurting self or others (e.g., suicide attempts without clear expectation of death; frequently violent; manic excitement)	20 Occasionally fails to maintain minimal personal hygiene, unable to function independently
10	10 Persistent danger of severely hurting self or others (e.g., recurrent violence)	10 Persistent inability to maintain minimal personal hygiene; unable to function without harming self or others or without considerable external support (e.g., nursing care and supervision)

This format of the GAF Scale permits the clinician to record the standard global score as well as separate scores for each subsection. Social and Occupational Functioning Assessment Scale (SOFAS) items are used in righthand column.

Source. Adapted with permission from Goldman HH, Skodol AE, Lave TR: "Revising Axis V for DSM-IV: A Review of Measures of Social Functioning." *American Journal of Psychiatry* 149:1148–1156, 1992; American Psychiatric Association: *Diagnostic and Statistical Manual of Mental Disorders*, 4th Edition. Washington, DC, American Psychiatric Association, 1994, pp. 760–761.

Appendix 2

Global Assessment of Relational Functioning (GARF) Scale

The GARF Scale permits the clinician to rate the degree to which a family or relational unit meets the affective or instrumental needs of its members in the following areas:

A. *Problem solving*—skills in negotiating goals, rules, and routines; adaptability to stress; communication skills; ability to resolve conflict
B. *Organization*—maintenance of interpersonal roles and subsystem boundaries; hierarchical functioning; coalitions and distribution of power, control, and responsibility
C. *Emotional climate*—tone and range of feelings; quality of caring, empathy, involvement, and attachment/commitment; sharing of values; mutual affective responsiveness, respect, and regard; quality of sexual functioning

The clinician should be familiar with the full criteria in DSM-IV before making these ratings.

81–100 *Overall:* Relational unit is functioning satisfactorily from self-report of participants and from perspectives of observers.

61–80 *Overall:* Functioning of relational unit is somewhat unsatisfactory. Over a period of time, many but not all difficulties are resolved without complaints.

41–60 *Overall:* Relational unit has occasional times of satisfying and competent functioning together, but clearly dysfunctional, unsatisfying relationships tend to predominate.

21–40 *Overall:* Relational unit is obviously and seriously dysfunctional; forms and time periods of satisfactory relating are rare.

1–20 *Overall:* Relational unit has become too dysfunctional to retain continuity of contact and attachment.

0 Inadequate information.

Appendix 3

Multiaxial Evaluation Report Form

This form is offered as one possibility for reporting multiaxial evaluations. In some settings, this form may be used exactly as is; in other settings, the form may be adapted to satisfy special needs.

AXIS I: *Clinical Disorders and*
  Other Conditions That May Be a Focus of Clinical Attention

Diagnostic code   DSM-IV name

— — —.— —   _____

— — —.— —   _____

— — —.— —   _____

AXIS II: Personality Disorders and Mental Retardation

Diagnostic code   DSM-IV name

— — —.— —   _____

— — —.— —   _____

AXIS III: General Medical Conditions

ICD-9-CM code   ICD-9-CM name

— — —.— —   _____

— — —.— —   _____

— — —.— —   _____

AXIS IV: Psychosocial and Environmental Problems   *Check:*
☐ **Problems with primary support group** *Specify:* _____
☐ **Problems related to the social environment** *Specify:* _____
☐ **Educational problems** *Specify:* _____
☐ **Occupational problems** *Specify:* _____
☐ **Housing problems** *Specify:* _____
☐ **Economic problems** *Specify:* _____
☐ **Problems with access to health care services** *Specify:* _____
☐ **Problems related to interaction with the legal system/crime** *Specify:*____
☐ **Other psychosocial and environmental problems** *Specify:*_____

AXIS V: Global Assessment of Functioning Scale   *Time frame:* _____

Overall score _____ Symptoms and psychological functioning score: ____
                                  Social and occupational functioning score: ____

Psychological Mindedness: 5 4 3 2 1 Quality of Relationships: 5 4 3 2 1

Source. Adapted from American Psychiatric Association: *Diagnostic and Statistical Manual of Mental Disorders,* 4th Edition. Washington, DC, American Psychiatric Association, 1994, p. 34. Copyright 1994, American Psychiatric Association. Used with permission.

Appendix 4

Psychological Mindedness Scale

Level 5: The patient is able to recognize the presence of defensive maneuvers and the extent to which they deal with the conflictual issue. "I know that all my relationships are going to fall apart, and I cannot bear to face that, so I make sure that I find some excuse to end the relationship early. At least then I'm the one who makes the move."

Level 4: The patient is able to identify a causal link between conflict, tension, or anxiety and the resulting expression; that conflict generates tension and attempts at resolution. "I'm beginning to understand how I get upset whenever I feel that I'm not being understood so that I just get out of the situation as fast as I can and end up being in a resentful state for days."

Level 3: The patient identifies conflictual elements or ambivalence and recognizes that internal impulses or wishes may come into conflict with the frustrating or nongratifying aspects of the outside world, or at least how the patient sees them, while the more rational part of the personality acts as mediator. "I know that it would not be proper to have a relationship with my instructor, but I can't get the idea out of my mind that he would be the ideal person for me."

Level 2: The patient recognizes that the internal state is motivating behavior and may contain aspects that are out of awareness (i.e., the idea of psychic determinism and unconscious mechanisms). "I'm upset because of the criticism I received."

Level 1: The patient is able to appreciate the existence of an internal psychological experience (i.e., "I'm angry"); even this may be difficult for patients with alexithymia.

Source. Adapted from Piper WE, McCallum M, Azim HFA: *Adaptation to Loss Through Short-Term Group Psychotherapy.* New York, Guilford Press, 1992. Copyright 1992, Guilford Press. Used with permission.

Appendix 5

Quality of Relationships Scale

Level	Behavior	Affect regulation	Self-esteem regulation	Definition of self identity
5. Mature	Maintains equitable "give and take" relations with both sexes	Capacity to experience breadth of appropriate emotion; tolerates loss	Realistic evaluation of self and others	Identity derived from equitable relationships
4. Triangular	Competes in relationships	Fear of success; anxiety and guilt over intimacy	Comparison of self to others	Identity depends on sense of triumph over others
3. Controlling	Controls or possesses (active or passive)	Anger and ambivalence	Maintenance through control and possession	Identity depends on control over others
2. Searching	Seeks, finds, and loses substitute others	Craving and longing; infatuation and dis-appointment	Dependent on availability of others	Identity depends on presence of relationships
1. Primitive	Becomes overattached; reacts with hypersensi-tivity to loss	Rage and fear of annihilation; emptiness	Idealization/ devaluation; inordinate reliance on others	Self-worth is labile and extreme; unstable self-identity

Source. Adapted from Azim HFA, Piper WE, Segal PM, et al.: "The Quality of Object Relations Scale." *Bulletin of the Menninger Clinic* 55:323–343, 1991. Copyright 1991. Used with permission.

Appendix 6

List of Important Relationships

The goal for this sheet is to identify the most important intimate relationships during your life. We begin with your parents. (**Note:** If your biological parents were not present during this age period, think of the most important female and male nurturing figures in your preadolescent years and write in their names.)

Mother (_____) when you were aged 5–10 years (elementary school):

Father (_____) when you were aged 5–10 years (elementary school):

Your parents' relationship when you were aged 5–10 years (elementary school):

The intent of the next selections is to identify important intimate relationships drawn from across major time periods: adolescence, early adult, middle years, as appropriate. These should include good as well as unsatisfactory relationships, and at least one of each sex. Try to include major marital or common-law partners. Consider any members of your extended family who were important at one time (siblings, grandparents, aunts, uncles). All relationships cannot be included, so variety and time spread should be used to make the final selections. For each of the people selected, write in the first name, or nickname, by which that person was known to you, and the type of relationship (former girlfriend from teens, best friend, co-worker, college friend, etc.). It is useful to review the list after it is completed to ensure that it represents a good cross section of important relationships of various types from throughout your life.

Current marital partner or most intimate current relationship:
Name: _____ Type: _____

Current closest friend of opposite sex to the above:
Name: _____ Type: _____

Name: _____ Type: _____
Name: _____ Type: _____
Name: _____ Type: _____
Name: _____ Type: _____

————

Appendix 7

Interpersonal Work Sheet

Introduction: This form is designed to begin the process of examining how important close relationships have influenced your life in a positive or a negative direction. There are often connections between psychological symptoms such as anxiety and depression and the nature of close relationships. This might happen in different ways. Did interpersonal stress lay the groundwork for you to get upset? Did a specific relationship issue or loss trigger your symptoms? Now that you are anxious or depressed, do relationship matters interfere with getting better? Have your symptoms produced a change in the nature of your close relationships? The bottom line is that relationships and psychological symptoms are often connected somehow. The following questions try to help clarify what these connections are for you.

1. **Name of person:** _____ **Type of relationship:** _____

2. Describe what this relationship is like NOW if that person is still in your life. You may want to use another sheet to rate it as it was at some time in the past as well. If the relationship is from the past, describe how you generally remember it. Remember that a relationship involves two people, so think about it in both directions.

3. Here are some useful ways of thinking about relationships. Make a guess where on each of the three lines you and this other person might be located. Circle a number from 1 to 10 on each line for YOU, and make a square from 1 to 10 on each line for the OTHER PERSON.

Negative/fear/ rejecting/angry	1 2 3 4 5 6 7 8 9 10	Positive/accepting/loving
Dominating and controlling	1 2 3 4 5 6 7 8 9 10	Submitting and passive
Distanced and almost out of the relationship	1 2 3 4 5 6 7 8 9 10	Overinvolved, almost lose a sense of self when with the other

4. Overall, how satisfactory or unsatisfactory is this relationship for you? What are the main issues in each direction for you? For the other?

5. What changes would improve or maximize the relationship? Changes you might make? Changes the other might make?

Appendix 8

Target Goals Form

Please describe three goals that will be of importance for your treatment. Try to describe each goal in terms of actual personal behavior or relationship issues, not just internal feelings. Using the Rating Scale as a guide, circle the number that best describes how much that goal is bothering you at present.	**RATING SCALE**
	0 not at all
	1 a little bit
	2 somewhat
	3 moderately
	4 quite a bit
	5 a great deal
Goal Description	6 extremely

Goal Description	
Goal 1:	
	0 1 2 3 4 5 6
Goal 2:	
	0 1 2 3 4 5 6
Goal 3:	
	0 1 2 3 4 5 6

Note: This form can also be used to rate Focus Areas as described in Chapter 5.

Appendix 9

Patient Information Handout

Information Regarding Group Therapy

Introduction

This information sheet is intended for people who are about to begin Group Therapy or who are considering it as a possible treatment. It is useful when starting Group Therapy to have some general ideas about how groups help people and how to get the most out of the experience. Group Therapy is different from individual therapy because many of the helpful events take place between the members and not just between the leader and the members. That is one reason why it is important that all of the members have a general introduction before beginning. Please read this material carefully and feel free to discuss any part of it with your group leader. The issues raised in this handout are also useful to talk about during the first few sessions in the group.

Do Groups Really Help People?

Group Therapy is widely used and has been a standard part of treatment programs for the last 40 to 50 years. Sometimes it is used as the main or perhaps the only treatment approach. This is especially true for outpatients. Sometimes it is used as part of a treatment approach that may include individual therapy, medications, and other activities. Group Therapy has been shown in research studies to be an effective treatment. Studies that have compared individual and group approaches indicate that both are about equally effective. The difference with groups, of course, is that a group has to form, and the members need to get to know each other a bit, before it can be of the greatest benefit. Most people have participated in some types of nontherapy groups, for example, as part of school, church, or community activities. Therapy groups will have many of the same features. The difference is that in a therapy group, the leader has a responsibility to ensure that the members stay focused on their treatment goals and that everyone participates in this.

How Group Therapy Works

Group therapy is based on the idea that a great many of the difficulties that people have in their lives can be understood as problems in getting along with other people. As children we learn ways of getting close and talking to others and ways of solving issues with others. Often, these early patterns are then applied in adult relationships. Sometimes these ways are not as effective as they might be, despite good intentions. Very often, symptoms such as anxiety or unhappiness, bad feelings about yourself, or a general sense of dissatisfaction with life reflect the unsatisfactory state of important relationships. Sometimes such symptoms result in interpersonal issues such as withdrawal or irritability. Groups offer an opportunity to learn more about these "interpersonal" patterns no matter how they got started.

There are many different kinds of groups. Some groups are designed to provide the members with information about some topic, such as eating disorders; others focus on a particular skill, such as assertiveness. Some groups are quite structured and may use a written manual, for example, cognitive-behaviorial groups, whereas others focus on understanding more about yourself and the nature of your important relationships. No matter what kind of group you are in, this information sheet is designed to let you know about how groups work and how you can get the most from your group experience.

Common Myths About Group Therapy

1. While it is true that groups offer an efficient way of treating several people at once, Group Therapy is not a cheaper or second-rate treatment in the sense that it has less power to help people than other treatments. As mentioned above, studies show that most of the "talking therapies" are about equally effective.
2. Some people are concerned that a therapy group will be like a forced confessional where they have to reveal all of the details of their life. This is not the case. Groups will progress at their own rate as members become more familiar with each other and can trust each other. In general, groups talk about the patterns in relationships and the meanings these have for

them. For this it is often not necessary to know specific details. Members will find their own level of comfort regarding how much they want to disclose about their personal lives. Details about where you live or work, even your last name, are not necessary for effective involvement in the group.

3. Some people worry that being in a room with other people with difficulties will make everyone worse. This idea of "the blind leading the blind" is understandable, but in practice people find that the process of talking about their problems is very helpful. Indeed, finding that others have had similar problems can be reassuring. Many Group Therapy patients are surprised to find that they have something to offer other people.

4. Some of the media presentation of groups suggests that people will lose control in groups and become so upset they can't function or maybe get so angry that they will be destructive. Very seldom is there any chance of this happening, and the group therapist will be alert and responsible to encourage the group if it gets too slow or to dampen things down if the tension gets too high.

5. When people picture being in a therapy group, they sometimes find themselves concerned that they may be rejected or excluded by the other group members, sometimes the fear is that they will be judged harshly by the other members, and sometimes they are afraid that they may lose their sense of themselves and be carried along by the group where they don't wish to go. All of these fears are perfectly understandable, and indeed, almost everyone experiences them to some extent when they enter a new social group situation. It is good to talk about these sorts of fears early in the group so that they can be understood and then put behind you.

How to Get the Most out of Group

1. The more you can involve yourself in the group, the more you will get out of it. In particular, try to identify the sorts of things that you find upsetting or bothersome. Try to be as open and honest as possible in what you say. Group time is precious; the group is a place to be working on serious issues, not just passing the time of day. Listen hard to what people are saying, think through what they mean, and try to make sense of it. You can help others by letting them know what you make of what they say and how it affects you. Many of the issues talked about in groups are general human matters with which we can all identify. At

the same time, listen hard to what others say to you about your part in the group. This process of learning from others is an important way to gain from the group experience. It takes time to appreciate how much a group can help you. So it is important that you commit yourself to come to a few sessions of the group before deciding if it's worthwhile for you. Discuss with your therapist before the group starts what the expectations are in terms of the length of your particular group.

2. One way of thinking about group is to view it as a "living laboratory" of relationships. It is a place where you can try out new ways of talking to people, a place to take some risks. You are a responsible member of the group and can help to make it an effective experience for everybody. A good way to think about how a group can help people is this. Consider a person risking a different way of talking about personal matters, getting some response from the other members that it sounds all right, and then trying to make sense of the experience.

3. Do your best to translate your inner reactions into words. Group is not a "tea party" where everything has to be done in a socially proper fashion. It is a place to try to explore the meaning of what goes on and the reactions inside that get stirred up.

4. Remember that how people talk is as important as what they say. As you listen to others and as you think about what you yourself have been saying, try to think beyond the words to the other messages being sent. Sometimes the meaning of the words does not match the tone of voice or the expression on the face.

5. Because the group is a place to learn from the experience itself, it is important to focus upon what is happening inside the group room between the members and between each member and the leader. Often, understanding these relationships throws new light on outside relationships. Many people have found it helpful to think about themselves in terms of the things they know and don't know about themselves, and the things that others know or don't know. The diagram below outlines this. One of the tasks in group is to try to make the box called "public knowledge" larger by three main methods: first, to talk about things that you normally keep hidden about yourself or speaking about your thoughts concerning others (self-disclosure); second, to listen to what others are saying about what might be your blind spots (receiving feedback); and third, to listen hard and think hard so that you can understand more about yourself (personal insight).

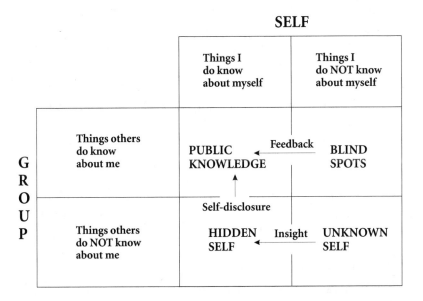

Common Stumbling Blocks

1. It is normal to feel anxious about being in groups. Almost everyone experiences it to some extent. One way of dealing with this is to talk about it at an early point in the group. This is a good model of the usefulness of talking about important issues so that they can be clarified and the anxiety related to them reduced.

2. It is the role of the leader to encourage members to talk with each other and to help keep the group focused on important tasks. The leader is not there to supply ready answers to specific problems. One of the things you will experience in group is learning to benefit from the process of talking with other people and not just getting pat answers.

3. Try hard to put into words the connection between how you are reacting or feeling and what is happening between you and other people both in the group and outside. It is all right to be emotional. This process of trying to understand reactions or symptoms in terms of relationships is important.

4. Many group members find themselves experiencing a sense of puzzlement or discouragement after the excitement of the first few group sessions. Please live through this stage. It almost always occurs, and it reflects the fact that it always takes groups some time to develop their full benefit for the members. Once the group has lived through this, it is in a much stronger position to be helpful.

5. From time to time in the group you may find yourself having negative feelings of disappointment, frustration, or even anger. It is important to talk about these reactions in a constructive fashion. Many people have difficulty with managing these sorts of feelings, and it is part of the group's task to examine them. Sometimes these negative feelings may be toward the leader. It is equally important that these also be talked about.

6. Try hard to apply what you learn in group to outside situations. Many group members have found it very useful to talk to the group about how they might go about applying what they are learning, and then to try it outside in their personal lives and report back to the group about how it went. Studies have shown that the more you can do this, the more therapy becomes "real" and the more you will get out of it. Many people report that keeping a regular personal journal is helpful in keeping on track with important issues between sessions. Remember that the rest of the world does not necessarily run the same way as a therapy group. Try out your ideas in the group first to test if your plans are well thought out.

7. Many people come to therapy groups because things have not been going well in their lives. There is a temptation to take the first advice you may hear and decide to make a big change. Please wait so that you have a chance to think about your ideas and talk about them in the group before making important life decisions.

Group Expectations

1. **Confidentiality:** It is very important that things that are talked about in the group do not get talked about outside. You may, of course, want to discuss your experience with people close to you, but even then it is important not to attach names or specific information to the talk. In our experience it is extremely uncommon for there to be any important break in confidentiality in therapy groups. Please be sure that you don't talk about others, just as you don't want them to talk about you outside the group.

2. **Attendance and punctuality:** It is very important that you attend all sessions and arrive on time. Once a group gets going, it functions as a group, and even if just one member is absent, it is not the same. So both for your sake and for the sake of all of the members, please be a regular attendee. If, for some reason, it is impossible for you to make

a session, then call in advance and discuss it with your therapist or at least leave the information. In that way the group will know you are not coming and won't find itself waiting to get down to work until you arrive. For outpatient groups, it is useful for the group to spend some time periodically talking about major absences such as trips or vacations and discuss how to plan for these as a group.

3. **Socializing with other group members:** It is important to think of groups as a treatment setting and not as a replacement for other social activities. Group members are strongly advised not to have outside contacts with each other. The reason for this is that if you have a special relationship with another group member, that relationship interferes with getting the most out of the group interaction. The two of you would find yourselves having secrets from the group or not addressing issues because of your friendship. If you should have some outside contact with group members, then it is important that this be talked about in the group so that the effects of such contact can be taken into account. You are asked to make a commitment to report such contacts within the group. (*Note:* Some groups that deal with learning and applying social skills may encourage members to practice together.)

4. **Contact between group sessions:** The therapist does not generally expect to have contact with group members outside of the group itself, unless it is something very urgent. All such contacts will be considered as part of the larger frame of the group experience, and the therapist may bring this material back into the group sessions. It is generally advisable not to engage in any other regular therapy while in the group with the exception of seeing your doctor for medication management. Any concerns or plans about seeing other therapists need to be discussed with the group leader before the group begins.

5. **Alcohol or drugs:** Groups are places for sensitive personal discussions. It is important that you not come to a session under the influence of alcohol or drugs except prescription medicines. This is not to say that it is good or bad to use alcohol or drugs, but only that they get in the way of making the most of the group experience. As a general rule, you will be asked to leave the session if your behavior is significantly affected. No food, drinks, or smoking is allowed in the group room. These tend to be distractions from the work of the group.

Appendix 10

Group Report Forms

Group Report Form

Group: _____ Date: _____ Session: _____

Therapist(s): _____

1. Major themes
2. Focal Incidents
3. Therapist issues
4. Supervision comments
5. For next session

Group Member Summary Form

Group: _____ Leader(s): _____

Member: _____

Quality/intensity of symptoms; participation in group; relevance to personal goals & external application

No.	Date	Comments	Initial
1			
2			
3			
4			
5			
6			
7			
8			
9			
10			

Signature	Initial	Signature	Initial

Group Session Summary Form

Group: _____ Leader(s): _____

Group cohesion and climate; major themes; critical incidents; therapist issues; notes for next session

No.	Date	Comments	Initial
1			
2			
3			
4			
5			
6			
7			
8			
9			
10			

Signature	Initial	Signature	Initial

Appendix 11

Model Confirmation Letter

[Substitute name and information for your group, and alter each paragraph to match your clinical situation.]

Therapists: Roy MacKenzie, M.D., and Mary Grant, Ph.D.

Welcome to the Wednesday Interpersonal Problems Group. The group will run for 20 sessions. The first session is 3 January 96 and the last session 22 May 96. The group will meet on Wednesdays from 4:30 to 6:00 P.M. in the Mental Health Clinic, Room 17, Main Floor. No food, drink, or smoking in the sessions, please.

There will be no session on 14 February 96.

Please check your calendars in detail and make arrangements so that you will be able to attend all sessions. Try to arrive on time, as even one person missing may hold the group back from getting into its discussion. It is very important that there be a sense of continuity to the group process. If you will be unable to make a session, be sure to let the group know well in advance. If you find on short notice that you cannot make a session, please leave a message so that the group can know what to expect. We would like to see you, even if you are under the weather and not keen on being very active in the session. If you must miss more than 3 of the 20 sessions for whatever reason, you will be asked to leave the group and shift to another treatment format.

Messages may be left at 999-1234.

The process of making personal changes is hard work. As part of the group task, you will be expected to apply what is being learned in the group to your outside circumstances. This includes keeping a Daily Journal and bringing it to the sessions.

As we discussed in pregroup interviews, it is important that all members make a commitment not to meet with each other outside of the group.

We would strongly discourage members even coming to the sessions together. The group is a place to work on important personal issues. If one or more members have a relationship outside of the group, it makes this much more difficult. If some of your personal goals include becoming more sociable or meeting more people, then that needs to be done by you in your own outside life, not as part of the group. It may be something you can talk about in the group and then apply as homework for yourself. If you should have contacts with other group members between sessions, we would ask you to make a commitment to discuss these in the next session.

[This is the stringent level of guidelines regarding extragroup socializing. Groups that are designed for a more supportive approach may want to temper these—perhaps just a word of caution and the request for reporting back to the group. Groups designed for development of social skills may actively encourage members to do activities together, and all that would be expected would be for the experiences to be shared with the group.]

The therapists do not generally expect to have contact with group members outside of the group itself. If there is something very pressing, you may contact us. However, all such contacts will be considered as part of the larger frame of the group experience. The therapists, at their discretion, may bring this material back into the group sessions. If you are receiving medication, this should be managed by your own doctor. We will not get into detailed discussion about your medications, although we may talk more generally about drugs and their benefits and side effects. Urgent situations should be managed through your regular medical resources or, if necessary, a hospital emergency department.

We are always trying to learn more about how groups can be most effective. We will be asking you to repeat part of the set of questionnaires during the group and the complete package a couple of weeks before the group ends. In addition, a brief questionnaire concerning the group itself will be answered at the end of some sessions. This will take only a couple of minutes. We appreciate your participation in this task. We will also be scheduling an individual follow-up appointment with you about 4 months after the group ends to review how things are progressing.

We look forward to seeing you at 4:30 on Wednesday 3 January 1996. Please allow extra time to get to this first meeting.

Appendix 12

Crisis Intervention Group Information Sheet

[Substitute name and information for your group, and alter each paragraph to match your clinical situation.]

The Rapid Access Group is one of a number of different groups offered by the Mental Health Center. The groups meets from 2:30 to 4:00 on Tuesday afternoons. [Add clear details about address and where to report.]

The Rapid Access Group provides a maximum of 8 sessions of treatment that you may use over a 12-week period. We recommend that new members attend each week for their first 3 or 4 sessions. After that time, you may spread your remaining sessions over the following 8- or 9-week period at your discretion.

The group will be led by Roy MacKenzie, M.D., and Karen Smith, M.S.W. Most of the work will be done through group discussion. The main focus will be on the current situation that is a problem for you and how you can best master it.

Please try to arrive on time. If you are unable to make a session that you had planned to attend, please leave a message so that the group can know what to expect. Messages may be left at 999-1234.

Most people referred to the Rapid Access Group will have had an intake interview by a clinician from the Mental Health Center. Many people find that the Rapid Access Group is all the treatment they need at this time. At the intake interview, some people may be referred to the Rapid Access Group until a space is available in one of the other ongoing treatment groups. If this is your situation, your attendance in the Rapid Access Group will end once you start another program. For others, the most appropriate plan for further therapy may not be clear at intake time and will be clarified while you are a member of the Rapid Access Group.

The therapists do not generally expect to have contact with group members outside of the group itself. If there is something very pressing, you should contact your family physician or, if necessary, call the Center at the above number and tell them you are a member of this group. In the event of a major problem, come to the Emergency Department.

We look forward to seeing you at your first session.

Appendix 13

Patient Change Measures

It is becoming increasingly more imperative that clinicians systematically document the effectiveness of their work. The following short list of commonly used brief and easily scored measures forms a reasonable starting point. The results of all of these measures can be readily shared and discussed with your patients. The Outcome Questionnaire and the Client Satisfaction Questionnaire would form a very basic level of assessment. The Symptom Checklist-90—Revised and the Brief Symptom Inventory cover symptom areas similar to those covered in the Outcome Questionnaire but in more detail. The Inventory of Interpersonal Problems and the Social Adjustment Scale add more depth. The Life Style Inventory is a checklist to identify general lifestyle issues. Most of these instruments use the same general style, so they form a simple package for patients to complete. A practical and well-documented survey is provided by Ogles and coworkers (1996).

Outcome Questionnaire (OQ-45.2) (45 items)

The OQ-45.2 is a recently developed questionnaire designed for use in a busy service setting (Burlingame et al. 1995; Lambert and Hill 1994). The results are reported as a global measure of distress and, at a more specific level, as subscores for subjective discomfort (symptoms), interpersonal relationships, and social role performance. Norms are available. The questionnaire also has screening questions for a number of common disorders such as substance abuse and panic attacks. The OQ-45.2 is copyrighted but is available for a nominal licensing fee from the following:

American Professional Credentialing Services LLC
10421 Stevenson Road, P.O. Box 346
Stevenson, Maryland 21153-0346
Telephone: (500) 488-2727
Fax: (410) 329-3777

Symptom Checklist–90—Revised (SCL-90-R) (90 items)

The SCL-90-R is a standard measure of psychological symptoms that is used in many outcome studies (Derogatis 1983; Derogatis and Melisaratos 1983). Results are expressed as mean item scores on each of nine subscales and an overall mean item score, or as standardized T-scores. The overall mean score correlates quite highly with the OQ-45.2 subjective discomfort score.

Brief Symptom Inventory (BSI) (53 items)

The BSI is a shorter form of the SCL-90-R and has the same subscales. There is a high correlation of the scores between the two instruments.

Both the BSI and the SCL-90-R are copyrighted. The instruments and scoring procedures can be obtained at the address below:

National Computer Systems Assessments
P.O. Box 1416
Minneapolis, Minnesota 55440
Telephone: 1-800-627-7271

Inventory of Interpersonal Problems (IIP) (64 items)

The IIP is a detailed measure of interpersonal style. It was first composed of 127 items, but this shorter version contains only the eight scales that form the Interpersonal Circumplex described in Chapter 5. The mean item score is a general measure of interpersonal problem distress that can be compared with the BSI mean score as a general measure of symptomatic distress. For clinical use, it is satisfactory to simply calculate the mean score on each subscale and think of the eight scales as forming a circle. The overall mean score correlates quite highly with the OQ-45.2 interpersonal subscale, but the IIP provides a more detailed description of the nature of relationships. A full description and more detailed scoring instructions are available (Alden et al. 1990; Horowitz et al. 1988). The IIP is copyrighted and available in versions of various lengths at the following address:

The Psychological Corporation
555 Academic Court
San Antonio, Texas 78204-2498
Telephone: 1-800-634-0424

Structural Analysis of Social Behavior (SASB)

The concepts of the SASB system are described in some detail in Chapter 5. They can be applied in a technical manner to transcript analysis or used in a questionnaire format to describe specific relationships. Appendix 7 contains a simplified format. The Intrex questionnaires and other information regarding the SASB can be obtained from

Dr. Lorna Benjamin
Department of Psychology
University of Utah
Salt Lake City, Utah 84112
Telephone: (801) 581-4463

Client Satisfaction Questionnaire (CSQ) (8 items)

The CSQ is a global measure of satisfaction (Nguyen et al. 1983). It could be augmented by questions concerning specific aspects of a treatment program. The CSQ is suitable for routine use at termination or follow-up visits in most clinical settings. An even shorter format is also available. The CSQ is published in Ogle et al. 1996. It may be obtained at the following address: Clifford Attkisson, Ph.D., Millberry Union, 200 West, 500 Parnassus Ave., University of California, San Francisco, California 94143-0244. Fax only: (415) 476-9690.

Life Style Inventory (LSI) (12 items)

The LSI is designed to stimulate a discussion of lifestyle issues and to track changes. When your lifestyle gets out of balance, most people experience a sense of being stressed or out of control. This may happen when there are too many obligations (too many "shoulds") and not enough pleasurable or satisfying components (not enough "haves"). When this occurs, it may lead to increased self-criticism ("I should be doing better" or "I'm a loser," or "I don't deserve any better," etc.). Sometimes the feeling of being deprived may lead to intensely wanting some sort of immediate gratification ("I owe it to myself")—for example, food, alcohol, buying sprees, or sex. This may result in impulsive decisions or actions that are not in your best interest and in fact may make things worse. They are then followed by more self-criticism or depression. Consider the list of general lifestyle issues below and rate each one in terms of how much of a problem it is for you currently. Add any additional items that are important for you.

Lifestyle activity	RATING SCALE 0 not at all 1 a little bit 2 somewhat 3 moderately 4 quite a bit 5 a great deal 6 extremely
1. Has there been a build-up of multiple stresses in your life?	0 1 2 3 4 5 6
2. Are obligations getting out of balance with satisfactions in your life at present?	0 1 2 3 4 5 6
3. Are you controlling your life too much so that there is no spontancity left?	0 1 2 3 4 5 6
4. Is your dieting or eating getting out of control; has your weight changed recently?	0 1 2 3 4 5 6
5. Has there been an increase in your use of alcohol, drugs, or tobacco?	0 1 2 3 4 5 6
6. Have your activities led to a persistent lack of sleep?	0 1 2 3 4 5 6
7. Is it hard to find enough opportunities for relaxation?	0 1 2 3 4 5 6
8. Has it been difficult for you to get enough exercise?	0 1 2 3 4 5 6
9. Has there been a decrease in your involvement with family or friends?	0 1 2 3 4 5 6
10. Have you been withdrawing from group social activities?	0 1 2 3 4 5 6
11. Have you been reducing or dropping activities and hobbies?	0 1 2 3 4 5 6
12. Has it been difficult for you to tell when your system is under increased stress?	0 1 2 3 4 5 6

Appendix 14

Group Process Measures

There are relatively few well-utilized measures of group process. The Group Climate Questionnaire is the most widely used member rating format. It asks the members to think of the whole group. The California Psychotherapy Alliance Scale for groups has not been widely used in the group literature, but it is well known as a measure of the therapeutic alliance in individual psychotherapy studies. The group members rate their own personal relationship to the group. These two measures thus offer the opportunity to tap into two different views of the group as experienced by the members. The Hill Interaction Matrix has been the most widely used measure for observer rating of group process.

Group Climate Questionnaire (GCQ) (12 items)

The GCQ, a 12-item measure (MacKenzie 1981; MacKenzie et al. 1987), contains three subscales:

- **Engaged:** a positive working climate comparable to the working alliance (items 1, 2, 4, 8, 11)
- **Conflict:** anger and rejection (items 6, 7, 10, 12)
- **Avoiding:** personal responsibility for group work (items 3, 5, 9)

Results are best shown as simply the mean item scores for each subscale. It should be noted that these scores will vary over time, so that sequential measures provide the most useful application of this instrument. (**Note:** Previously published norms are not recommended because they shift considerably depending on the nature of the group population.)

Group Climate Questionnaire

Name: _____ **Date:** _____

Read each statement carefully and try to think of the group as a whole. Using the Rating Scale as a guide, circle the number for each statement that best describes the group during today's session. Please mark only ONE answer for each statement.	**RATING SCALE** 0 not at all 1 a little bit 2 somewhat 3 moderately 4 quite a bit 5 a great deal 6 extremely

1. The members liked and cared about each other	0 1 2 3 4 5 6
2. The members tried to understand why they do the things they do, tried to reason it out	0 1 2 3 4 5 6
3. The members avoided looking at important issues going on between themselves	0 1 2 3 4 5 6
4. The members felt what was happening was important and there was a sense of participation	0 1 2 3 4 5 6
5. The members depended on the group leader(s) for direction	0 1 2 3 4 5 6
6. There was friction and anger between the members	0 1 2 3 4 5 6
7. The members were distant and withdrawn from each other	0 1 2 3 4 5 6
8. The members challenged and confronted each other in their efforts to sort things out	0 1 2 3 4 5 6
9. The members appeared to do things the way they thought would be acceptable to the group	0 1 2 3 4 5 6
10. The members rejected and distrusted each other	0 1 2 3 4 5 6
11. The members revealed sensitive personal information or feelings	0 1 2 3 4 5 6
12. The members appeared tense and anxious	0 1 2 3 4 5 6

Please describe briefly the event that was most personally important to you during today's session. This might be something that involved you directly, or something that happened between other members but that made you think about yourself. Explain what it was about the event that made it important for you personally.

California Psychotherapy Alliance Scales (CALPAS)

The CALPAS comprises a more recent group of therapeutic alliance scales that are in wide use in the psychotherapy research community (Gaston 1991; Marmar et al. 1989). This group of scales includes a 24-item group alliance measure as well as several different versions for individual therapy. The CALPAS can be obtained from the following:

Alliance Scales
Langley Porter Psychiatric Institute
Box F-0984
University of California
401 Parnassus Avenue
San Francisco, California 94143-0984
Telephone: (415) 476-7562

Hill Interaction Matrix (HIM)

The HIM is an observer rating system that uses four content and five process categories (Hill 1977). It is based on the theory that the group is most effective when personal issues are discussed in a confrontational manner by all group members. It is expected, therefore, that successful groups will eventually be working in the lower-right work/member-centered area. The process categories are defined as follows:

1. **Responsive:** Members' responding to therapist suggestions
2. **Conventional:** Social conversation about general topics
3. **Assertive:** Argumentative or assertive statements revealing biases, beliefs, or prejudices without attempts to solicit or accept help from other members
4. **Speculative:** Interest in exploring interactional topics in a cooperative and task-oriented manner
5. **Confrontive:** A higher level of risk taking and tension around content material that is usually avoided

The Responsive and Conventional styles are common during the engagement stage, and the Assertive style is typical of the differentiation stage. The two work categories, Speculative and Confrontive, predominate when the group matures in its working capacity. The HIM uses the term *pre-work* for the first three interactional process categories, but it should be noted that the term addresses a technical aspect of the group process only. The members will receive considerable therapeutic benefits from these early "pre-work" stages.

Content Categories

		Non-member centered		Member centered	
		Topic I	Group II	Personal III	Relationship IV
Pre-Work	Responsive **A**	IA	IIA	IIIA	IVA
	Conventional **B**	IB (1)	IIB (2)	IIIB (9)	IVB (10)
	Assertive **C**	IC (3)	IIC (4)	IIIC (11)	IVC (12)
Work	Speculative **D**	ID (5)	IID (6)	IIID (13)	IVD (14)
	Confrontive **E**	IE (7)	IIE (8)	IIIE (15)	IVE (16)

Process Categories

The HIM is also available as a 72-item rating scale, the HIM-G, that can be scored by an observer or therapist after a session. The HIM-G serves as an excellent way to train students or staff to look critically at what is transpiring in a group. Within the HIM-G, 32 items address leader behavior. These may be used to develop a leader profile that can help beginning leaders to conceptualize their activities.

Appendix 15

Current Books

The last few years have seen a remarkable flourishing of books regarding group psychotherapy. The following is a selective list of books chosen because of their prominence and wide coverage of the field.

Alonso A, Swiller HI (eds): Group Therapy in Clinical Practice. Washington, DC, American Psychiatric Press, 1993

Bergin AE, Garfield SL (eds): Handbook of Psychotherapy and Behavior Change, 4th Edition. New York, Wiley, 1994

Bernard HS, MacKenzie KR (eds): Basics of Group Psychotherapy. New York, Guilford, 1994

Brabender V, Fallon A: Models of Inpatient Group Psychotherapy. Washington, DC, American Psychological Association, 1993

Flores PJ: Group Psychotherapy With Addicted Populations, 2nd Edition. New York, Haworth Press, 1996

Fuhriman A, Burlingame GM (eds): Handbook of Group Psychotherapy: An Empirical and Clinical Synthesis. New York, Wiley, 1994

Halperin DA, Kymissis P: Group Therapy With Children and Adolescents. Washington, DC, American Psychiatric Press, 1996

Kaplan HI, Sadock BJ (eds): Comprehensive Group Psychotherapy. Baltimore, MD, Williams & Wilkins, 1993

Klein RH, Bernard HS, Singer DL (eds): Handbook of Contemporary Group Psychotherapy. Madison, CT, International Universities Press, 1992

MacKenzie KR (ed): Classics in Group Psychotherapy. New York, Guilford, 1992

Marziali E, Munroe-Blum H: Interpersonal Group Psychotherapy for Borderline Personality Disorder. New York, Basic Books, 1994

McKay M, Paleg K (eds): Focal Group Psychotherapy. Oakland, CA, New Harbinger, 1992

Piper WE, McCallum M, Azim HFA: Adaptation to Loss Through Short-Term Group Psychotherapy. New York, Guilford, 1992

Rutan JS, Stone WN: Psychodynamic Group Psychotherapy. New York, Guilford, 1993

Stone WN: Group Psychotherapy for People With Chronic Mental Illness. New York, Guilford, 1966

Yalom ID: Theory and Practice of Group Psychotherapy, 4th Edition. New York, Basic Books, 1995

Source Notes

1. The scope of managed healthcare programming began to widen rapidly in the late 1980s, and the quoted passage is from one of the earlier books devoted to the topic (Goodman et al. 1996).

2. Ken Howard and colleagues, from Northwestern University in Evanston, have contributed a series of important papers on psychotherapy outcome and time. The authors popularized the use of the term *dose-response relationship* to psychotherapy studies (Howard et al. 1986, 1992).

3. Utilization rates tend to be reasonably stable in a given system over time and will be related to the demographic characteristics of the population served (Howard et al. 1993; S. Shapiro et al. 1984).

4. The lower curve in Figure 1–1 is based on a large service delivery system database derived from mental health center and general hospital outpatient programs (Phillips 1987). Two studies have looked specifically at outpatient programs that purported to offer primarily longer-term psychodynamic treatment but had quite brief actual mean utilization rates in the range of 3 to 4 months (Garfield and Kurz 1952; Sledge et al. 1990).

5. The most widely quoted meta-analytic study of the psychotherapy efficacy research is that by Smith and colleagues (1980). Lambert and Bergin (1994) have provided a comprehensive update.

6. There is nearly universal agreement that no difference in outcome is found between the same sort of treatment provided in an individual and group format (Lambert and Bergin 1994; Orlinsky and Howard 1986; Piper and Joyce 1996; Tillitski 1990; Toseland and Siporin 1986).

7. These randomized studies were designed specifically to compare group and individual treatment (Budman et al. 1988; Pilkonis et al. 1984; Piper et al. 1984).

8. Much of this chapter is based on the American Group Psychotherapy Association Presidential Address, delivered in February 1994 (MacKenzie 1994c), entitled "Where Is Here and When Is Now? The Adaptational Challenge of Mental Health Reform for Group Psychotherapy." At the time of this event, an extensive Congressional debate regarding health-care legislation was taking place.

9. A comprehensive history of group psychotherapy in the United States is found in the chapter by Scheidlinger and Schamess (1992) in the book *Classics in Group Psychotherapy* (MacKenzie 1992), where the authors refer to Menninger's statement of 1946. This book also contains a selection of important original papers from 1900 to 1980 by senior group theoreticians and practitioners assembled in honor of the 50th anniversary of the American Group Psychotherapy Association.

10. The *Handbook of Psychotherapy and Behavior Change*, now in its fourth edition (Bergin and Garfield 1994), has been the bible of psychotherapy researchers ever since the publication of the first edition in 1971. It provides a comprehensive survey of available clinical research along with extensive integrative commentary. Fortunately, most of the contributing authors are also clinicians, so the material has a distinctly applied flavor. The fourth edition arrived in late 1994, just in time for this book.

11. The term *generic model* was used by Orlinsky and Howard (1987) to describe a complex mix of therapeutic ingredients that had been shown to be correlated with psychotherapy outcome. An updated version of this model is presented in the chapter on process and outcome in the fourth edition of the *Handbook of Psychotherapy and Behavior Change* (Orlinsky et al. 1994), which contains a summary of the voluminous literature now available on this subject and is an excellent current resource for those wishing to explore this literature. It has been long recognized that common factors account for many of the benefits of psychotherapy. Jerome Frank wrote in 1961 of the importance of hope in psychotherapy and presaged many aspects of the generic model. His provocative book is now available in a new, third edition (Frank and Frank 1991). A parallel literature also suggests that the theoretical orientation adopted by a clinician is not a very good predictor of what that clinician is actually doing in therapy sessions (Lambert 1989). There is a strong suspicion that the sensible clinician, in fact, provides a rich mixture of the common therapeutic ingredients but then justifies them post hoc using the language of his or her own

theoretical model. The important feature of the generic model is that it is based on only those process and outcome findings that are replicated across a broad cross section of studies.

12. Winston and Muran (1996), in a recent review of the literature, identified six common factors: 1) expression of feelings and thoughts, 2) self-examination and self-understanding, 3) provision of a rationale that includes a plausible system of explanation of the patient's problems and distress, 4) strengthening of the patient's expectations of help and arousal of hope, 5) encouragement of mastery efforts and testing of different approaches and solutions, and 6) existence of a patient-therapist or helping relationship. This review article also includes a thorough discussion of the therapeutic alliance.

13. The quoted passage is from the chapter on process and outcome in the fourth edition of the *Handbook of Psychotherapy and Behavior Change* (Orlinsky et al. 1994, p. 278).

14. Ed Bordin was a major contributor to the early theoretical understanding of therapeutic alliance (Bordin 1979). He also stimulated and supported a generation of psychotherapy researchers who put his ideas to the test.

15. A recent publication, *Handbook of Group Psychotherapy: An Empirical and Clinical Synthesis* (Fuhriman and Burlingame 1994), provides a comprehensive survey of existing studies for the field of group psychotherapy. This is the first such compilation in recent times and is a good source both for information about clinical investigations into groups and for an orientation as to how such studies might be conducted.

16. This chapter is an abridged version of the first section of my earlier text, *Introduction to Time-Limited Group Psychotherapy* (MacKenzie 1990). It is presented here as a synopsis for quick reference.

17. A succinct overview of general systems theory applied to small groups, as well as a good cross section of relevant references, is found in Agazarian and Janoff (1993).

18. MacKenzie (1979) provides an introduction to the concept of norms in therapy groups.

19. The two-by-two matrix used in this section for consideration of specific normative dimensions was developed by Bond (1983).

20. A discussion of the effects of group size on participation can be found in Mullen and Goethals 1987. My discussion of the various categories of group size is based in part on Hare 1976.

21. A comprehensive review of the literature concerning group development is found in MacKenzie 1994a. In that discussion, the conclusion was reached that there is substantial empirical evidence for the development of an initial group climate characterized by increasing cohesion and self-disclosure followed by the emergence of a period of intragroup tension and conflict. Group-level measures of positive and negative emotional tone identify these two early stages. Beyond that point, the nature of group interaction becomes more complex and requires more attention to specific interpersonal dimensions and individual cognitive styles. In a seminal contribution, Beck (1974) described nine stages of group development, particularly focusing on identifying transition markers between the stages.

22. Beck (1974), using the term *distributed leadership,* has described in detail the functional importance of role behaviors in the mastery of group developmental stages. These ideas have been developed in greater detail, and sociometric data have been presented, by Brusa and associates (1994). Livesley and MacKenzie (1983) applied a similar orientation to the concept of social role, with some modification of the details. There are some minor discrepancies between the labels used by Beck and those used in this book, although the concepts are similar. The Sociable Role is closely related to Beck's "Emotional Leader." The Structural Role is assumed by Beck to be fulfilled by the "Designated Leader" and is given a broader role definition that includes many of the attributes of positive leadership. The Divergent Role corresponds to "the Scapegoat" in Beck's system. The Cautionary Role corresponds to Beck's "Defiant Member," with Beck stressing the challenge side of the role more than the underlying sense of social alienation. Beck describes a member who assumes this role as managing a compromise solution to group membership by aligning with the leader in a special relationship.

  In some of the sociology literature, the assumption is made that only one member can be a role leader. This assumption unnecessarily restricts use of the role concepts. A potential liability of thinking in terms of only one person fulfilling each role is that a subtle process of role stereotyping may be encouraged that can make it difficult for the person so identified to try out alternative behaviors. Promoting each member to be active in multiple roles is in keeping with the idea of psychological maturity being characterized by role flexibility. In clinical situations, it is useful to think of the sum of role resources available in the total group membership.

23. A comprehensive review of the concept of cohesion and of how it can be assessed is provided by Drescher and co-workers (1985). The effects of group cohesion on outcome have been reviewed by Budman and colleagues (1989).

24. Budman and his colleagues in Boston developed a rating scale to be used by an observer (Budman et al. 1987). The subscale headings are listed in Table 3–4 (see Budman et al. 1987 for detailed descriptions of the subscales).

25. Corsini and Rosenberg (1955) provided the first major discussion of therapeutic factors, and Yalom (1970) incorporated these concepts as a major portion of the first edition of his standard text, now in its fourth edition (Yalom 1995). An updated review of the research literature on therapeutic factors in group therapy has been provided by Crouch and co-workers (1994).

26. The question of whether or how well one can predict how a patient will participate in a group has been discussed by Piper and McCallum (1994).

27. See American Psychiatric Association 1994.

28. See World Health Organization 1992.

29. See American Psychiatric Association 1987.

30. The GAF Scale was modified by Goldman and colleagues (1992) to separate symptoms and psychological functioning from social and occupational functioning, with the result that each category is rated separately. The format shown in Appendix 1 also allows a simple global rating.

31. Considerable evidence suggests that OCD is related to dysregulation in the serotonergic system. However, there is a high relapse rate after cessation of pharmacological treatment. Cognitive-behavioral strategies of in vivo exposure and response prevention appear to have satisfactory effectiveness and to be associated with a lower rate of relapse (Emmelkamp 1994).

32. As an example of overlap in Axis II categories, Widiger and colleagues (1987) found an average of 3.75 Axis II diagnoses per person, and Skodol and colleagues (1988) found 4.6. Marziali and Munroe-Blum (1994) provided a comprehensive review of the diagnosis of borderline personality disorder and reported a 40%–60% overlap of BPD with Axis I disorders. Oldham and colleagues (1992) identified an even greater overlap of BPD with other Axis II disorders. Indeed, it is hard to find a patient with a diagnosis of BPD who does not have symptomatology

that also meets the criteria for several other Axis I and Axis II categories. A thorough review of the issues surrounding the diagnosis of personality disorder is found in Livesley 1995.

33. Eysenck's system has received wide attention. The dimension of psychoticism in his system is defined as a tendency toward cognitive distortions, not psychosis per se (Eysenck 1987).

34. Biological interventions, such as use of serotonin reuptake inhibitors for impulsivity, operate on the biological "hardware" that in many cases has genetic loading. The talking therapies work at the "software" level, attempting to foster self-mastery and acting on internal constructs about self and relationships. This computer analogy also reflects the mutual dependence between hardware and software; a fast computer can perform only as well as its software, and clever software cannot get good results from a slow computer. This perspective suggests that a multimodal approach incorporating both "hardware" and "software" is important in understanding human behavior.

35. The American psychologist George Kelly (1955) described in some detail the process by which the individual creates a personal view of reality. The use of Kelly's "repertory grid" technique to determine patterns of construct usage has been elaborated on by a number of authors. An introduction to this literature can be found in Bannister and Fransella 1982 and Neimeyer 1993. These ideas are now merging with the growing interest in cognitive mediating mechanisms reflected, for example, in the brief psychotherapy literature (Horowitz 1994) and in cognitive treatment of depression (Beck et al. 1990). This perspective is quite compatible with psychodynamic concepts and forms a bridge to cognitive-behavioral theory. Recently, the *International Journal of Personal Construct Psychology* had its title changed to the *Journal of Constructivist Psychology*. This change in title is aligned with the "postmodern" emphasis on the role of language and narrative in constructing social realities (White and Epston 1990).

36. The best single reference in regard to the Big Five personality dimensions is Costa and Widiger 1994. This book contains both technical and clinical review articles applying the dimensional concepts. An introduction to this material is found in Costa and McCrae 1990.

37. McCallum and Piper (1990) have operationalized the measurement of psychological mindedness in a unique manner. They use a brief 3-minute video of an actress describing a scene in which she sees her

ex-husband at a jewelry counter. Every psychological defense mechanism imaginable is worked into the tape. The patient being assessed is simply asked to describe what he or she thinks is troubling this woman. The resulting brief description is then analyzed with the Psychological Mindedness Scale (see Appendix 4), with a particular focus on the ideas of wishes, anxiety, and defenses. The usefulness of the measure in predicting group dropout was fully reviewed by Piper and colleagues (1992).

38. The Quality of Relationships Scale will be familiar to most clinicians (see Appendix 5). It codifies individual development in terms of increasingly sophisticated object relations (Azim et al. 1991). Piper, Azim, and colleagues have followed the current trend in psychotherapy research by defining their scale in terms of the nature of real interpersonal relationships as revealed in an assessment interview. This focus on the interpersonal realm improves reliability in assessment. As with the Psychological Mindedness Scale (see note 37 above), the Piper group has welded clinical investigation techniques into terms that the clinician can understand and use. DSM-IV contains the Defensive Functioning Scale as a measure for further study (American Psychiatric Association 1994, pp. 751–757). This scale covers some of the same ground as the Psychological Mindedness Scale. However, there is some controversy over the hierarchy of the scale. For example, denial is at the fourth level of seven, even though some studies have suggested that the use of denial is a positive coping technique unless it seriously distorts overall adaptation. The general descriptions of the defense mechanisms are imprecise, so there is likely to be difficulty in agreement among clinicians.

39. The expanded concept of psychopathy is captured well in the Psychopathy Checklist (Hare et al. 1990).

40. Much of the material in this chapter concerning behavioral goal setting has been adapted from Rose 1989, a useful reference for behavioral and cognitive-behavioral group work.

41. Cognitive-behavior therapy has an important role in the therapeutic armamentarium of today's psychotherapist. The original concepts of Ellis (1962, 1980) and Beck (see Beck et al. 1979, 1990) have been well researched and applied to an increasing list of disorders, most of which are in the depression and anxiety categories. A review is found in a special section of the *Journal of Consulting and Clinical Psychology*, edited by Mahoney (1993).

In their book *Cognitive Therapy of Depression,* Beck and colleagues (1979) include a chapter on the use of groups. Current advances in the use of cognitive group therapy have been reviewed by Covi and Primakoff (1988), Neimeyer and Feixas (1990), and Robinson and colleagues (1990). Ellis (1992) leads the reader through a demonstration of his colorful therapeutic style.

42. A comprehensive approach to the theoretical integration of the psychotherapy literature is provided by Norcross and Goldfried (1992). An introduction to a review of transference-related measures is found in Luborsky and Barber 1994. This fills an entire issue of *Psychotherapy Research: Journal of the Society for Psychotherapy Research* (Vol. 4, Nos. 3–4). Segal and Blatt (1993) offer an extended discussion of the interface between cognitive and psychodynamic perspectives.

43. Personality disorders can be usefully thought of as dysfunctional interpersonal behaviors (McLemore and Benjamin 1979; Sullivan 1953). Benjamin (1993) has provided a detailed application of interpersonal concepts to the entire range of DSM-IV personality disorder categories. The high relapse rate for the treatment of depression with either pharmacological or psychological approaches remains a major problem, often involving the combination of depressive illness and personality pathology. A series of scholarly reviews is provided in M. H. Klein et al. 1993. Hoyt (1994) has described a variety of methods to identify the goals of treatment in terms of seeking solutions and solving problems.

44. The Inventory of Interpersonal Problems (IIP; Horowitz et al. 1988) is a clinically meaningful measure of interpersonal pathology (Alden et al. 1990). The structure of the IIP questions is identical to that of the questions in the Brief Symptom Inventory (Derogatis and Melisaratos 1983) (see note 45 below) or the Outcome Questionnaire–45 (Burlingame et al. 1995) (see note 46 below), so that when these inventories are used together, one can readily compare distress expressed as symptoms or as interpersonal problems. See Appendix 13 for more detailed descriptions of these inventories. An adjective checklist version of the interpersonal circumplex is also available (Wiggins et al. 1988).

45. The Brief Symptom Inventory (Derogatis and Melisaratos 1983) is a short version of the Symptom Checklist–90 (SCL-90), which in turn is the most recent version of the Hopkin's Symptom Checklist, which was based on the original Cornell Medical Index psychology section (Derogatis 1983). See Appendix 13 for more detailed descriptions of these measures.

46. The Outcome Questionnaire–45 is a relatively new instrument designed for routine use in clinical settings as a measure of symptomatic change (Burlingame et al. 1995). See Appendix 13 for a more detailed description of this questionnaire.

47. Attachment pathology has been steadily increasing in importance as a way of conceptualizing psychological difficulties (Bowlby 1977; also see Ainsworth et al. 1978). Linehan (1993) and Marziali and Munroe-Blum (1994) provide complementary in-depth reviews of attachment and severe personality disorders.

48. I am indebted to Lorna Benjamin for the opportunity to discuss with her on numerous occasions the clinical use of SASB. While I take responsibility for the final text, the material in this book has been significantly shaped by these discussions. SASB offers a theoretically sound yet practical map on which to locate interpersonal behavior. Quite apart from specific measurement instruments that she has developed, Benjamin's ideas in the SASB system make immediate sense to a clinician and help to organize understanding of the interpersonal world. There is a long historical tradition of describing interpersonal behavior as the interaction of a small number of core dimensions. The first popular system was developed by Leary (1957) in the Interpersonal Circle (IPC), from which the IIP was developed. A somewhat similar system was developed by Schaefer (1965), with the same horizontal Affiliation dimension but Psychological Autonomy Giving substituting for the vertical dimension rather than Control/Submission. The Schaefer system has been used extensively in the family therapy field. The SASB system integrates these two models into a single theoretical system (Benjamin 1993). The SASB system can be used in many different ways. Later in this chapter, its use as an assessment self-report questionnaire is described. It can also be used to analyze interactional transcripts or simply as a way of thinking about the ongoing interaction of a therapy session (see Appendix 13).

49. To become familiar with the three faces of the model, it might be helpful to draw the three circles separately and write in the cluster names around each one. The advantage of the composite model in Figure 5–5 is that the complementary links between behaviors in any given segment are immediately recognizable; for example, Blame elicits Sulk and vice versa and may be internalized as Self-Blame as well. Another way of thinking about these connections is that negative elicits negative and control elicits submission and vice versa.

50. A detailed description of the use of groups in day treatment programs is presented by Melson (1995). Crisis Intervention Group programs are described by Lonergan (1985) and Cross (1995). A comprehensive review of inpatient group psychotherapy is provided by Brabender and Fallon (1993), and a review of the empirical literature is presented by R. H. Klein and colleagues (1994).

51. A critical review of the empirical literature on client characteristics and group psychotherapy is provided by Piper (1994). In a comprehensive chapter, Garfield (1994) reviews the same area for psychotherapy in general, and the findings would be equally applicable to group therapy. MacKenzie (1994b) discusses the application of the Big Five personality dimensions to clinical practice.

52. The effects of homogeneity have not been well studied. A review of the issues is provided by Piper and colleagues (1992).

53. Roller and Nelson (1991, 1993) have reviewed cotherapy issues.

54. Kaul and Bednar (1994) surveyed the literature concerning pretherapy preparation and concluded that there is strong evidence for its effectiveness. They link pretherapy with the idea of providing early structure in a group to enhance the development of cohesion. The issue of providing early structure is somewhat contentious because early structure would to some extent go against the grain of the psychodynamically oriented group psychotherapist. Nonetheless, the available evidence suggests that structure helps, and personal experience has shown that the group can move on into less structure quite comfortably—that the early structure does not necessarily impede group development (Bednar et al. 1974). Pretherapy preparation is particularly important for time-limited formats in that it encourages a rapid entry into work material. It can also be used, as exemplified in this book, to develop a working focus for each member.

55. Pregroup workshops for education of patients and for gathering of further information on which to base final selection decisions have been described by Piper and colleagues (1982) and Budman and colleagues (1981).

56. See note 54.

57. The therapist might find it helpful to think of the work in this stage in terms of the Structural Analysis of Social Behavior (SASB) system as being primarily that of Protect/Trust, corresponding to the lower-right quadrant of the SASB system shown in Figure 5–5.

58. The dominance hierarchy (MacKenzie and Kennedy 1989) is a fundamental property of primate social systems. It serves to regulate power and aggression so that they do not become destructive forces. The hierarchy is to some extent based on physical strength, but kinship support and negotiated coalitions play an important part as well. Position in the hierarchy is a major determinant of sexual access. Interestingly, dominance has not been systematically studied in therapy groups.

59. Gabbard (1993) provides a review of projective identification and countertransference. The features of projective mechanisms and scapegoating in groups have been expanded by Scheidlinger (1982), Horwitz (1983), and Wright and colleagues (1988). van der Kolk (1993) discussed the tendency for some patients with posttraumatic stress disorder to idealize the leader and to demonstrate a compulsive care-giving role. Other patients, especially males, may reenact their own victimization. Such phenomena are pervasive in therapy groups, and the references above are recommended when the therapist is confronted with the need to address such issues. These phenomena are always accompanied by considerable affective arousal, and the therapist is best prepared with a solid cognitive introduction to the issues.

60. The Hill Interaction Matrix (Hill 1965, 1977) is one of the more widely used systems for analyzing group interaction. It is described in more detail in Appendix 14.

61. Alexander and French (1946/1980) coined the term *corrective emotional experience* to refer to a type of relationship in the therapy setting in which the patient is both supported and challenged regarding areas of distortion or overreaction in the actual relationship with the therapist. Their work is commonly cited as the first major publication on brief psychotherapy.

62. The Encounter Group study (Lieberman et al. 1973) drew attention to the importance of cognitive integration of affectively powerful group experience. For many years this study of 18 encounter groups at Stanford University was the most comprehensive study of groups that had many of the features of a therapy group. Piper and colleagues (1992) conducted a study of similar proportions with more contemporary measurements on actual psychotherapy groups.

   Dies (1983) reviewed the literature in regard to the relative effectiveness of affective versus cognitive dimensions. Luborsky and colleagues (1988) and Horowitz and co-workers (1993) demonstrated the importance of maintaining a consistent work focus for effective individual therapy. This idea is also the essence of the Therapeutic Operations portion of the generic model discussed in Chapter 2. A more recent review is found in a special section of the *Journal of Consulting and Clinical Psychology* edited by Luborsky, Barber, and Beutler (1993).

63. The Johari Window (Luft 1970) was described by, and named after, Joseph Luft and Harry Ingram. It was initially developed for use in T-groups but can be applied just as effectively to therapy groups.

64. Jacobs and co-workers (1973) have provided a review of the technical dimensions of feedback. The principles involved in the feedback process are continuously operative. It is helpful for the therapist to use them knowledgeably rather than by accident.

65. See note 35.

66. The idea of Focal Incidents has a lengthy history in the group literature. In the first major study of group process and outcome, Frank looked at group sessions in terms of clusters of events, a process he called "situation analysis" (Powdermaker and Frank 1953). The Encounter Group study (Lieberman et al. 1973) used a more formalized approach through a questionnaire, the Critical Incident Questionnaire. A version of this questionnaire is included in the Group Climate Questionnaire in Appendix 14. Yalom (1995) described this process of learning through critical incidents as the enactment of a corrective emotional experience. Leszcz (1992) presented a thoughtful summary of the interpersonal approach to group psychotherapy. The label of "Critical Incident" from the research literature has been replaced here with the more generic term Focal Incident to avoid the impression that only really major events count.

67. Agazarian uses a modified systems approach to managing groups that mobilizes issues through a process of polarization into subgroups (Agazarian and Janoff 1993). The use of subgroups offers the individual a supportive subgroup context with which to identify and, at the same time, encourages confrontation between subgroups over issues of intimacy and conflict. Although still undergoing development, these concepts offer some provocative ways of understanding and using group dynamics.

68. Ekman and colleagues (1972) presented a sophisticated analysis of facial behavior very much in keeping with Darwin's original observations

(Darwin 1872). Ekman concluded that basic affect states are "hard wired" into facial responses to form an innate communication system.

69. Bion (1959) used somewhat obscure language, but his concepts are quite useful. The three "basic assumption" states can be located around the lower pole in the SASB circle, with dependency at the bottom, fight/flight in the lower-left quadrant, and pairing in the lower-right quadrant. These concepts are associated today with "Tavistock" training experiences, often sponsored in the United States by the A. K. Rice Institute.

70. Laws (1989) has provided a full introduction to the relapse prevention literature.

71. The idea of a firm time limit extends back into the early days of psychotherapy, to the writings of Rank (1929/1973) and Alexander and French (1946/1980).

72. Virtually all of the original contributors to the time-limited literature emphasized the importance of establishing a clear focus for treatment. Key figures in this area (with their most recent publication) are Mann (1991), Malan (1979), Sifneos (1987), and Davanloo (1980). A major comparative survey is found in Barber and Crits-Christoph 1995.

73. More recent contributions to the time-limited literature include those by Ryle (1990), Gustafson (1986, 1995), Bauer and Kobos (1987), and D. Shapiro (1989). A special section of the *International Journal of Group Psychotherapy* (Volume 46, Number 1, January 1996) comprises a series of articles on termination that have direct application to time-limited approaches.

74. This quotation is from Mann 1991, p. 43, and was adapted from Mann and Goldman 1987.

75. The general text by Budman and Gurman (1988) has been influential and contains a detailed description of time-limited group psychotherapy techniques.

76. The quoted passage is from Budman and Gurman 1988, p. 6.

77. This material concerning setting a time limit is taken from my review article surveying the time-limited literature (MacKenzie 1988).

78. Yalom (1980) discusses psychotherapy in the context of existential philosophy. Interestingly, little mention is made of termination issues.

79. Numerous authors have discussed the issues involved in deciding on the termination date of an individual member of an ongoing group (Lothstein 1993; Rutan and Stone 1993; Yalom 1995).

80. Foulkes (1975), in his excellent book *Group-Analytic Psychotherapy: Method and Principles,* discusses the role of time in psychotherapy.

81. We are at the mercy of language here. Neither "supportive" nor "interpretive" really captures the essence of the two positions. The description "supportive" is technically correct in that one tries to support the patient's defenses and usual coping style unless they are seriously dysfunctional. However, the inclusion of active focusing, problem identification, and challenge does not quite fit the usual image of pure support. "Interpretive" focuses on the linking of internal affective states to relationship themes, but the focusing and challenging activities of the supportive mode often have a clear interpretive quality, with the intent being to change the patient's frame of reference. Luborsky (1984), in his research studies, prefers the term "expressive" to "interpretive," but again a specialized meaning of the word is intended, because almost all psychotherapy expects some expressiveness from the patient. Frank and Frank (1991) use the more accurately descriptive term "evocative." A more general term might be "intrusive," in that the therapist attempts to disrupt established patterns, be they behavioral, cognitive, interpersonal, or intrapsychic in nature. "Insight-oriented" is another term used to imply the interpretive end of the spectrum. This term again is inadequate, because patients in supportive therapy regularly obtain important insight into the nature of their relationships even though intrapsychically directed interpretations may not be used. It seems unjustified to assume that these interpersonal interventions are of lesser importance. Supportive therapy may certainly be anxiety-provoking. Asking patients to try out more assertive behavior, for example, may trigger a strong affective response. Insight is commonly described as producing anxiety, when what is being described is actually resistance to acknowledging the interpretive message, another unfortunate example of linguistic confusion. Benjamin (1994) argues that the identification of a defense is really only a part of the diagnostic process and that psychological change comes from the social learning experience of recognizing interpersonal patterns and learning from the therapeutic context that these patterns can be altered. Piper (1996) provides a thoughtful discussion of these issues and includes a list of 12 characteristics of supportive-interpretive continua that has considerable overlap with that presented in this book.

82. The renewed interest in supportive dimensions is reflected in works by Pinsker and colleagues (1991), Rockland (1992), Winston and co-workers (1994), and Hellerstein and co-workers (1994). These authors suggest that a psychodynamic understanding of the patient may be inappropriately converted into an abstinent and sterile interpretive therapeutic style that impedes rather than enhances compliance with therapeutic work.

83. The use of treatment manuals has now become widespread. Luborsky and DeRubeis (1984) provide an introduction to the idea of manuals. Manuals for cognitive-behavior therapy (Beck et al. 1979) and interpersonal psychotherapy (Klerman et al. 1984) are in wide use. Psychodynamic therapy manuals came into use during the 1980s (Laikin and Winston 1988). A variety of manual-derived protocols are pulled together in an excellent book by Crits-Christoph and Barber (1991). Winston and colleagues (1994) demonstrate how two manual-driven time-limited psychotherapies can be used effectively for patients with personality disorders. Many treatment systems now have a series of manuals for more structured and time-limited groups. These vary considerably in the degree of detail. The models in the last section of this book suggest how the generic group can be adapted to various conditions and populations. A general discussion of the use of manuals has been presented by Kazdin (1994) and Lambert and Bergin (1994).

84. The manual by Piper and colleagues (1992) for treating patients with person loss is the most elaborate group psychotherapy manual. Neimeyer and Feixas (1990) describe a cognitive-behavioral group treatment for depression. A thorough review of group therapy manuals is provided by Dies (1994).

85. The Encounter Group Study (Lieberman et al. 1973) identified the first four style characteristics. Subsequent studies of the impact of group leadership have largely confirmed these findings.

86. Carl Rogers' book *Client-Centered Therapy* (1951), in which Rogers presented his ideas of "necessary and sufficient" therapist qualities, has had a profound effect on clinical practice. The theoretical basis of Rogers' ideas lay in the belief that given the right opportunity, people will grow and develop. This optimistic stance has been modified through a greater understanding of the Therapeutic Bond referred to in Chapter 2. It has been identified that once a minimal level of therapist interest is available, it is the contribution of the patient that plays the major role in determining the quality of the alliance.

87. A variety of ways of using clarification and interpretive techniques have been presented by Crits-Christoph and Barber (1991).

88. Porter (1993) provides a review of the issues involved in the use of two therapists.

89. A major review of the literature on negative effects of psychotherapy is provided by Lambert and Bergin (1994). Negative effects have been found in all types of psychotherapy, and the incidence of such effects appears to be about 10%, a finding fairly consistent across studies (Doherty et al. 1986 [charismatically led marital therapy]; Lieberman et al. 1973 [encounter groups]; Stone 1990 [borderline personality disorder]; Sachs 1983 [general psychotherapy]). One of the interesting findings in the National Institute of Mental Health Treatment of Depression Collaborative Research Program (see note 93 below) is that interpersonal psychotherapy had virtually no negative effects, whereas the cognitive model was reported to have negative effects in about 10% of patients (Ogles et al. 1993).

    Highly disturbed patients are more likely to have a negative experience, especially if they receive a therapeutic approach that encourages the challenging of their usual coping strategies. Failure to provide structure for the disturbed patient, and failure to quickly address negative attitudes toward the therapy or the therapist, also are correlated with a higher incidence of negative effects.

    Therapist characteristics that are consistently associated with higher levels of negative effects have been identified. They include impatience, authoritarian interventions, and difficulty in establishing a positive working alliance. These characteristics are often associated with the therapist's experiencing personal emotional difficulties.

    Studies of premature termination and unplanned termination late in the group's life often cite early conflict as a precipitant (Dies and Teleska 1985). Early conflict is often associated with a negative or hostile therapeutic style (Hartley et al. 1976; Lieberman et al. 1973) or a failure to develop supportive group norms (Bond 1983).

90. Crosby and Sabin (1996) give a brief introduction to developing group psychotherapy programs. They base their article on their experience in two of the larger and well-established programs in the United States. The Group Program Readiness Checklist presented in this chapter is adapted from a model developed by Greg Crosby and used with permission. Spitz (1996) provides a review of the use of groups in a man-

aged care context. A special section of the *International Journal of Group Psychotherapy* (Volume 46, Number 3, July 1996) provides a series of articles dealing with group psychotherapy in the managed care service context. The division of time categories for determining length of treatment follows that used in this book: lower severity but high-volume problems (crisis intervention), intensive alternatives to hospital care (formal time-limited format), and severe and persistent disorders (longer term) (Piper and Joyce 1996; Steenbarger and Budman 1996).

91. This list of ethical issues that apply in specific ways to the group psychotherapy context is adapted from the *Guidelines for Ethics* statement of the American Group Psychotherapy Association. The complete document can be obtained from

> American Group Psychotherapy Association
> 25 East 21st Street, 6th Floor
> New York, NY 10010
> Telephone: (212) 477-2677
> Fax: (212) 979-6627

The National Registry of Certified Group Psychotherapists is found at the same address (Telephone: [212] 477-1600).

92. Lonergan (1994) describes a single group critical incident from seven different theoretical viewpoints. This sort of comparative perspective is helpful for the trainee.

93. The National Institute of Mental Health (NIMH) Treatment of Depression Collaborative Research Program remains the most ambitious attempt to compare various psychotherapy treatment approaches, although legitimate criticisms have been raised about various aspects of the study. The results were first presented by Elkin and colleagues (1989), and the entire study has been well reviewed by Elkin (1994).

The results of the study pleased no one. They serve as a reminder of the general trend to less striking efficacy reports as a treatment is studied over time and in settings removed from where the particular treatment originated. In addition, differential efficacy decreases when there is careful blinding conditions, random allocation, monitoring of the treatment actually provided, and an active control condition. The NIMH study was designed to address most of these conditions.

In the NIMH study, there was little evidence for differential effectiveness in the treatment of major depression with antidepressive medication (imipramine), interpersonal psychotherapy (IPT, Klerman model), and cognitive-behavior therapy (CBT, Beck model). The control treatment consisted of a pill-placebo plus a weekly supportive brief office visit where no attempt was made to do formal psychotherapy. This is a considerably more active control condition than is usually utilized. This simple regular contact was quite effective—indeed, equal to the active treatment—for patients in the lower end of the severity scale. At the high end of severity, the control condition was clearly less effective, and IPT was better than CBT on some measures and statistically not inferior to imipramine. Imipramine was associated with an earlier response and was somewhat more effective in the most severely depressed group of patients. In short, all three active treatments had a good response initially. All treatment conditions had a high relapse rate: fewer than one-third of the patients remained without relapse at 18-month follow-up.

94. Milieu concepts regarding day treatment programs have been reviewed by Kennedy (1993) and Azim (1993).

95. Riester and Kraft (1986) and Schamess (1993) address the treatment of children, and Cramer-Azima and Richmond (1989) and Kymissis and Halperin (1996) the treatment of adolescents. van der Kolk (1993) discusses the management of patients with histories of catastrophic trauma. Ganzarain and Buchele (1988) address the problems of childhood incest.

96. Spiegel and colleagues (1989) found a substantial reduction in mortality from breast cancer in those receiving a year of outpatient group therapy. More sophisticated technology for studying the immune system has made this an exciting area of contemporary research. Frasure-Smith (1991) reported a threefold increase in mortality for patients with high stress levels following myocardial infarction; a stress management program virtually eliminated this increased risk. These reports are a sample from an area of the treatment literature that is undergoing rapid expansion.

97. The book by Klerman, Weissman, and colleagues (1984) is an excellent example of a clinical manual for providing psychotherapy. Cognitive-behavior therapy (CBT) manuals are also available for the treatment of depression (Beck et al. 1979; Padesky and Greenberger 1995). Inter-

personal psychotherapy (IPT) has been used in numerous studies regarding the treatment of major depression with well-documented effectiveness. In many cases, this modality was compared with CBT. These "horse race" studies vary back and forth regarding which of the two is more effective. A conservative position would be that both have been clearly shown to be effective. The question of matching individual patients to specific treatment modality is as yet unresolved. The American Psychiatric Association's practice guideline for major depressive disorder provides a full review of treatment options (American Psychiatric Association 1993b). See note 93.

98. In a recent survey of over 8,000 adults, Blazer and colleagues (1994) reported that the prevalence of major depression was 4.9% and the lifetime prevalence was 17.1%. Simon and colleagues (1995) found that patients with depressive and anxiety disorders incurred almost twice the overall healthcare costs compared with those without such diagnoses. Depression is by far the most commonly diagnosed psychiatric condition.

99. Otto and colleagues (1993) review the use of cognitive-behavioral strategies for panic disorder, and Rose (1993) discusses cognitive-behavioral group psychotherapy.

100. Burns's popular *The Feeling Good Handbook* (1990) and *Ten Days to Self-Esteem* (1993) provide an easily understood approach to the use of cognitive-behavioral strategies. It is useful to caution patients that the title of the first book is a bit of a misnomer. The goal is not eternal bliss, but rather learning to use somewhat difficult techniques to regain mastery for oneself. A companion workbook is also available for the second book that can be used as a manual for patients to use in the sessions. McKay and Fanning (1992) also focus on self-esteem issues. Bourne (1990) has developed a manual with many work sheets for patient use. Craske and colleagues (1994) provide a detailed manual for a range of anxiety disorders with versions for both the patient and the therapist.

101. There is a large literature concerning the cognitive-behavior therapy of depression, with numerous examples of group application. See note 41. Rice (1995) provides a detailed outline of a structured 12-session group for lower-functioning outpatients that uses a range of techniques.

102. Fals-Stewart and Lucente (1994) provide an excellent summary of treatment approaches to obsessive-compulsive disorder and a detailed outline of a group format for behavioral treatment.

103. A current review of the outcome literature concerning phobias has been provided by Emmelkamp (1994). The principles of treatment can be applied in homogeneous groups, where there will be an abundant source of interpersonal support in addressing the feared situation.

104. Imber and colleagues (1979) and Lonergan (1985) have described crisis intervention groups.

105. Mitchell (1988) has described a protocol for critical incident stress debriefing.

106. Brabender and Fallon (1993) provide a comprehensive review of inpatient group work. Maxmen's (1984) educative model describes a pragmatic approach. Yalom (1983) uses an interpersonal approach. Rice and Rutan (1987) apply a psychodynamic framework. Kibel (1993) discusses the management of inpatient groups with a focus on adaptation to the ward milieu. The empirical literature, reviewed by R. H. Klein and co-workers (1994), notes the value placed by inpatients on altruism.

107. Borderline personality disorder (BPD) is reported in close to 15% of psychiatric outpatients and 20% of inpatients. More recent reports of outcome with individual therapy indicate a high number of early dropouts and limited gains for completers (Clarkin et al. 1991). The question has been raised as to whether intensive treatment for this patient population may do more harm than good (Vaillant 1992). Marziali and Munroe-Blum (1994) provide a comprehensive review of the literature regarding both diagnostic and etiologic issues. Livesley and colleagues (Livesley and Jackson 1992; Livesley et al. 1994) argue for the use of a dimensional diagnostic approach similar to that used in this book. Neurobehavioral defects, separation-individuation blocks, early loss or severe abuse, affective disorder, and models of attachment relationships have all been implicated in the etiology of BPD.

   Linehan and colleagues (Linehan 1993; Linehan et al. 1991) use a model referred to as *dialectical behavior therapy* (DBT), which is based on two complementary strategies. A behavioral component focuses on self-mastery techniques through detailed behavioral analysis of problematic incidents, with an emphasis on affect management. These techniques are accompanied by constant efforts to validate what the patient is experiencing. These strategies are conceptualized as representing a state of dialectical tension rooted in Eastern philosophy combined with components of feminist theory. A combination of individual and group components is used, with treatment lasting 1 to

2 years. Linehan et al.'s comparison group was treatment-as-usual in the community. Outcome assessments indicated a reduction in parasuicidal behaviors and fewer days in hospital. It is interesting to note that there was no effect on suicidal ideation or depression.

Marziali and Munroe-Blum (1994) use a 30-session interpersonal group model based on relationship management strategies (Dawson and Macmillan 1993). They compared this group model with individual psychodynamic psychotherapy, the most commonly recommended treatment approach to BPD. Both approaches had positive but similar outcomes. The group format was considerably more efficient than individual therapy, and the therapists reported greater satisfaction with the group format, noting that it was easier to align empathetically with patients in the group context. Marziali and Munroe-Blum include a training manual.

The model presented in this book is a combination of self-mastery techniques borrowed from the Linehan protocol and interpersonal strategies that form the core of the Dawson/Marziali approach. Other, more recent articles concerning psychodynamic group psychotherapy with BPD patients include those by Horwitz (1987) and Leszcz (1992) and those in collections edited by Roth and colleagues (1990) and R. H. Klein and co-workers (1992).

108. Kanas (1993, 1996) has reviewed the literature regarding the use of groups for schizophrenic patients. Detailed descriptions of outpatient medication clinics based on group principles are provided by Brook (1993) and W. N. Stone (1996).

109. There is considerable evidence that negative *expressed emotion* (EE) in the family environment is correlated with a higher rate of relapse for schizophrenic patients (Tarrier and Barrowclough 1990). The measure of EE has two components: criticism and anger, and intrusiveness. Techniques to modify these are focused on family communication style and can be conducted in a group format.

110. The use of group psychotherapy in the full spectrum of treatments of eating disorders is the central focus of a volume edited by Harper-Giuffre and MacKenzie (1992, 1993). An excellent review of treatment for bulimia nervosa has been provided by Yager (1992). A carefully developed psychoeducational program, The Road to Recovery, is described in detail by Davis and colleagues (1992) in an appendix to the Harper-Giuffre and MacKenzie book. The American Psychiatric Association's

practice guideline for eating disorders provides a full review of treatment options (American Psychiatric Association 1993a).

111. More detailed descriptions of psychotherapy groups for substance abuse patients have been provided by Flores (1996) and Vannicelli (1989, 1992).

112. The role of shame in group psychotherapy is well addressed by Alonso and Rutan (1988).

113. Lieberman (1990) has provided a comprehensive perspective on self-help groups.

References

Agazarian YM, Janoff S: Systems theory and small groups, in Comprehensive Group Psychotherapy, 3rd Edition. Edited by Kaplan HI, Sadock BJ. Baltimore, MD, Williams & Wilkins, 1993, pp 32–44

Ainsworth MDS, Blehar MC, Waters E, et al: Patterns of Attachment: A Psychological Study of the Strange Situation. Hillsdale, NJ, Lawrence Erlbaum, 1978

Alden LE, Wiggins JS, Pincus AL: Construction of circumplex scales for the Inventory of Interpersonal Problems. J Pers Assess 55:521–536, 1990

Alexander F, French TM: Psychoanalytic Therapy: Principles and Application (1946). Lincoln, University of Nebraska Press, 1980

Alonso A, Rutan JS: The experience of shame and the restoration of self-respect in group therapy. Int J Group Psychother 38:3–14, 1988

Alonso A, Swiller HI (eds): Group Therapy in Clinical Practice. Washington, DC, American Psychiatric Press, 1993

American Psychiatric Association: Diagnostic and Statistical Manual of Mental Disorders, 3rd Edition, Revised. Washington, DC, American Psychiatric Association, 1987

American Psychiatric Association: Practice guideline for eating disorders. Am J Psychiatry 150:207–228, 1993a

American Psychiatric Association: Practice guideline for major depressive disorder in adults. Am J Psychiatry 150(No 4, Suppl):1–26, 1993b

American Psychiatric Association: Diagnostic and Statistical Manual of Mental Disorders, 4th Edition. Washington, DC, American Psychiatric Association, 1994

421

Azim HFA: Group psychotherapy in the day hospital, in Comprehensive Group Psychotherapy, 3rd Edition. Edited by Kaplan HI, Sadock BJ. Baltimore, MD, Williams & Wilkins, 1993, pp 619–634

Azim HFA, Piper WE, Segal PM, et al: The Quality of Object Relations Scale. Bull Menninger Clin 55:323–343, 1991

Bannister D, Fransella F: Inquiring Man: The Psychology of Personal Constructs, 2nd Edition. Malabar, FL, Krieger, 1982

Barber JP, Crits-Christoph P (eds): Dynamic Therapies for Psychiatric Disorders. New York, Basic Books, 1995

Bauer GP, Kobos JC: Brief Therapy: Short-Term Psychodynamic Intervention. Northvale, NJ, Jason Aronson, 1987

Beck AP: Phases in the development of structure in therapy and encounter groups, in Innovations in Client-Centered Therapy. Edited by Wexler DA, Rice LN. New York, Wiley, 1974, pp 421–463

Beck AT, Rush AJ, Shaw BF, et al: Cognitive Therapy of Depression. New York, Guilford, 1979

Beck AT, Freeman A, and Associates: Cognitive Therapy of Personality Disorders. New York, Guilford, 1990

Bednar RL, Melnick J, Kaul TJ: Risk, responsibility, and structure: a conceptual framework for initiating group counseling and psychotherapy. Journal of Counseling Psychology 21:31–37, 1974

Benjamin LS: Interpersonal Diagnosis and Treatment of Personality Disorders. New York, Guilford, 1993

Benjamin LS: Good defenses make good neighbors, in Ego Defenses: Theory and Practice. Edited by Conte HR, Plutchik R. New York, Wiley, 1994, pp 53–78

Bergin AE, Garfield SL (eds): Handbook of Psychotherapy and Behavior Change, 4th Edition. New York, Wiley, 1994

Bernard HS, MacKenzie KR (eds): Basics of Group Psychotherapy. New York, Guilford, 1994

Bion WR: Experiences in Groups and Other Papers. New York, Basic Books, 1959

Blazer DG, Kessler RC, McGonagle KA, et al: The prevalence and distribution of major depression in a national community sample: The National Comorbidity Survey. Am J Psychiatry 151:979–986, 1994

Bond GR: Norm regulation in therapy groups, in Advances in Group Psychotherapy: Integrating Research and Practice (AGPA Monogr 1). Edited by Dies RR, MacKenzie KR. New York, International Universities Press, 1983, pp 171–189

Bordin ES: The generalizability of the psychoanalytic concept of the working alliance. Psychotherapy: Theory, Research and Practice 16:252–260, 1979

Bourne EJ: The Anxiety & Phobia Workbook. Oakland, CA, New Harbinger Publications, 1990

Bowlby J: The making and breaking of affectional bonds, I: aetiology and psychopathology in the light of attachment theory. Br J Psychiatry 130:201–210, 1977

Brabender V, Fallon A: Models of Inpatient Group Psychotherapy. Washington, DC, American Psychological Association, 1993

Brook DW: Medication groups, in Group Therapy in Clinical Practice. Edited by Alonso A, Swiller HI. Washington, DC, American Psychiatric Press, 1993, pp 155–170

Brusa JA, Stone MH, Beck AP, et al: A sociometric test to identify emergent leader and member roles: Phase I. Int J Group Psychother 44:79–100, 1994

Budman SH, Gurman AS: Theory and Practice of Brief Therapy. New York, Guilford, 1988

Budman SH, Clifford M, Bader L, et al: Experiential pregroup preparation and screening. Group 5:19–26, 1981

Budman SH, Demby A, Feldstein M, et al: Preliminary findings on a new instrument to measure cohesion in group psychotherapy. Int J Group Psychother 37:75–94, 1987

Budman SH, Demby A, Redondo JP, et al: Comparative outcome in time-limited individual and group psychotherapy. Int J Group Psychother 38:63–86, 1988

Budman SH, Soldz S, Demby A, et al: Cohesion, alliance and outcome in group psychotherapy. Psychiatry 52:339–350, 1989

Burlingame GM, Lambert MJ, Reisinger CW, et al: Pragmatics of tracking mental health outcomes in a managed care setting. Journal of Mental Health Administration 22:226–236, 1995

Burns DD: The Feeling Good Handbook. New York, Plume, 1990

Burns DD: Ten Days to Self-Esteem. New York, William Morrow, 1993

Clarkin JF, Marziali E, Munroe-Blum H: Group and family treatments for borderline personality disorder. Hosp Community Psychiatry 42:1038–1043, 1991

Corsini R, Rosenberg B: Mechanisms of group psychotherapy: processes and dynamics. Journal of Abnormal and Social Psychology 51:406–411, 1955

Costa PT, McCrae RR: Personality disorders and the five-factor model of personality. Journal of Personality Disorders 4:362–371, 1990

Costa PT, Widiger TA (eds): Personality Disorders and the Five-Factor Model of Personality. Washington, DC, American Psychological Association, 1994

Covi L, Primakoff L: Cognitive group therapy, in American Psychiatric Press Review of Psychiatry, Vol 7. Edited by Frances AJ, Hales RE. Washington, DC, American Psychiatric Press, 1988, pp 608–626

Cramer-Azima FJ, Richmond LH (eds): Adolescent Group Psychotherapy. Madison, CT, International Universities Press, 1989

Craske MG, Meadows E, Barlow DH: Therapist's Guide for the Mastery of Your Anxiety and Panic II + Agoraphobia Supplement. San Antonio, TX, Psychological Corporation/Graywind Publications, 1994

Crits-Christoph P, Barber JP: Handbook of Short-Term Dynamic Psychotherapy. New York, Basic Books, 1991

Crosby G, Sabin JE: Developing and marketing time limited therapy groups. Psychiatr Serv 46:7–8, 1996

Cross CD: Organizing group psychotherapy programming in managed care settings, in Effective Use of Group Therapy in Managed Care. Edited by MacKenzie KR. Washington, DC, American Psychiatric Press, 1995, pp 27–41

Crouch EC, Bloch S, Wanless J: Therapeutic factors: interpersonal and intrapersonal mechanisms, in Handbook of Group Psychotherapy: An Empirical and Clinical Synthesis. Edited by Fuhriman A, Burlingame GM. New York, Wiley, 1994, pp 269–315

Darwin C: The Expression of the Emotions in Man and Animals. London, J Murray, 1872

Davanloo H: Short-Term Dynamic Psychotherapy. New York, Jason Aronson, 1980

Davis R, Dearing S, Faulkner J, et al: The Road to Recovery: a manual for participants in the psychoeducational group for bulimia nervosa, in Group Psychotherapy for Eating Disorders. Edited by Harper-Giuffre H, MacKenzie KR. Washington, DC, American Psychiatric Press, 1992, pp 281–310

Dawson DL, Macmillan HL: Relationship Management of the Borderline Patient: From Understanding to Treatment. New York, Brunner/Mazel, 1993

Derogatis LR: SCL-90: Administration, Scoring and Procedures Manual for the Revised Version. Baltimore, MD, Clinical Psychometric Research, 1983

Derogatis LR, Melisaratos N: The Brief Symptom Inventory: an introductory report. Psychol Med 13:595–605, 1983

Dies RR: Clinical implications of research on leadership in short-term group psychotherapy, in Advances in Group Psychotherapy: Integrating Research and Practice (AGPA Monogr 1). Edited by Dies RR, MacKenzie KR. New York, International Universities Press, 1983, pp 27–78

Dies RR: Therapist variables in group psychotherapy research, in Handbook of Group Psychotherapy: An Empirical and Clinical Synthesis. Edited by Fuhriman A, Burlingame GM. New York, Wiley, 1994, pp 114–154

Dies RR, Teleska PA: Negative outcome in group psychotherapy, in Negative Outcome in Psychotherapy and What to Do About It. Edited by Mays DT, Franks CM. New York, Springer, 1985, pp 118–141

Doherty WJ, Lester ME, Leigh GK: Marriage encounter weekends: couples who win and couples who lose. Journal of Marital and Family Therapy 12:49–61, 1986

Drescher S, Burlingame GM, Fuhriman A: Cohesion: an odyssey in empirical understanding. Small Group Behavior 16:3–30, 1985

Ekman P, Friesen WV, Ellsworth P: Emotion in the Human Face. New York, Pergamon, 1972

Elkin I: The NIMH Treatment of Depression Collaborative Research Program: where we began and where we are, in Handbook of Psychotherapy and Behavior Change, 4th Edition. Edited by Bergin AE, Garfield SL. New York, Wiley, 1994, pp 114–139

Elkin I, Shea MT, Watkins JT, et al: National Institute of Mental Health Treatment of Depression Collaborative Research Program: general effectiveness of treatments. Arch Gen Psychiatry 46:971–982, 1989

Ellis A: Reason and Emotion in Psychotherapy. New York, Lyle Stuart, 1962

Ellis A: Rational-emotive therapy and cognitive behavior therapy: similarities and differences. Cognitive Therapy and Research 4:325–340, 1980

Ellis A: Group rational-emotive and cognitive-behavioral therapy. Int J Group Psychother 42:63–80, 1992

Emmelkamp PMG: Behavior therapy with adults, in Handbook of Psychotherapy and Behavior Change, 4th Edition. Edited by Bergin AE, Garfield SL. New York, Wiley, 1994, pp 379–427

Eysenck HJ: The definition of personality disorders and the criteria appropriate for their description. Journal of Personality Disorders 1:211–219, 1987

Fals-Stewart W, Lucente S: Behavioral group therapy with obsessive-compulsives: an overview. Int J Group Psychother 44:35–51, 1994

Flores PJ: Group Psychotherapy With Addicted Populations, 2nd Edition. New York, Haworth Press, 1996

Foulkes SH: Group-Analytic Psychotherapy: Method and Principles. London, Gordon & Breach, 1975

Frank JD, Frank JB: Persuasion and Healing: A Comparative Study of Psychotherapy, 3rd Edition. Baltimore, MD, Johns Hopkins, 1991

Frasure-Smith N: In-hospital symptoms of psychological stress as predictors of long-term outcome after acute myocardial in men. Am J Cardiol 67:121–127, 1991

Fuhriman A, Burlingame GM (eds): Handbook of Group Psychotherapy: An Empirical and Clinical Synthesis. New York, Wiley, 1994

Gabbard GO: An overview of countertransference with borderline patients. Journal of Psychotherapy Practice and Research 2:7–18, 1993

Ganzarain R, Buchele BJ: Fugitives of Incest. Madison, CT, International Universities Press, 1988

Garfield SL: Research on client variables in psychotherapy, in Handbook of Psychotherapy and Behavior Change, 4th Edition. Edited by Bergin AE, Garfield SL. New York, Wiley, 1994, pp 190–228

Garfield SL, Kurz M: Evaluation of treatment and related procedures in 1216 cases referred to a mental hygiene clinic. Psychiatr Q 26:4124–4424, 1952

Gaston L: Reliability and criterion-related validity of the California Psychotherapy Alliance Scales—Patient Version. Psychological Assessment: A Journal of Consulting and Clinical Psychology 3:68–74, 1991

Goldman HH, Skodol AE, Lave TR: Revising Axis V for DSM-IV: a review of measures of social functioning. Am J Psychiatry 149:1148–1156, 1992

Goodman M, Brown JA, Deitz PM: Managing Managed Care II: A Handbook for Mental Health Professionals, 2nd Edition. Washington, DC, American Psychiatric Press, 1996

Gustafson JP: The Complex Secret of Brief Psychotherapy. New York, WW Norton, 1986

Gustafson JP: The Dilemmas of Brief Psychotherapy. New York, Plenum, 1995

Hare AP: Handbook of Small Group Research, 2nd Edition. New York, Free Press, 1976

Hare RD, Harpur TJ, Hakstian AR, et al: The Revised Psychopathy Checklist: reliability and factor structure. Psychological Assessment: A Journal of Consulting and Clinical Psychology 2:338–341, 1990

Harper-Giuffre H, MacKenzie KR (eds): Group Psychotherapy for Eating Disorders. Washington, DC, American Psychiatric Press, 1992

Harper-Giuffre H, MacKenzie KR: Group psychotherapy for eating disorders, in Comprehensive Group Psychotherapy, 3rd Edition. Edited by Kaplan HI, Sadock BJ. Baltimore, MD, Williams & Wilkins, 1993, pp 443–459

Hartley D, Roback HB, Abramowitz SI: Deterioration effects in encounter groups. Am Psychol 31:247–255, 1976

Hellerstein DJ, Pinsker H, Rosenthal RN, et al: Supportive psychotherapy as the treatment model of choice. Journal of Psychotherapy Practice and Research 3:300–306, 1994

Hill WF: Hill Interaction Matrix Manual and Supplement (1965), Revised Edition. Los Angeles, CA, Youth Studies Center, University of Southern California, 1965

Hill WF: Hill Interaction Matrix: the conceptual framework, derived rating scales, and updated bibliography. Small Group Behavior 8:251–268, 1977

Horowitz LM: Pschemas, psychopathology, and psychotherapy research. Psychotherapy Research 4:1–19, 1994

Horowitz LM, Rosenberg SE, Baer BA, et al: Inventory of Interpersonal Problems: psychometric properties and clinical applications. J Consult Clin Psychol 56:885–892, 1988

Horowitz LM, Rosenberg SE, Bartholomew K: Interpersonal problems, attachment styles, and outcome in brief dynamic psychotherapy. J Consult Clin Psychol 61:549–560, 1993

Horwitz L: Projective identification in dyads and groups. Int J Group Psychother 33:319–330, 1983

Horwitz L: Indications for group psychotherapy with borderline and narcissistic patients. Bull Menninger Clin 51:248–260, 1987

Howard KI, Kopta SM, Krause MS, et al: The dose-effect relationship in psychotherapy. Am Psychol 41:159–164, 1986

Howard KI, Lueger R, Schank D: The psychotherapeutic service delivery system. Psychotherapy Research 2:164–180, 1992

Howard KI, Lueger RJ, Maling MS, et al: A phase model of psychotherapy: causal mediation of outcome. J Consult Clin Psychol 61:678–685, 1993

Hoyt MF (ed): Constructive Therapies. New York, Guilford, 1994

Imber SD, Lewis PM, Loiselle RH: Uses and abuses of the brief intervention group. Int J Group Psychother 29:39–49, 1979

Jacobs M, Jacobs A, Feldman G, et al: Feedback II—the credibility gap: delivery of positive and negative emotional and behavioral feedback in groups. J Consult Clin Psychol 41:215–223, 1973

Kanas N: Group psychotherapy with schizophrenia, in Comprehensive Group Psychotherapy, 3rd Edition. Edited by Kaplan HI, Sadock BJ. Baltimore, MD, Williams & Wilkins, 1993, pp 407–418

Kanas N: Group Therapy for Schizophrenic Patients. Washington, DC, American Psychiatric Press, 1996

Kaplan HI, Sadock BJ (eds): Comprehensive Group Psychotherapy, 3rd Edition. Baltimore, MD, Williams & Wilkins, 1993

Kaul TJ, Bednar RL: Pretaining and structure: parallel lines yet to meet, in Handbook of Group Psychotherapy: Empirical and Clinical Synthesis. Edited by Fuhriman A, Burlingame G. New York, Wiley, 1994, pp 155–188

Kazdin AE: Methodology, design, and evaluation in psychotherapy research, in Handbook of Psychotherapy and Behavior Change, 4th Edition. Edited by Bergin AE, Garfield SL. New York, Wiley, 1994, pp 19–71

Kelly GA: The Psychology of Personal Constructs. New York, WW Norton, 1955

Kennedy LL: Groups in the day hospital, in Group Therapy in Clinical Practice. Edited by Alonso A, Swiller HI. Washington, DC, American Psychiatric Press, 1993, pp 137–154

Kibel HD: Inpatient group psychotherapy, in Group Therapy in Clinical Practice. Edited by Alonso A, Swiller HI. Washington, DC, American Psychiatric Press, 1993, pp 93–111

Klein MH, Kupfer DJ, Shea MT (eds): Personality and Depression. New York, Guilford, 1993

Klein RH, Bernard HS, Singer DL (eds): Handbook of Contemporary Group Psychotherapy. Madison, CT, International Universities Press, 1992

Klein RH, Brabender V, Fallon A: Inpatient group therapy, in Handbook of Group Psychotherapy: An Empirical and Clinical Synthesis. Edited by Fuhriman A, Burlingame GM. New York, Wiley, 1994, pp 370–415

Klerman GL, Weissman MM, Rounsaville BJ, et al: Interpersonal Psychotherapy of Depression. New York, Basic Books, 1984

Kymissis P, Halperin DA (eds): Group Therapy With Children and Adolescents. Washington, DC, American Psychiatric Press, 1996

Laikin M, Winston A: A Short-Term Dynamic Psychotherapy (STDP) Manual. Social and Behavioral Science Documents 18, No 2, 1988

Lambert MJ: The individual therapist's contribution to psychotherapy process and outcome. Clinical Psychology Review 9:469–485, 1989

Lambert MJ, Bergin AE: The effectiveness of psychotherapy, in Handbook of Psychotherapy and Behavior Change, 4th Edition. Edited by Bergin AE, Garfield SL. New York, Wiley, 1994, pp 143–189

Lambert MJ, Hill CE: Assessing psychotherapy outcomes and process, in Handbook of Psychotherapy and Behavior Change, 4th Edition. Edited by Bergin AE, Garfield SL. New York, Wiley, 1994, pp 72–113

Laws DR: Relapse Prevention With Sex Offenders. New York, Guilford, 1989

Leary T: Interpersonal Diagnosis of Personality. New York, Ronald Press, 1957

Leszcz M: Group psychotherapy of the borderline patient, in Handbook of Borderline Disorders. Edited by Silver D, Rosenbluth M. Madison, CT, International Universities Press, 1992

Leszcz M: The interpersonal approach to group psychotherapy. Int J Group Psychother 42:37–62, 1992

Lieberman MA: A group therapist perspective on self-help groups. Int J Group Psychother 40:251–278, 1990

Lieberman MA, Yalom ID, Miles MB: Encounter Groups: First Facts. New York, Basic Books, 1973

Linehan MM: Cognitive-Behavioral Treatment of Borderline Personality Disorder. New York, Guilford, 1993

Linehan MM, Armstrong HE, Suarez A, et al: Cognitive-behavioral treatment of chronically parasuicidal borderline patients. Arch Gen Psychiatry 48:1060–1064, 1991

Livesley WJ (ed): DSM-IV Personality Disorders. New York, Guilford, 1995

Livesley WJ, Jackson DN: Guidelines for developing, evaluating, and revising the classification of personality disorders. J Nerv Ment Dis 180: 609–618, 1992

Livesley WJ, MacKenzie KR: Social roles in psychotherapy groups, in Advances in Group Psychotherapy: Integrating Research and Practice (AGPA Monogr 1). Edited by Dies RR, MacKenzie KR. New York, International Universities Press, 1983, pp 117–135

Livesley WJ, Schroeder ML, Jackson DN, et al: Categorical distinctions in the study of personality disorder: implications for classification. J Abnorm Psychol 103:6–17, 1994

Lonergan EC: Utilizing group process in crisis-waiting-list groups. Int J Group Psychother 35:355–372, 1985

Lonergan EC: Using theories of group therapy, in Basics of Group Psychotherapy. Edited by Bernard HS, MacKenzie KR. New York, Guilford, 1994, pp 189–216

Lothstein LM: Termination processes in group psychotherapy, in Comprehensive Group Psychotherapy, 3rd Edition. Edited by Kaplan HI, Sadock BJ. Baltimore, MD, Williams & Wilkins, 1993, pp 115–124

Luborsky L: Principles of Psychoanalytic Psychotherapy: A Manual for Supportive-Expressive Treatment. New York, Basic Books, 1984

Luborsky L, Barber JP: Perspectives on seven transference-related measures applied to the interview with Ms. Smithfield. Psychotherapy Research 4:152–154, 1994

Luborsky L, DeRubeis RJ: The use of psychotherapy treatment manuals: a small revolution in psychotherapy research style. Clinical Psychology Review 4:5–14, 1984

Luborsky L, Crits-Christoph P, Mintz J, et al: Who Will Benefit From Psychotherapy? Predicting Therapeutic Outcomes. New York, Basic Books, 1988

Luborsky L, Barber JP, Beutler L (eds): Special section: Curative factors in dynamic psychotherapy. J Consult Clin Psychol 61·539–610, 1993

Luft J: Group Processes: An Introduction to Group Dynamics. Palo Alto, CA, National Press, 1970

MacKenzie KR: Group norms: importance and measurement. Int J Group Psychother 29:471–480, 1979

MacKenzie KR: Measurement of group climate. Int J Group Psychother 31:287–295, 1981

MacKenzie KR: Recent developments in brief psychotherapy. Hosp Community Psychiatry 39:742–752, 1988

MacKenzie KR: Introduction to Time-Limited Group Psychotherapy. Washington, DC, American Psychiatric Press, 1990

MacKenzie KR (ed): Classics in Group Psychotherapy. New York, Guilford, 1992

MacKenzie KR: Group development, in Handbook of Group Psychotherapy: An Empirical and Clinical Synthesis. Edited by Fuhriman A, Burlingame GM. New York, Wiley, 1994a, pp 223–268

MacKenzie KR: Using personality measurements in clinical practice, in Personality Disorders and the Five-Factor Model of Personality. Edited by Costa PT, Widiger TA. Washington, DC, American Psychological Association, 1994b, pp 237–250

MacKenzie KR: Where is here and when is now? The adaptational challenge of mental health reform for group psychotherapy. Int J Group Psychother 44:407–428, 1994c

MacKenzie KR: Rationale for group psychotherapy in managed care, in Effective Use of Group Therapy in Managed Care. Edited by MacKenzie KR. Washington, DC, American Psychiatric Press, 1995, pp 1–25

MacKenzie KR, Kennedy JW: Primate ethology and group dynamics, in Psychoanalytic Group Theory and Therapy: Essays in Honor of Saul Scheidlinger (AGPA Monogr 7). Edited by Tuttman S. New York, International Universities Press, 1989, pp 357–377

MacKenzie KR, Livesley WJ: A developmental model for brief group therapy, in Advances in Group Psychotherapy: Integrating Research and Practice. Edited by Dies RR, MacKenzie KR. New York, International Universities Press, 1983, pp 101–116

MacKenzie KR, Dies RR, Coche E, et al: An analysis of AGPA Institute groups. Int J Group Psychother 37:55–74, 1987

Mahoney MJ: Special section: Recent developments in cognitive and constructivist psychotherapies. J Consult Clin Psychol 61:187–275, 1993

Malan DH: Individual Psychotherapy and the Science of Psychodynamics, 2nd Edition. London, Butterworth, 1979

Mann J: Time-limited psychotherapy, in Handbook of Short-Term Dynamic Psychotherapy. Edited by Crits-Christoph P, Barber JP. New York, Basic Books, 1991, pp 17–43

Mann J, Goldman R: A Casebook in Time-Limited Psychotherapy (1982). Washington, DC, American Psychiatric Press, 1987

Marmar CR, Weiss DS, Gaston L: Towards the validation of the California Therapeutic Alliance Rating System. Psychological Assessment: A Journal of Consulting and Clinical Psychology 1:46–52, 1989

Marziali E, Munroe-Blum H: Interpersonal Group Psychotherapy for Borderline Personality Disorder. New York, Basic Books, 1994

Maxmen JS: Helping patients survive theories: the practice of an educative model. Int J Group Psychother 34:355–368, 1984

McCallum M, Piper WE: The psychological mindedness assessment procedure. Psychological Assessment: A Journal of Consulting and Clinical Psychology 2:412–418, 1990

McKay M, Fanning P: Self-Esteem. Oakland, CA, New Harbinger Publications, 1992

McKay M, Paleg K (eds): Focal Group Psychotherapy. Oakland, CA, New Harbinger Publications, 1992

McLemore C, Benjamin LS: Whatever happened to interpersonal diagnosis? A psychosocial alternative to DSM-III. Am Psychol 34:17–34, 1979

Melson SJ: Brief day treatment for nonpsychotic patients, in Effective Use of Group Therapy in Managed Care. Edited by MacKenzie KR. Washington, DC, American Psychiatric Press, 1995, pp 113–128

Mitchell JT: Stress: development and functions of a critical incident stress debriefing team. Journal of Emergency Medical Services 13:43–46, 1988

Mullen B, Goethals GR: Theories of Group Behavior. New York, Springer-Verlag, 1987

Neimeyer RA: An appraisal of constructivist psychotherapies. J Clin Consult Psychol 61:221–234, 1993

Neimeyer RA, Feixas G: The role of homework and skill acquisition in the outcome of group cognitive therapy for depression. Behavior Therapy 21:281–292, 1990

Norcross JC, Goldfried MR (eds): Handbook of Psychotherapy Integration. New York, Basic Books, 1992

Nguyen TD, Attkisson CC, Stegner BL: Assessment of patient satisfaction: development and refinement of a service evaluation questionnaire. Evaluation and Program Planning 6:299–313, 1983

Ogles BM, Lambert MJ, Sawyer D: Clinical significance of the NIMH Treatment of Depression Collaborative Study. Paper presented at annual meeting of the Society for Psychotherapy Research, Pittsburgh, PA, June 1993

Ogles BM, Lambert MJ, Masters KS: Assessing Outcome in Clinical Practice. Boston, MA, Allyn & Bacon, 1996

Oldham JM, Skodol AE, Kellman HD, et al: Diagnosis of DSM-III-R personality disorders by two structured interviews: patterns of comorbidity. Am J Psychiatry 149:213–220, 1992

Orlinsky DE, Howard KI: Process and outcome in psychotherapy, in Handbook of Psychotherapy and Behavior Change, 3rd Edition. Edited by Bergin AE, Garfield SL. New York, Wiley, 1986, pp 311–381

Orlinsky DE, Howard KI: A generic model of psychotherapy. Journal of Integrative and Eclectic Psychotherapy 6:6–27, 1987

Orlinsky DE, Grawe K, Parks BK: Process and outcome in psychotherapy—Noch einmal, in Handbook of Psychotherapy and Behavior Change, 4th Edition. Edited by Bergin AE, Garfield SL. New York, Wiley, 1994, pp 270–376

Otto MW, Pollack MH, Sachs GS, et al: Discontinuation of benzodiazepine treatment: efficacy of cognitive-behavioral therapy for patients with panic disorder. Am J Psychiatry 150:1485–1490, 1993

Padesky CA, Greenberger D: Clinician's Guide to Mind Over Mood. New York, Guilford, 1995

Phillips EL: The ubiquitous decay curve: delivery similarities in psychotherapy, medicine and addiction. Professional Psychology: Research and Practice 18:650–652, 1987

Pilkonis PA, Imber SD, Lewis P, et al: A comparative outcome study of individual, group, and conjoint psychotherapy. Arch Gen Psychiatry 41:431–437, 1984

Pinsker H, Rosenthal R, McCullough L: Dynamic supportive psychotherapy, in Handbook of Short-Term Dynamic Psychotherapy. Edited by Crits-Christoph P, Barber JP. New York, Basic Books, 1991, pp 220–247

Piper WE: Client variables, in Handbook of Group Psychotherapy: An Empirical and Clinical Synthesis. Edited by Fuhriman A, Burlingame GM. New York, Wiley, 1994, pp 83–113

Piper WE: Psychodynamic psychotherapy, in American Psychiatric Press Review of Psychiatry, Vol 15. Edited by Dickstein LJ, Riba MB, Oldham JM. Washington, DC, American Psychiatric Press, 1996, pp 109–128

Piper WE, Joyce AS: A consideration of factors influencing the utilization of time-limited, short-term group therapy. Int J Group Psychother 46:311–328, 1996

Piper WE, McCallum M: Selection of patients for group interventions, in Basics of Group Psychotherapy. Edited by Bernard HS, MacKenzie KR. New York, Guilford, 1994, pp 1–34

Piper WE, Debbane EG, Bienvenu JP, et al: A study of group pretraining for group psychotherapy. Int J Group Psychother 32:309–325, 1982

Piper WE, Debbane EG, Bienvenu JP, et al: A comparative study of four forms of psychotherapy. J Consult Clin Psychol 52:268–279, 1984

Piper WE, McCallum M, Azim HFA: Adaptation to Loss Through Short-Term Group Psychotherapy. New York, Guilford Press, 1992

Porter K: Combined individual and group psychotherapy, in Group Therapy in Clinical Practice. Edited by Alonso A, Swiller HI. Washington, DC, American Psychiatric Press, 1993, pp 309–341

Powdermaker FB, Frank JD: Group Psychotherapy: Studies in Methodology of Research and Therapy. Cambridge, MA, Harvard University Press, 1953

Rank O: The Trauma of Birth (1929). New York, Harper & Row, 1973

Rice AH: Structured groups for the treatment of depression, in Effective Use of Group Therapy in Managed Care. Edited by MacKenzie KR. Washington, DC, American Psychiatric Press, 1995, pp 61–96

Rice CA, Rutan JS: Inpatient Group Psychotherapy: A Dynamic Perspective. New York, Macmillan, 1987

Riester AE, Kraft IA (eds): Child Group Psychotherapy: Future Tense (AGPA Monogr 3). Madison, CT, International Universities Press, 1986

Robinson LA, Berman JS, Neimeyer RA: Psychotherapy for the treatment of depression: a comprehensive review of controlled outcome research. Psychol Bull 108:30–49, 1990

Rockland LH: Supportive Therapy for Borderline Patients: A Psychodynamic Approach. New York, Guilford, 1992

Rogers CR: Client-Centered Therapy. London, Constable, 1951

Roller B, Nelson V: The Art of Co-Therapy: How Therapists Work Together. New York, Guilford, 1991

Roller B, Nelson V: Cotherapy, in Comprehensive Group Psychotherapy, 3rd Edition. Edited by Kaplan HI, Sadock BJ. Baltimore, MD, Williams & Wilkins, 1993, pp 304–312

Rose SD: Working With Adults in Groups: Integrating Cognitive-Behavioral and Small Group Strategies. San Francisco, CA, Jossey-Bass, 1989

Rose SD: Cognitive-behavioral group psychotherapy, in Comprehensive Group Psychotherapy, 3rd Edition. Edited by Kaplan HI, Sadock BJ. Baltimore, MD, Williams & Wilkins, 1993, pp 205–214

Roth BE, Stone WN, Kibel HD (eds): The Difficult Patient in Group: Group Psychotherapy With Borderline and Narcissistic Disorders. Madison, CT, International Universities Press, 1990

Rutan JS, Stone WN: Psychodynamic Group Psychotherapy, 2nd Edition. New York, Guilford, 1993

Ryle A: Cognitive-Analytic Therapy: A New Integration in Brief Psychotherapy. New York, Wiley, 1990

Sachs JS: Negative factors in brief psychotherapy: an empirical assessment. J Consult Clin Psychol 51:557–564, 1983

Schaefer ES: Configurational analysis of children's reports of parent behavior. Journal of Consulting Psychology 29:552–557, 1965

Schamess G: Group psychotherapy with children, in Comprehensive Group Psychotherapy, 3rd Edition. Edited by Kaplan HI, Sadock BJ. Baltimore, MD, Williams & Wilkins, 1993, pp 560–576

Scheidlinger S: Presidential address: On scapegoating in group psychotherapy. Int J Group Psychother 32:131–143, 1982

Scheidlinger S, Schamess G: Fifty years of AGPA 1942–1992: an overview, in Classics in Group Psychotherapy. Edited by MacKenzie KR. New York, Guilford, 1992, pp 1–22

Segal ZV, Blatt SJ (eds): The Self in Emotional Distress. New York, Guilford, 1993

Shapiro D: Psychotherapy of Neurotic Character. New York, Basic Books, 1989

Shapiro S, Skinner EA, Kessler LG, et al: Utilization of health and mental health services: three Epidemiologic Catchment Area sites. Arch Gen Psychiatry 41:971–978, 1984

Sifneos PE: Short-Term Dynamic Psychotherapy, 2nd Edition. New York, Plenum, 1987

Simon G, Ormel J, VonKorff M, et al: Health care costs associated with depressive and anxiety disorders in primary care. Am J Psychiatry 152: 352–357, 1995

Skodol AE, Rosnick L, Kellman HD, et al: Validating structured DSM-III-R personality disorder assessments with longitudinal data. Am J Psychiatry 145:1297–1299, 1988

Sledge WH, Moras K, Hartley D, et al: Effect of time-limited psychotherapy on patient dropout rates. Am J Psychiatry 147:1341–1347, 1990

Smith ML, Glass GV, Miller TI: The Benefits of Psychotherapy. Baltimore, MD, The Johns Hopkins University Press, 1980

Spiegel D, Bloom JR, Kraemer HC, et al: Effect of psychosocial treatment on survival of patients with metastatic breast cancer. Lancet 8668:888–891, 1989

Spitz HI: Group Psychotherapy and Managed Mental Health Care: A Clinical Guide for Providers. New York, Brunner/Mazel, 1996

Steenbarger BN, Budman SH: Group psychotherapy and managed behavioral health care: current trends and future challenges. Int J Group Psychother 46:297–311, 1996

Stone MH: Treatment of borderline patients: a pragmatic approach. Psychiatr Clin North Am 13:265–285, 1990

Stone WN: Group Psychotherapy for the Chronically Mentally Ill. New York, Guilford, 1996

Sullivan HS: The Interpersonal Theory of Psychiatry. New York, WW Norton, 1953

Tarrier N, Barrowclough C: Family interventions for schizophrenia. Behavior Modification 14:408–440, 1990

Tillitski CJ: A meta-analysis of estimated effect size for group vs individual vs control treatments. Int J Group Psychother 40:215–224, 1990

Toseland RW, Siporin M: When to recommend group treatment: a review of the clinical and group literature. Int J Group Psychother 36:171–201, 1986

Vaillant GE: The beginning of wisdom is never calling a patient a borderline. Journal of Psychotherapy Practice and Research 1:117–134, 1992 van der Kolk BA: Group psychotherapy with posttraumatic stress disorder, in Comprehensive Group Psychotherapy, 3rd Edition. Edited by Kaplan HI, Sadock BJ. Baltimore, MD, Williams & Wilkins, 1993, pp 550–560

Vannicelli M: Group Psychotherapy With Adult Children of Alcoholics. New York, Guilford, 1989

Vannicelli M: Removing the Roadblocks: Group Psychotherapy With Substance Abusers and Family Members. New York, Guilford, 1992

Weissman MM, Bothwell S: The assessment of social adjustment by patient self-report. Arch Gen Psychiatry 33:1111–1115, 1976

White M, Epston D: Narrative Means and Therapeutic Ends. New York, WW Norton, 1990

Widiger TA, Trull TJ, Hurt S, et al: A multidimensional scaling of the DSM-III personality disorders. Arch Gen Psychiatry 44:557–563, 1987

Wiggins JS, Trapnell P, Phillips N: Psychometric and geometric characteristics of the revised Interpersonal Adjective Scales (IAS-R). Multivariate Behavioral Research 23:517–530, 1988

Winston A, Muran JC: Common factors in the time-limited psychotherapies, in American Psychiatric Press Review of Psychiatry, Vol 15. Edited by Dickstein LJ, Riba MB, Oldham JM. Washington, DC, American Psychiatric Press, 1996, pp 43–68

Winston A, Laikin M, Pollack J, et al: Short-term psychotherapy of personality disorders. Am J Psychiatry 151:190–194, 1994

World Health Organization: The ICD-10 Classification of Mental and Behavioral Disorders: Clinical Descriptions and Diagnostic Guidelines. Geneva, World Health Organization, 1992

Wright F, Hoffman XH, Gore EM: Perspectives on scapegoating in primary groups. Group 12:33–44, 1988

Yager J: Psychotherapeutic strategies for bulimia nervosa. Journal of Psychotherapy Practice and Research 1:91–102, 1992

Yalom ID: Theory and Practice of Group Psychotherapy. New York, Basic Books, 1970

Yalom ID: Existential Psychotherapy. New York, Basic Books, 1980

Yalom ID: Inpatient Group Psychotherapy. New York, Basic Books, 1983

Yalom ID: Theory and Practice of Group Psychotherapy, 4th Edition. New York, Basic Books, 1995

Index

Page numbers printed in **boldface** type refer to tables or figures, page numbers <u>underlined</u> refer to appendixes, and page numbers printed in *italics* refer to source notes.